Women's Health Care

Women's Health Care

Activist Traditions and Institutional Change

Carol S. Weisman

Department of Health Management and Policy
School of Public Health
The University of Michigan
Ann Arbor, Michigan

The Johns Hopkins University Press

Baltimore and London

© 1998 The Johns Hopkins University Press
All rights reserved. Published 1998
Printed in the United States of America on acid-free paper
9 8 7 6 5 4 3 2 1

The Johns Hopkins University Press
2715 North Charles Street, Baltimore, Maryland 21218-4319
The Johns Hopkins Press Ltd., London

Library of Congress Cataloging-in-Publication Data will be
found at the end of this book.
A catalog record for this book is available from the British Library.

ISBN 0-8018-5825-9
ISBN 0-8018-5826-7 (pbk.)

To my mother, sister, and daughter

Contents

Acknowledgments

My work on this book would not have been possible without the help of colleagues, several organizations, and a first-rate social support system.

The Robert Wood Johnson Foundation provided an Investigator Award in Health Policy Research that supported my time to work on the book and provided the opportunity for meetings and conversations with other investigators. I am particularly grateful to Sol Levine, who directed the investigators' program until his death, for nurturing this work. The Commonwealth Fund, and in particular Karen Davis and Karen Scott Collins, provided access to the 1993 Survey of Women's Health as well as grant support for a study of women's health centers. The Jacobs Institute of Women's Health, and in particular Martha Romans and Warren Pearse, provided the opportunity to participate in work on women's health and managed care. The discussion of these projects in this book, however, reflects my conclusions and opinions and not those of these organizations or individuals. The Department of Health Policy and Management at the Johns Hopkins University School of Hygiene and Public Health provided a minisabbatical that allowed time to spend many hours alone with my personal computer.

Colleagues who helped me, whether they know it or not, by sharing information and insights, include Barbara Bartman, Karen Carlson, Carolyn Clancy, Kay Dickersin, Elizabeth Fee, Bernard Guyer, Eileen Hoffman, Anne Kasper, Patricia Looker, Mary Mahowald, Constance Nathanson, Robert Ross, Diane Rowland, Sheryl Burt Ruzek, and Donna Strobino. Others are acknowledged for specific contributions in endnotes. I would also like to thank those whom I interviewed as knowledgeable informants about recent episodes in women's health policymaking.

I am fortunate to have worked with extraordinary students at Johns Hopkins. I would like to thank the students in my course, "Women's Health, Health Care, and Policy," who helped me articulate many of the ideas in this book. In addition, the following current and former doctoral students deserve special thanks for their contributions over the years: Sandra D. Cassard, Christopher Cassirer, Tracy L. Johnson, Amal J. Khoury, Stacey B. Plichta, Virginia Poole, Martha A. Teitelbaum, and Christine Vogeli.

I would also like to thank my longtime assistant, Mary Wisniewski, whose skills and loyalty always made my work easier, and Wendy Harris at The Johns Hopkins University Press, who was unerringly supportive of this project and a pleasure to work with.

Finally, family. My husband, Gary Chase, deserves special thanks for putting up with lost weekends and for providing a critical reading and many suggestions (some of which I even took). Our daughter, Sarah Weisman, was an insightful consultant on American history, and our son, Sandy Chase, provided some interesting distractions in the world of dance. This group has never failed to remind me to "get a life" and to give me one.

Women's Health Care

Introduction

WOMEN'S HEALTH became a prominent public issue around 1990. A coalition of women in Congress and their staffs, government officials, women physicians and biomedical researchers, associations of health care professionals, and women's health advocacy and interest groups sought to change federal policy on women's health research and to improve the quality of women's health care. The next four years witnessed an unprecedented spate of legislative and programmatic activity, including a large commitment of federal funds to biomedical research on the health problems of women. In the public discourse surrounding these events, including wide coverage in the national media, the issues were framed as a matter of gender equity. The major claim was that both biomedical research and medical practice reflected an "androcentric bias" by focusing on the bodily experiences and diseases of men and either neglecting those of women or narrowly construing them in terms of reproduction. A paradigm shift to "women-centered" health care required some fundamental changes in how health care was defined and delivered. Women's health advocates called for changes in policies that had limited women's participation as subjects in clinical research, for a reallocation of public resources to support new research initiatives and programs on women's health, for programs to support the career development of women in the biomedical sciences, and for reforms in the training of physicians. They achieved policy successes in all of these areas.

This was an extraordinary episode of women's health policymaking that seemed to demonstrate new political possibilities for women, both inside and outside of government, and to represent a unique historical confluence of participants and problems in women's health. The events also overlapped with a resurgence of national debate on health care reform, which heightened public attention to health care issues generally and provided an opportunity for a women's health coalition to forge a position on such issues as universal access to health care and the elements of a basic health insurance benefits package for women. By 1994, when the Clinton administration's health care reform proposal failed and the political climate changed dramatically, the momentum of the women's health agenda appeared to slow as well.

Another way of looking at this episode, however, is to see it as the latest installment in a long American tradition of organized efforts by groups of primarily middle-class women to draw public attention to their health problems and to reshape health care institutions. These efforts have waxed and waned across the nineteenth and twentieth centuries and show no signs of disappearing as we enter the twenty-first. Indeed, health care could be viewed as a key social arena in which gender issues surface and are contested, with important consequences for women's social status and well-being. Historically and today, the ways in which women experience their health and health care form a prism through which a variety of gender-based concerns are revealed.

The relationship between women and health care institutions—particularly how they experience health care and seek to change it—is the subject of this book. The specific objectives are to examine the social and historical context of women's health as a recurring public issue in the United States, to investigate current health care delivery issues for women and models for change, and to consider how women's health issues can be incorporated in health care policymaking. Because U.S. health care is undergoing a major market-driven transformation, it is an opportune time both to recognize the legacies of women's health movements and institution building and to identify women's concerns that need to be addressed within the changing health care delivery system.

SOME KEY IDEAS

Women's health was neither invented nor resolved as a public issue in the 1990s. The United States has experienced a series of episodes of intense public attention to women's health spanning the last two centuries, and these could be regarded as waves in a women's health "megamovement." (These waves, which are described in chapter 2, include the women's health component of the Popular Health Movement, which peaked in the 1830s and 1840s; the post–Civil War women's medical movement and campaigns against contraception and abortion; Progressive Era movements in maternal and child health and for legalization of birth control; the Women's Health Movement of the 1960s and 1970s; and the women's health agenda of the early 1990s.) Because these waves occurred in different historical eras, they were conditioned by different conceptions of women's social roles and health problems. Yet they were all concerned with changing the social conditions affecting health, with reshaping health care institutions, or with formulating public policy to improve the health (and sometimes the social status) of women. An aspect of this latest wave of women's health activism that has not yet been explored is how it is embedded in this tradition of American women's health movements.

A central thesis of this book is that women's health has been the subject of recurring social movement activity because of the deeply rooted and continuously evolving cultural relationship between women and American health care institutions. In considering why women, rather than men or some other social group, have been perennial health reformers, it is tempting to revert to a biological explanation. Some have argued, for example, that because women have the capacity to get pregnant and men do not, women are more vulnerable physically and have greater health care needs than men. Further, because society depends for its survival upon the reproductive health of women, society must be, at some level, attentive to women's health needs and receptive to their demands. Whether women or men are more biologically vulnerable has been debated for some time, however, and a strong case can be made that the risks to women's health posed by pregnancy and childbirth are at least as much culturally as biologically determined. A related reductionistic appeal to biological factors might argue that the bodily experiences shared by most women (e.g., menstruation, pregnancy, and menopause) have provided the basis for gender solidarity that cuts across socioeconomic, racial, ethnic, and religious groups and gives voice to women's universal health concerns. Cultural differences in the meanings of reproductive experiences have been observed, however, and all women do not agree on whether or how medical interventions should be used in connection with their reproductive or other bodily functions.

The argument made here depends upon understanding how culture elaborates biology and, in particular, the reproductive role of women. Because women, historically, have been purveyors of domestic medicine, including midwifery, and have been expected to be caregivers for their children and other family members, they have been uniquely culturally situated as both providers and consumers of health care. As American health care institutions became more formalized and male dominated and as the health care marketplace became more complex, inevitable gender-based tensions arose over who had authority to define and control health care practices—particularly in the realms of fertility control and childbearing, which have always been central to women's status—and who would provide for the poor and vulnerable. The working out of these issues in one historical era, furthermore, often set the stage for another round of contention in a subsequent era, particularly as women's social and economic roles underwent major transformations throughout the nineteenth and twentieth centuries.

Health care has never been simply the rational application of biomedical science or technology to the problems of the human body. It is also a negotiated social arrangement for providing personal services that are perceived to be needed and appropriate by providers, consumers, insurers, policymakers, and others. These groups have diverse interests and do not always agree, and perceptions change over time. The historical development of U.S. health care institutions, furthermore, has been particularly contentious and has involved major rivalries among competing medical paradigms as well as struggles by women to attain legitimacy as health care professionals, particularly within medicine. Gender has provided a basis both for the elaboration of health care roles and for the design of health care delivery organizations. In consequence, women and men experience basic health care in substantially different ways. Women not only consume more health services than men throughout most of the life span, they also establish more regular patterns of health care and receive basic care from a different array of providers and organizations and through a variety of publicly funded programs that serve a large proportion of the female population. Women also tend to be responsible for the health care of their children and other family members, which involves both informal (unpaid) home care and interacting with the health care system on the family's behalf. Finally, although most health care workers and consumers in the United States today are women, and although women are increasingly represented within the institutions that formulate health care policies and practices, many health care institutions are dominated by male physicians and administrators, and health care policy is formulated largely by men.

Contrary to conventional wisdom, however, women have not been passive victims of medical control. Historically, women have provided a key market for health services and products; they have incited some important changes in medical practice through their power as consumers; and at times they have been prominent and highly influential providers of health care. In addition, they have formed associations and fomented social movement activity that has resulted in the creation of new organizations for women's health care and has influenced national health care policy. In consequence, the current configuration of health care institutions is the product of multiple factors and is not simply a reflection of androcentric bias. It is also a legacy, in part, of women's organized efforts over the years to generate new services and organizations to meet needs that were not being addressed by mainstream providers.

Acknowledging the influences of women's health movements does not imply that they have been uniformly beneficial to women. Although there have been a number of important innovations in U.S. health care that were the work of women—such as the introduction of prenatal care and the first federal funding for maternal and child health care programs under the Sheppard-Towner Act of 1921—not all changes brought about by women activists of earlier eras would be viewed as positive ones in light of current feminist sensibilities. The movement history does, however, permit an understanding of the political possibilities of women's health activism as well as the enduring concerns that have mobilized women in different eras. Some of these concerns, which need to be recognized by providers and policymakers today, include women's demands for health and body information relevant to their own and their families' health; women's preferences for gender-appropriate health care and, in at least some circumstances, for care by women providers; and women's determination to understand and control their fertility and the conditions of childbearing.

Policymaking with respect to women's health also has a history. At times health policymaking has been gender specific, and at times it has sought to be gender neutral. American culture is quite conflicted about gendered approaches to social problems in general, not only in the health arena. The current dominant ideology of gender equality in some ways has blinded policymakers to differences in the health care experiences and needs of women and men, as, for example, when debates about restructuring Medicaid and Medicare fail to acknowledge the differential impact of policy options on women and men. On the other hand, demands for gender equity in the allocation of public resources, sometimes to redress past inequities, have been used to justify gender-specific programs and policies, such as recent allocations of federal funds earmarked for women's health research. Indeed, health care policy that is gender neutral in intent is not likely to be gender neutral in impact, and some gender-specific policies may carry costs that in the long run are not beneficial to women. One of the challenges is to find ways to incorporate gender-based concerns in health care policymaking in such a way as to simultaneously eliminate gender-based disadvantages and attend to women's specific needs. Organized women's health advocacy provides one mechanism for incorporating women's viewpoints and strategies for change in health care policymaking.

CULTURAL CONTEXT

The focus of this book is on women's health in the United States and within the context of evolving U.S. health care institutions. Currently, however, women's health issues are receiving nearly global attention. The Fourth World Conference on Women held in Beijing in 1995 asserted in a declaration unanimously adopted by 189 countries that "the right of all women to control all aspects of their health, in particular their own fertility, is basic to their empowerment," and the conference identified access to health care and related services as one of twelve "critical areas of concern" for women's advancement (United Nations 1996:650). Some of the trends in women's health care, such as attempts to expand its scope beyond maternal health to include both a multirole and a life span perspective, are evident to varying degrees in both developed and developing countries (Koblinsky, Timyan, and Gay 1993; Smyke 1991). In addition, women's health movements are not unique to the United States and often have contemporaneous international counterparts associated with waves of feminist or other social movements (Bolt 1993; Calhoun 1995; Chafetz, Dworkin, and Swanson 1990; Doyal 1983).

While it is beyond the scope of this book to provide comprehensive international comparisons of women's health care issues or movements, several apparently distinctive aspects of the U.S. context suggest how women's health might be constructed as a public issue in this country. To begin with, American society has frequently been characterized as particularly fertile ground for voluntary associations organized around a variety of social issues, including health. This was first commented upon by Alexis de Tocqueville in the 1830s (Mayer 1988) and has also been noted in relation to the founding and impact of voluntary associations on a variety of personal and public health issues (many of which did not focus on women's health exclusively) during the nineteenth and early twentieth centuries. Voluntary action, moreover, frequently has goaded governmental action. In his history of public health, for example, George Rosen points out that voluntary action by private individuals and groups frequently stimulated government action to promote the health of the community and that "the voluntary health movement has had its fullest flowering in the United States" (Rosen 1993:358–359). He notes the proliferation of U.S. voluntary associations organized to combat specific diseases (e.g., tuberculosis), disorders of specific organs (e.g., the heart), health problems of specific groups (e.g., mothers and babies), and health problems of the community as a whole (e.g., sanitary reform). Rosen attributes the "voluntary health movement" in the United States to industrialization and rapid urbanization, which simultaneously created problems of poverty and privation and produced the resources and leisure time necessary to found new organizations.

In addition, the prominent historical role and organizing skills of middle-class U.S. women in voluntary associations for moral reform and social welfare issues has been described by numerous scholars, especially since the 1970s (Baker 1990; Cott 1977; Ginzberg 1990; Muncy 1991; Rothman 1978; Skocpol 1992; West and Blumberg 1990). The activism of U.S. women throughout the nineteenth and early twentieth centuries has been attributed to such factors as shifts in gender role ideology and changing conceptions of citizenship following the Revolutionary War; rapid urbanization and industrialization, which among other things brought women into contact with each other and with the problems of immigrants and the poor; and expanding educational opportunities for women. While it is debatable whether U.S. women have been, overall, more influential than their counterparts in Britain, with whom American women have been frequently compared, health-related movements provide some of the examples of U.S. women's distinctive identity-based politics and organizational strategies (Bolt 1993; Doyal 1995; Shryock 1966; Skocpol 1995).

Finally, the development of the U.S. medical profession followed a distinctive path, despite the considerable influences of European medicine during the eighteenth and nineteenth centuries. American medicine's early development was characterized by a period of intense competition among rival practitioners and among alternative medical paradigms, in a relatively open market for health services and products (Rothstein 1992). In the late nineteenth and early twentieth centuries, the medical profession consolidated its authority and grew to dominate U.S. health care's financial and organizational structure to a degree unparalleled in other nations (Freidson 1973; Starr 1982). Paul Starr (1982:196), for example, describes how the American principle "that the state should not compete with private business" enabled physicians in private practice to limit public health activities perceived as competitive and to elevate the status of private clinical medicine over public health. The proliferation of medical specialties and the absence of a national health care system, furthermore, have created opportunities for local variation and experimentation in health care practices and for the emergence of new and increasingly diverse organizational forms. Applying the lens of gender to this history reveals not only that women have always provided a key client base for the American medical profession but also that there are many instances in which women, as both consumers and providers, have helped shape the content of medical practice and the nature of U.S. health care institutions.

PLAN OF THE BOOK

Chapter 1 presents some concepts and theoretical perspectives guiding this sociohistorical consideration of women's health as a public issue and of gender as an attribute of health care. The chapter considers the topics of gender as a social cause of health and illness; the social construction of health and body issues; the concept of human agency in the shaping of health care institutions; the concepts of social problems and social movements and the continuity of women's health movements; and an argument about the cultural significance of women's health in the United States.

Chapter 2 provides a historical overview of five episodes of public attention to women's health issues that constitute waves in the women's health "megamovement." Each wave is described with regard to its sociohistorical context and precipitating factors, the contemporary state of health care institutions, the specific women's health issues addressed, and the strategies used by women activists to change the conditions of their health and health care. The legacies and unintended consequences of each episode for women's health care and health care institutions in general are noted, as are the recurring themes and unresolved issues that to some extent still concern women's health advocates today.

Chapter 3 considers one of the key claims of the 1990s women's health movement episode, namely, that women are disadvantaged because of inequitable access to the benefits of health care. Current evidence for gender differences in health status and in health care utilization patterns is examined, and alternative explanations for observed gender differences in utilization are explored, with particular emphasis on issues of access to care. The nature of women's health care is discussed, and evidence is presented that women's basic health care is configured differently from that of men. Women's basic health care is fragmented; that is, reproductive health care often is separated from other components of care for sociohistorical reasons including medical specialization, the organizational and financial separation of services, and the politics of women's reproductive health services. Recent data on women's patterns of health care are presented, and the implications of the growth of managed care for women's health are considered.

Chapter 4 addresses one of the recurring themes and unresolved issues in women's health movements, namely, whether women's health care ought to be delivered by women providers or in separate organizations for women. The historical origins of concerns about gender-congruent care for women and of separate organizations for women's health care are discussed. The recent growth in the proportion of women physicians, particularly in primary care, and of various types of women's health centers provides an unprecedented opportunity to investigate the evidence for the possible benefits and costs of gender-congruent and gender-segregated models of health care for women. Although many questions remain, it is apparent that the issues are alive in the health care marketplace and that some types of women's health centers have developed innovative models for women-centered health care.

Chapter 5 provides a discussion of how women's concerns can be incorporated into health care policymaking. American society is conflicted about approaches for dealing with gender in public policy, yet the growing number and level of influence of women's health advocacy and interest groups provide a basis for influencing health care decisions made by both governmental and nongovernmental bodies. Breast cancer activism and women's health advocacy during the recent episode of health care reform activity provide case studies of the influence of women's health groups. Three areas of policymaking that will challenge women's health advocates in the changing health care environment include ensuring women's access to care, designing women-centered models of care delivery, and empowering women to maintain or improve their health.

1

The Social and Historical
Context of Women's Health Care

Women's health has been a recurring topic of public debate in the United States for nearly two centuries and has been the focus of multiple social movements. The concerns raised in these movements, however, are not just about health and illness, and they cannot be explained by appealing only to epidemiological evidence of health problems in the population. More importantly, they are about the relationship between women and the health care institutions that affect their social status and well-being. Several theoretical perspectives and key concepts provide a basis for a sociohistorical understanding of women's health care as a public issue and as a focus of women's social action.

SOCIAL CAUSATION AND GENDER

A basic premise in medical sociology is that health and illness are affected by social as well as biological factors. "Social causation" refers to the idea that individuals' locations within the social structure and the nature of social relations are important determinants of health status. Accordingly, the causes of sex differences in health and illness cannot be attributed exclusively to genetic factors, hormones, metabolism, immune system function, or body size or composition. Although women and men are not the same biologically, the principle of social causation directs attention to how biology interacts with sociocultural factors to produce sex differences in health and illness. (Conceptions of health and illness also are influenced by culture, as discussed below.)

Gender can be regarded as one of the underlying "social causes" of health and illness (Brown 1995; Link and Phelan 1995). The term "gender" currently is used by social scientists in at least two ways: it refers to the socially prescribed roles and statuses that attach to the sexes within a given cultural and historical context, and it refers to an organizing principle by which societies define sex-linked roles and statuses, relationships, and self-conceptions or gender identities.[1] In either of these meanings, prevailing societal conceptions of gender, or gender role ideologies, are understood to be normative, rather than descriptive, depictions of behavior. In addition, they reflect the views of dominant social groups, rather than a consensus among members of a social system, and they evolve in response to changing social conditions and changing patterns of behavior. Nevertheless, gender conceptions can be powerful influences on behavior and institutions, and gender can play a pivotal role in structuring individuals' relationships with health care institutions and with other health-producing resources.

The relationships among sex, gender, and health are complex and vary by social and historical context. Gender also interacts with other social causes of health and illness, such as age, socioeconomic status, race, and ethnicity.[2] To the extent that social and economic resources are differentially allocated by gender, or that gender conceptions vary by subcultural context, specific subgroups of women may have health experiences that are quite different from those of other women. This notion is often lost in discussions of women's health, sometimes because of the presumption that health is totally biologically determined and sometimes because information is not available on relevant subgroups. Poor or low-income women and women who are members of disadvantaged racial or ethnic minorities often obtain fewer or different health services than do more affluent women, and they often experience different risks to health and worse health status. In addition, minority women may not experience their health problems as a function of gender, but as problems of poverty, racism, or other factors. It would be misleading, however, to assume that the existence of social inequalities among women negates the importance of the "main effect" of gender. On the contrary, prevailing conceptions of health and health care are highly gendered, and there are important commonalities in how women are viewed medically and in how they are treated by health care providers. Minority women, furthermore, are increasingly involved in women's health advocacy and have articulated important interactions between gender and race/ethnicity that have an impact on health.

In theory, gender may affect health through several pathways. Differential social value assigned to the sexes and gender-linked cultural rituals affect exposure to health risks. Societal conceptions of "masculinity" and "femininity" may produce differences in lifestyle behaviors that expose the sexes to different risks to health. Allocation of women and men to different social roles also may result in different exposures, role stresses, or inequalities in access to health-producing resources (e.g., education, income). Learned illness-related behaviors may produce differences in how individual women and men experience stress and bodily problems and in how they interact with health care providers. Finally, health care providers may respond to or treat women and men differently, producing differences in use of services, the process of care, or health outcomes. Each of these pathways has implications for both males and females.

First, the relative status or social value assigned to each sex within a specific sociocultural context may affect life chances or health status (Doyal 1995; Jacobson 1993). In cultures where male children are preferred, for example, practices such as female infanticide or prenatal sex-selection favor the survival of males. Similarly, female children may receive fewer resources, especially food and health care, leading to nutritional and other deficiencies that affect current and subsequent health status, including reproductive capacity and maternal mortality. Differences in social value as well as power differentials between men and women mean that female children and adults may be exposed to more domestic violence, including sexual abuse, than males (Campbell and Landenburger 1995). Power differentials also may impede women's access to health care in cultures where a male relative's permission is required for provision of services.

Second, cultural rituals associated with gender may produce differential risks to health. For example, male and female circumcision carry the immediate risks of infection and trauma, but female genital mutilation carries the longer-term risks of sexual dysfunction and reproductive health problems (Doyal 1995). Male initiation rites involving physical risk-taking carry the risks of injury or death. Female rituals associated with menstruation or childbirth that label women as "unclean" or isolate them from support networks can be dangerous to women's physical and mental health. (On the other hand, gender-based bonding rituals may provide a source of social support that is protective of health.) Cultural taboos regarding communication about such matters as menstruation, conception, and nonconsensual sexual relations may expose adolescent women to unintended pregnancies and sexually transmitted diseases.

Third, differences between women and men's lifestyles and social roles also may affect health by exposing women and men to different risks. These factors have been examined frequently in studies of gender and health in the United States. Sociologists and psychologists often conclude that acquired risks associated with lifestyle and social roles account for much of the observed differences in morbidity and mortality between women and men (Rodin and Ickovics 1990; Verbrugge 1989, 1990; Walsh, Sorensen, and Leonard 1995). This view, however, tends to downplay the role of health care institutions in structuring the experience of illness differently for women and men, as is explored below.

Gender-linked lifestyle differences tend to be associated with cultural notions of "masculinity" and "femininity." In American society, gender-linked behaviors that currently produce risks to health include men's more frequent use of tobacco, alcohol, and illicit drugs and their more frequent physical risk taking (including aggressive sports and fast driving); they also include women's less frequent participation in regular vigorous exercise and more frequent dieting and use of over-the-counter diet medications (Rodin and Ickovics 1990). Men's patterns of substance use and other physical risk taking have been interpreted as major contributors to their higher overall mortality (Waldron 1995). Other gender-related behaviors that are not always recognized as having health implications include the use of certain fashions (e.g., women's high-heeled shoes) or beauty products.

Social role differences between women and men are thought to affect health primarily by influencing access to health-producing resources such as nutrition, shelter, education, paid employment, supportive social networks, health care insurance, and health care services. Gender stratification theorists have shown how societies structure access to such resources along gender lines (Chafetz 1991; Dunn, Almquist, and Chafetz 1993). Women in the United States are more likely than men to be economically disadvantaged, for several reasons. Women are less likely than men to work for pay or, if they are employed, to work full-time; women earn less income than men, even for the same work; women are less likely than men to have health insurance through their own employment and more likely than men to be insured through a family member's insurance or through public programs, especially Medicaid;

and women are more likely to be responsible for the care of children or other dependents.[3] Lower socioeconomic status is persistently associated with poorer health (Feinstein 1993; Marmot, Bobak, and Smith 1995).

Women's labor force participation also is associated with their health. Overall, despite earlier concerns that rising female labor force participation in the United States would expose women to more stress because of the demands of multiple roles (Nathanson 1975), employed women generally report better health status than do women who are not employed. This probably reflects both selection of healthier women into the work force (the "healthy worker effect") and the psychosocial and material benefits that accrue from employment. Some scholars therefore interpret women's lower rates of paid employment, relative to men, as a risk factor for health (Hartmann, Kuriansky, and Owens 1996; Ross and Bird 1994; Ross and Mirowsky 1995; Verbrugge 1989). Ross and Bird (1994) attribute gender differences in perceived health status to a combination of social roles and lifestyle; they argue that if women had the same level of labor force involvement and of leisure time physical activity as men, their perceived health would equal or exceed that of men by midlife (i.e., after age 54). On the other hand, the allocation of women and men to different types of jobs, and such gender-related workplace issues as exposure to sexual harassment and availability of childcare, raise questions about overall gender differences in work-related stresses that could have important effects on health (Hall 1991; Walsh, Sorensen, and Leonard 1995).

Fourth, learned illness behaviors associated with gender may affect health. These behaviors pertain to how people experience and act upon illness or other bodily conditions; they include women's presumed greater willingness to seek health-related information from a number of sources, to acknowledge bodily signs and symptoms, to report signs and symptoms to health professionals or in health surveys, to engage in health promotion activities, to seek health care in a timely fashion when symptoms occur, and to convalesce appropriately (Hibbard and Pope 1986; Mechanic 1978). Indeed, by all available indicators, women consume more health products and services than men. Some argue that the weight of current evidence suggests that gender-linked care-seeking behaviors are more likely to occur in relation to minor health problems than for major, life-threatening ones (Walsh, Sorensen, and Leonard 1995). However, another explanation for observed gender differences in care-seeking is that health care institutions may structure care differently for women and men. For instance, physicians may be likely to interpret women's symptoms or bodily experiences, more so than men's, as treatable conditions and to encourage greater use of services by women than by men.

Gender affects both health risks and individuals' interactions with the health care system. While the overall calculus of gender effects may not favor the health of one sex or the other, awareness of some of the ways in which gender might affect health is important in considering health care issues for both women and men.[4] Recognizing the relationships between gender and health is also key to understanding why the "biomedical" model of health, which neglects the psychosocial context of health and illness, is criticized by feminists as too narrowly focused and incapable of providing the solutions to women's health problems.

THE SOCIAL CONSTRUCTION OF HEALTH

It is now a truism within social science that conceptions of health and illness are socially constructed and historically changeable. "Social constructionism" contrasts with the view that knowledge proceeds incrementally from the discovery of objective "facts" or the progress of science. Instead, definitions of health and the labeling of specific conditions as "diseases" or "health problems" are understood as the products, at least in part, of shifting social and cultural factors and of the competing views of multiple social actors, including both professional and lay persons (Lupton 1994). Socially constructed conceptions of health and illness, furthermore, help structure social reality, as when these conceptions are used to provide rationales for the social position of a particular group or to control what is perceived as morally deviant behavior (Hubbard 1990).

The understanding of disease definition, or the identification and acceptance of diagnostic categories, as a sociopolitical process is an important example of the social constructionist perspective (Brown 1995). Women's health problems have frequently been discussed within this perspective, in connection with the phenomenon of "medicalization." Medicalization is the process of labeling conditions as diseases or disorders as a basis for providing medical treatment of some kind, and the medicalization of many of women's biological functions, such as menstruation and pregnancy, frequently has been cited to illustrate both the social construction of disease and the general expansion of medical control into everyday life (Conrad 1992; Zola 1972). That society generally, and women in particular, sometimes desire and encourage medicalization has been less frequently acknowledged.

The case of menopause provides an interesting illustration of the social construction of women's health and illness. Research reveals how conceptions of menopause vary in different cultural contexts and over time within the same culture. The anthropologist Margaret Lock (1993) has shown that in Japan in the 1980s, where women's average life expectancy at birth was about four years longer than in the United States, menopause was not regarded as a medical condition by either women or physicians. Further, Japanese women reported significantly fewer, and different, menopausal symptoms than women in Canada and the United States: the most frequently reported symptom among Japanese women was shoulder stiffness, whereas hot flushes (for which there is no word in Japanese) were the most common symptom among Canadian and American women.

In the United States, conceptions of menopause have undergone several transformations, reflecting changes in both scientific knowledge and gender ideology. Despite conventional wisdom that menopause has only recently been identified as a major women's health issue, considerable attention was addressed to it over a century ago. In the late nineteenth century, consistent with the medical beliefs that a woman's health was controlled by her reproductive organs and that her moral purpose resided in maternity, physicians began to view menopause as a "physiological crisis" and major risk to health. Carroll Smith-Rosenberg (1985) points out that physicians of the period tended to attribute all diseases of aging females to menopause and to believe that the moral propriety of women's sexual and social behavior affected their adaptation to the postreproductive phase of life; women, however, often viewed menopause as freedom from the demands of childbearing and child rearing. In the 1930s and 1940s, scientific advances in sex endocrinology and the ability to synthesize estrogen provided the opportunity for a medical redefinition of menopause as a hormone "deficiency disease" and for the use of estrogen replacement therapy to treat symptoms of the menopausal transition such as hot flushes, menstrual irregularities, and depression (Bell 1987). In the 1960s, estrogen replacement therapy was promoted by some physicians and by the pharmaceutical industry as a lifelong treatment for postmenopausal women to preserve their "femininity," rather than as a short-term treatment to alleviate menopausal symptoms (Wilson 1966; Coney 1994).

By the 1990s, as the post–World War II "baby-boom" generation of women approached midlife, their demands for information and treatments were expected to inundate the health care delivery system and to provide marketing opportunities for pharmaceutical companies and providers. A new "prevention paradigm" began to guide both medical and lay conceptions of menopause. Menopause had come to be regarded as a normal part of female aging that does not produce bothersome symptoms in all women. Indeed, some women's health advocates referred to the "signs" rather than "symptoms" of menopause, to emphasize that it is not a disease (Doress-Worters and Siegal 1994) and to "hormone therapy," rather than "hormone replacement therapy," to dispel the notion that postmenopausal women suffer a deficiency of hormones. Nevertheless, lifelong hormone therapy or nonhormonal treatments began to be promoted by health professionals for symptomless menopausal women as a means of preventing heart disease and osteoporosis (Worcester and Whatley 1992). Thus the "perimenopause" was being redefined as an opportune time in healthy women's lives for a medical evaluation and initiation of therapy to prevent future disease and disability. This therapy, furthermore, requires a long-term relationship, including reassessments and follow-up, with health care providers.

Another case of social construction of women's heath and illness is the formulation of an official psychiatric diagnosis for premenstrual syndrome. Attaching mental health labels or diagnoses to normative female gender-role behavior has been identified as a problem by women's health advocates since the 1970s, and there have been several recent cases that have stirred controversy. (An example is a proposed diagnosis of self-defeating personality disorder, which included criteria such as "excessive self-sacrifice that is unsolicited by the intended recipients" and "fails to accomplish tasks crucial to his or her personal objectives" [American Psychiatric Association 1987:216–217] that could be regarded as components of normal female caregiving.) Premenstrual syndrome was first described as a hormonal condition by an American gynecologist in the 1930s, and it became the subject of a proposed psychiatric diagnosis when, in 1985, an advisory committee to the American Psychiatric Association recommended that it be included in the Diagnostic and Statistical Manual of Mental Disorders (DSM) used by mental health providers and insurers. Called "premenstrual dysphoric disorder," this proposed diagnosis aroused a campaign of opposition led by women psychiatrists, psychologists, and social workers, joined by women's health advocacy groups. These women were concerned that the proposed diagnosis was based on weak science, reflected male bias about female behavior, and could stigmatize and cause harm to all women. (Not all women opposed the diagnosis, however, and some found that it validated their bodily experiences.) The diagnosis was debated, renamed twice, and modified, and it was finally included in DSM-IV in 1994. In her recent case study of the social structuring of this psychiatric disorder, Anne Figert (1996) describes the process as a struggle for "ownership" of premenstrual syndrome among various health and mental health professionals, scientists and biomedical researchers, and women, as both expert professionals and persons who had experienced premenstrual symptoms.

The view that medicine reinforces women's dependency by creating normative definitions of health, disease, and behavior—and by enforcing these conceptions through diagnosis and treatment—has been widely accepted among feminist critics of the health care system since the 1960s. For example, Barbara Ehrenreich and Deirdre English (1973a:83) have called the medical system "a powerful instrument of social control, replacing organized religion as a prime source of sexist ideology and an enforcer of sex roles." Susan Sherwin (1992:180) argues that "classifying the ordinary events of women's lives as illnesses licences wide-scale medical management of women under claims of beneficence."

Emerging definitions of women's health attempt to balance the desire to limit medical intrusion in matters of personal behavior with the need for a more holistic view of health that takes social causation into account. The new "biopsychosocial" conceptions of women's health focus on the whole woman (mind and body) through the life span and acknowledge the social, economic, and cultural conditions that produce health. The emphasis is not only on how women's health differs from men's but also on how health can be understood from a women-centered perspective. Rodriguez-Trias (1992), for example, proposes two concepts for defining women's health: centrality (i.e., using women's experiences as the basis for health research, services, and policy) and totality (i.e., health understood holistically and in the context of women's lives.) Sheryl Ruzek (1993) argues for a more "inclusive social model" of health that recognizes the diversity of women's social circumstances and targets the community, as well as the body, as a place to intervene to improve health. Intervening in the community might include, for example, improving the living standards of women, reducing exposure to environmental contaminants, or reducing domestic violence or other threats to personal safety. A social definition of women's health was adopted in the Platform for Action of the Fourth World Conference on Women in Beijing, based on the World Health Organization's definition of health as "a state of complete physical, mental and social well-being and not merely the absence of disease or infirmity" (United Nations 1996:667). However, while biomedical definitions of women's health are criticized for their focus on disease rather than wellness and for their biological essentialism, social definitions also have their critics. The bioethicist Laura Purdy (1996), for example, is concerned that notions of social health might encourage the extension of medical authority into social and behavioral realms in which medical professionals have no special expertise.

Social well-being, defined with respect to some standard of social justice, might be more appropriately conceptualized as both a cause and a consequence of health.

To the extent that the medical profession currently enjoys the cultural authority to identify diseases and other conditions requiring medical treatment, to define normative health-seeking behavior, and to control access to important health information or effective services, it has the capacity to affect individuals' health status, quality of life, pursuit of personal objectives, and full participation in the life of the community. There are a number of problems, however, with the simplistic view of medicalization as the social control of women. For one thing, the power of the medical profession to prescribe women's lives has often been overstated. The medical profession is not the only institution that influences gender role conceptions or affects how individuals "practice" gender in their daily lives. R. W. Connell (1987) discusses, for example, how educational institutions, the family, the workplace, the church, and the state reproduce society's gender order through routinized practices he calls "gender regimes." In addition, physicians themselves are educated and practice within a social and historical context, and they are subject to the same prevailing gender role ideologies and gender power relations that affect other members of society. Moreover, medicine clearly provides some effective treatments for conditions that would otherwise limit individuals' life chances or capacities to realize their personal objectives, and not all treatments of female-specific conditions can be regarded as attempts to oppress women or to exploit them as patients. Finally, an overemphasis on medical control neglects the historical role women themselves have played in demanding medical attention for their problems and in creating markets for new services. Women often have contributed to the identification of health problems requiring treatment, and they often have demanded new medical services in response to their experiences of bodily symptoms, such as the discomforts that may accompany menstruation, childbirth, or the menopausal transition.

Catherine Riessman (1983) argues that women are more likely than men to have their bodily experiences defined and treated as medical conditions. In her view, this occurs because women's reproductive function, social responsibility for the family's health care and consequent greater contact with the health care system, and subordination to male control within health care institutions make them a convenient market for the expansion of medicine's domain. Yet she also perceptively points out that the medicalization of women's problems may sometimes serve the needs of women to have their bodily experiences acknowledged and validated and that women may "collaborate in the medicalization process" (Riessman 1983:3). Historically, women from the relatively privileged classes, who were most able to afford medical care, were particularly influential in the medicalization of experiences that were central to their lives, such as pregnancy and childbirth. As we shall see, women are not always passive participants in the medicalization process, nor are they necessarily "controlled" by medical diagnoses or treatments.

HUMAN AGENCY

Institutions have been defined as the "cognitive, normative, and regulative structures and activities that provide stability and meaning to social behavior" (Scott 1995:33). Institutions both provide a context for human activities and are the products of those activities. Human "agency" refers to the purposive actions of individuals who intervene in events and to the production, or reproduction, of social structure through human actions (Giddens 1979, 1986). In this conception, human actions are not viewed as totally controlled by social structure, but rather as occurring within the context of structure and as continuously reinventing that structure.

These concepts point to mutual influences between individuals and health care institutions. They direct us to consider not only how women have been affected by health care institutions but also how women have attempted to shape conceptions of their health and the nature of their health care. Women's political agency with respect to social welfare issues has recently been explored by a number of historians and social scientists, but activism with respect to health and body issues has received less attention. Earlier scholarship of the relationship between women and health care institutions typically took the view that the male-dominated medical profession has controlled and oppressed women, first by usurping women's traditional role as midwife and domestic healer, and then by attempting to control women's behavior (particularly reproductive behavior) and to secure their patronage by defining their bodily functions (especially pregnancy and childbirth) as diseases (Ehrenreich and English 1973a, 1978). Sheila Rothman (1978:7) argues that the medical profession is one of several institutions that have "shaped attitudes toward womanhood and exerted a profound influence on women's sense of self." Without denying that there are power differentials between women and men and that many institutions, including health care institutions, are typically male dominated, it is nevertheless possible to identify ways in which women, as both consumers and providers, have taken actions to influence the development of American health care practice and policy.

The perspective of women's agency—in contrast to the perspective emphasizing the social control or oppression of women—can be unsettling, however, because it illuminates some instances in which women's participation in the development of social policies and institutions may not have contributed to an expansion of women's rights or to an improvement of women's social condition. Identifying women's agency in health care does not imply that women have always been successful in their attempts to influence health institutions or that they have always been feminist in their intent or that progress has been linear. Some attempts to influence health care fail, some have unintended consequences, and some result in what might be perceived as regressions, rather than progressions, from the perspective of improving women's health or social well-being. Theda Skocpol (1992:38), for example, points out that women's groups may achieve legislative victories in their promotion of social welfare policies targeted to women, "but then may be unable to control the implementation of social policies, so that they end up doing harm rather than good to many women." In another example pertaining to health care innovation, Ruzek (1995a) observes that women's health advocacy groups in the 1990s sometimes lobbied for increased access to new biotechnologies whose efficacy had not been demonstrated; when they succeeded, they inadvertently exposed women to increased iatrogenic risks. Despite these dynamics, or perhaps because of them, it is important to consider the ways in which women's agency has played out not only to better understand the current status of women's health care but also as a basis for considering women's political capacities and future change strategies.

To begin with, the process of medicalization results not only from medical expansionism and entrepreneurship but also from consumers' demands for recognition of their bodily symptoms as legitimate health problems that may cause discomfort or inhibit normal social functioning. Medical recognition of problems holds the promise of a number of benefits to individuals, including liberation from attributions of blame; validation of experienced symptoms; an understanding of how to prevent health problems; access to safe and effective treatments for conditions that are painful, debilitating, or inconvenient; access to health insurance for these treatments; and socially sanctioned excuses to withdraw from regular social activities and duties because of illness. There are numerous examples of American women's efforts, sometimes against substantial medical resistence, to gain recognition and treatment for specific bodily problems, including pain during childbirth, menstrual and premenstrual symptoms, infertility, and the side effects of drugs or devices, such as intrauterine devices and silicone breast implants (Brown 1995; Conrad 1992; Marsh and Ronner 1996; Riessman 1983). There have also been attempts by women to "demedicalize" bodily experiences, especially childbirth, and to attain lay control over medical procedures, such as abortion and artificial insemination (Conrad 1992).

The ways in which lay (i.e., nonprofessional) persons exercise influence on the social construction of health and illness and, by extension, on the nature of health care institutions and policy is a seriously underresearched topic. This may be a by-product of social scientists' preoccupation with understanding the development of the distinctive cultural authority of the American medical profession and its influence on the nature of U.S. health care. There has also been a tendency to interpret the historical development of the health professions and of specific health institutions, such as the hospital, largely as a function of scientific discoveries or advances in biomedical technology. Longstanding and recurring efforts by women to influence health care have not yet been conceptualized within a framework that might provide some insight into lay influence processes generally or the dynamic relationship between women and health care institutions specifically.

Theoretically, the influence of lay persons can be considered at two levels of analysis: at the microlevel, within the context of health care encounters, and at the macrolevel, through collective action. Another way of thinking about these levels of influence is as markets and movements—that is, as interactions between purchasers and providers of health care versus the dynamics of organized social action. At the microlevel, the influence of consumers on the definition of health and illness and on the practices of their health care providers may be exercised within the context of patient-provider exchanges. In most health care encounters, the individual practitioner (or the employing organization) has an incentive to satisfy the patient so that the patient will remain in the practice or recommend the practice to others. Freidson (1973) points out that in "client-dependent" medical practices, in which physicians rely on lay referrals rather than on referrals from colleagues (or, today, on contracts with insurers), physicians have a strong incentive to be responsive to consumers' demands for specific services, even if those services are not professionally sanctioned. This is an important point because client-dependent practices predominated in American health care prior to the growth of medical specialization and the widespread practice of referral-based medicine, beginning around 1900. To some extent, the dynamics of client dependence continue today, even in managed care, since plans may compete, in part, on the basis of patient satisfaction and retention levels.

A classic case of consumers' influence on the practices of their personal physicians is American women's growing demand, against considerable medical opposition, for pain relief in childbirth during the second half of the nineteenth century. Anesthesia had been introduced in the 1840s, but many physicians were reluctant to use it in childbirth for a variety of reasons. These included religious beliefs that women were meant to suffer in childbirth; moral concerns for propriety, which were already heightened by the presence of male physicians in the birthing chamber; and medical uncertainty about safe dosages (Duffy 1993; Wertz and Wertz 1989). At the time, childbirth occurred in the home and was controlled by the woman and her attendants. Because physicians competed with lay midwives for women's patronage, they had an incentive to provide the new services women wanted. American women's demands for pain relief apparently grew after Queen Victoria used chloroform in childbirth in 1853, and the written accounts of contemporary physicians include reports of using anesthesia only if their patients demanded it. Thus women's demands are thought to have been the major factor in physicians' wider adoption of ether and chloroform in childbirth (Leavitt 1986). The medical use of anesthesia, in turn, may have accelerated women's use of physicians rather than midwives as childbirth attendants.

At the macrolevel, organized groups of consumers may engage in collective action to advocate or implement changes in health care delivery or policy. At different points in time, American women have organized to educate themselves about their health and health care, to advocate for new medical treatments or technologies, to provide services not otherwise available to women, to infuse women's values into mainstream health care organizations, to extend care to underserved groups, to advocate for public health programs, and to change public policy governing health care delivery, health care financing, or health research. Women's collective action has taken the form of direct action protests, self-help groups, patient advocacy groups, single-issue or multi-issue political action organizations, and the creation of alternative (sometimes consumer-controlled) health care institutions. Health care organizations created by and for women include maternity hospitals, prenatal care services, birth control clinics, self-help women's clinics, freestanding birth centers, abortion clinics, and multidisciplinary women's health centers.

Women's health advocacy groups have a long history. An early example from the 1910s—again related to pain relief in childbirth—was the organization of middle- and upper-class clubwomen, joined eventually by working-class women, to pressure the reluctant medical profession to adopt "twilight sleep," a combination of scopolamine and morphine that had been developed in Germany. Following publicity stemming from a 1914 article in *McClure's* magazine, an estimated 4 to 5 million women became involved in local advocacy activities. The National Twilight Sleep Association (NTSA), founded in New York in 1915, included prominent society women, suffragists, and women physicians among its leaders. In the face of sustained opposition to twilight sleep by the medical profession and its rejection by prestigious hospitals such as Johns Hopkins, as well as the death of a member of the NTSA executive committee during a twilight-sleep delivery, this organization of advocates failed in its objective and was disbanded. It did, however, succeed in promoting the increased use of pain relief technology in childbirth by compelling physicians to respond to women's demands. It also contributed to changes in the conditions of childbirth by accelerating the trends toward hospital-based delivery and the decline of lay midwifery (Leavitt 1986; Miller 1979).

Current women's health advocacy and interest groups include organizations of patients with a specific disease (most notably, breast cancer survivors), single-issue and multi-issue public-interest and educational groups, political action organizations, and associations of health professionals. Women physicians and nurses have been particularly prominent participants in organized efforts to change health care institutions. These organizations maintain vigilance on women's health problems, establish communication networks, and can quickly mobilize people and other resources when an opportunity for public action arises.

Political action on behalf of women's health also has had some profound influences on health policy. For example, women social reformers were in the forefront of efforts to improve the public health during the late 1800s and early 1900s; their activism encompassed a variety of issues including municipal sanitation, preventive medicine, and health education of the population through publicly funded programs. Progressive Era women reformers who organized effective political action in the days before women had the right to vote were responsible for the first federal government financing for women's health care programs in the United States. The Sheppard-Towner Maternity and Infancy Act of 1921 established publicly funded maternal and child health services that not only set a precedent for federally subsidized health care services through grants-in-aid to the states but also created incentives for the medical profession to incorporate prenatal care and other preventive services (for both women and men) into mainstream practice (Ladd-Taylor 1990;

Lesser 1985; Rothman 1978). Skocpol (1992:481) refers to the act as "America's first explicit federal social welfare legislation."

Thus there is an impressive historical record of the impact of women's health activism on the adoption of new medical technologies and on American health care institutions and policy.

SOCIAL PROBLEMS AND SOCIAL MOVEMENTS

That women's health emerged as a public issue in the United States around 1990 is well known; that it has been a recurring public issue over two centuries is less well recognized. The "social problems" and "social movement" literatures provide a framework for understanding the continuing prominence of women's health as a public issue. "Social problems" scholars tend to be interested in how social conditions become defined as social problems and compete for a place on the public agenda. "Social movement" scholars tend to be interested in how collective action to change some aspect of the social system is mobilized, what happens to these movements over time, and the extent to which movement goals become institutionalized or transform the culture.

A "social problem" is a social condition that has been collectively defined as a problem requiring public attention and corrective action. (Gusfield [1981:5] refers to a condition so defined as a "public problem.") Social scientists point out that social conditions such as poverty or gender inequality are not inherently problematic or objectively identifiable as problems demanding action (Blumer 1971; Spector and Kitsuse 1987). Rather, problem definition is the result of a process of social construction—or "claims-making activities" (Spector and Kitsuse 1987)—in which a dominant perception emerges that a given social condition merits both public attention and public solutions.

Hilgartner and Bosk (1988:55) define a social problem as "a putative condition or situation that is labeled a problem in the arenas of public discourse and action." The public arenas in which problems are labeled include, for example, the executive and legislative branches of government, the courts, the media, political campaigns, and social action and advocacy groups. The process of labeling a problem is the work of individuals or groups who identify and champion specific problems and specific solutions. These actors are sometimes called "issue entrepreneurs" or "policy entrepreneurs." Different groups may vie, furthermore, over problem definition in order to garner public attention or resources for their cause. For example, is abortion a moral issue, a civil rights issue, or a health issue? Is domestic violence a criminal justice problem or a women's health problem?

Since public attention is a scarce resource, at any point in time many potential problems compete with each other for public attention and commitments to action. Those problems that successfully compete tend, for example, to be related to broad cultural concerns (such as health), to be easily dramatized and communicated, and to be supported by dominant social groups. John Kingdon (1995), a political scientist who has studied how problems capture the attention of individuals in and around government, emphasizes the importance of shared beliefs that something can and should be done to solve the problem. Nevertheless, no social problem can sustain a high level of salience and public attention for long, and if solutions to the problem are attempted, an impression may be created that the problem has been addressed, and it may recede from public attention. Some social problems, furthermore, "grow, decline, and later reemerge, never vanishing completely, but receiving greatly fluctuating quantities of public attention" (Hilgartner and Bosk 1988:57).

Some social problems become the focus of sustained collective actions that are perceived as "social movements." (Social problems do not inevitably generate social movements.) Social movements are generally regarded as collective actions to change some specific aspect of the social system that becomes perceived as problematic. According to Sidney Tarrow (1994:3–4), social movements are "collective challenges by people with common purposes and solidarity in sustained interaction with elites, opponents and authorities." Social movements both respond to opportunities for action in the environment and create opportunities for mobilization. The earliest theories of social movements viewed them as the product of shared grievances and shared beliefs about the means of resolving these grievances, within a social class or other collectivity (Smelser 1962; Turner and Killian 1987). Later theories emphasized the importance of the strategic mobilization of resources—primarily people's time and money—by social movement organizations in order for collective action to develop out of a shared preference for change (McCarthy and Zald 1977). More recently, analyses of the so-called *new* social movements (e.g., student movements, peace movements, environmental movements) have emphasized cultural factors and the search for collective identity as key components in movement formation (Johnston, Laraña, and Gusfield 1994). There is active debate about whether these latter movements are really "new," and one of the points on which this debate turns is the issue of social movement continuity (Tarrow 1994).[5]

Social movement theorists have recognized for some time that movements often emerge together in clusters or "movement families" and in periods of heightened collective activity known as "cycles of protest" (McAdam 1995; Tarrow 1993). In a sense, these clusters reflect a growing social consensus on the need and opportunity for institutional change. For example, the 1960s were characterized by a rash of social movements including civil rights, student, antiwar, and women's rights movements—all of which challenged key institutions. Snow and Benford (1992) attribute the emergence of a cycle of protest to the development of an innovative "master frame" that serves to define the social problems and the possible solutions for the participants. The "civil rights master frame" is said to have characterized the various social movements of the 1960s, which tended to be based on rights claims by various social groups (McAdam 1994). Tarrow (1994) argues that the "rights" frame arose in the civil rights movement and then spread to other groups, including women, who used it to mobilize a following. These concepts also suggest the possibility of "waves" *within* a specific social movement—that is, cyclical periods of movement ascendancy, decline, dormancy, and resurgence—prompted, in part, by shifts in master frames.

Yet the problem of continuity in social movements has not received much attention by scholars (Johnston, Laraña, and Gusfield 1994). One reason for this neglect might be that it is difficult to recognize and account for the decline and resurgence of public attention to a problem area as waves in a larger social movement, particularly when the episodes are separated by a great expanse of time. Longer periods of dormancy between waves make it difficult to account for continuity in either the issues publicly raised (since they may be reframed in different historical eras) or the participation of individuals or organizations. Furthermore, one of the ways in which problem entrepreneurs capture public attention is by defining a new problem category or emphasizing the novelty of an issue (Hilgartner and Bosk 1988; Kingdon 1995); thus, these individuals may have an interest in obscuring cultural or historical antecedents of the problem they are promoting, even if movement participants are aware of such antecedents.

Social movement scholars recently have begun to consider the types of conditions or mechanisms that might sustain movements through repeated waves. Continuity in both material resources (such as formal organizations, meeting houses, mailing lists, newsletters, and volunteer activity) and cultural resources (such as collective identities and traditions of activism) has been considered. Tilly (1995) first introduced the concept of a "repertoire of contention" to refer to the set of routines that people use in collective actions to pursue their shared interests. He also described some routines as "modular," in the sense that they were used by different groups in different times and places. Tarrow (1994:18) has pointed out that "contention by convention" occurs when "particular groups have a particular history—and memory—of collective action." The Parisian tradition of barricades is a classic example of a repertoire of contention that became culturally inscribed (Traugott 1995); women banging pots and pans in social protest is an example of a cross-national repertoire (West and Blumberg 1990). Modularity and cultural repertoires can be advantages to movement organizers, furthermore, because they enable actors to mobilize without bearing the costs of inventing new symbols or techniques of contention. McAdam (1994:43), for example, refers to "long-standing activist subcultures" as providing "repositories of cultural materials" (e.g., ideas, metaphors, activist traditions) that succeeding generations of activists can draw upon to revitalize a movement. The importance of the latter point is that it helps account for continuity of a movement across longer expanses of time.

An example of recurrence in the American women's rights movement illustrates continuity across generations. The women's rights movement experienced a period of quiescence between the end of the suffrage movement (with ratification of the Nineteenth Amendment in 1920) and the emergence of the women's rights movement of the 1960s. Leila Rupp and Verta Taylor (1987) demonstrate the historical continuity of the women's movement by tracing how a combination of women who had participated in the suffrage movement and of women's organizations that adopted new goals (such as passage of the Equal Rights Amendment) sustained the movement's social networks, meeting houses, goals and tactics, and collective identity through a period that was generally hostile to feminism. Because of movement "abeyance structures" (Taylor 1989), the organizational and ideological resources of the movement were available to the new activists who emerged in the 1960s.

Women's health is another area in which there have been recurring movement episodes.

WOMEN'S HEALTH MOVEMENTS

Women's health is an example of an enduring "social problem" that has been the subject of multiple episodes of public attention and social movement activity within the United States spanning the last two centuries. (These episodes are discussed in chapter 2.) These recurring waves typically cluster with other social movements, including peaks in the women's rights movement, and they are multi-issue in the sense that they address a number of women's health and body concerns, sometimes within different movement organizations. Because the waves occurred over an expanse of time in which women's social roles and available avenues for collective action changed dramatically, the continuity of the health "theme" characterizing these episodes tends to be obscured. In addition, the impact that these waves of activism have had on evolutionary shifts in the nature of health care institutions has not previously been emphasized.

Previous scholarship on women's health movements has tended to focus either on a single wave, as exemplified by Sheryl Ruzek's (1978) definitive study of the Women's Health Movement of the 1960s and 1970s, or on the history of single-issue movements, such as the birth control movement (Gordon 1990a) or the abortion rights movement (Staggenborg 1991). Occasionally scholars allude to historical antecedents of movement waves. For example, Marieskind (1975) noted some similarities between the Women's Health Movement and the Popular Health Movement of the mid-nineteenth century, and Howes and Allina (1994) located the origins of the 1990s episode in women's health activism in the earlier Women's Health Movement. In contrast, Auerbach and Figert (1995) minimized this connection and stressed the "new" policy aspects of the 1990s episode.

Nevertheless, the recurring episodes of multi-issue women's health activism could be viewed as waves in a women's health "megamovement." This megamovement is a series of movement episodes in which women's health and body concerns have emerged into public discourse and evoked collective action by successive generations of activists intent on changing some aspect of women's health care or policy. As previously suggested, conceptualizing this megamovement does not depend on demonstrating that the health and body issues raised in each wave were identically framed, that activists in the various waves shared the same philosophy or an explicitly feminist perspective, or that there was continuity in individual participants. With regard to framing, changes in collective consciousness and the ways in which issues are framed would be expected in different historical periods, particularly if the earlier episode had successfully altered the discourse on women's health. With regard to points of view, no women's movement yet identified, including the American suffrage movement, has reflected unanimity among participants, and despite their shared biology, women do not always agree on interpretations of illness or bodily issues, such as reproductive control. American women may differ on health and bodily issues on the basis of racial or ethnic background, socioeconomic status, religious ideology, sexual orientation, or age group. During movement waves, however, dominant perspectives emerge that capture the public debate, at least temporarily, and may indeed transform prevailing viewpoints. With regard to continuity, activist traditions and networks of women's health advocacy groups help provide the resources and cultural repertoires connecting the waves.

Similarly, Calhoun (1995:181) observes that tracing the roots of social movements to the late eighteenth or early nineteenth centuries "is not necessarily the identification of a linear, unidirectional process of development." Using the women's rights movement as an example, he points out that claims making in the early nineteenth century was based on beliefs about essential differences between women and men and of the moral superiority of women, whereas later claims for women's rights would become based on notions of equality of the sexes. Consequently, to modern eyes, claims of the earlier movement might not appear "feminist." In the women's health megamovement, a clear example of this occurs with respect to women's demands for reproductive control. Nineteenth-century framings of this issue were based on assumptions of women's asexuality and moral purity and of men's greater sexual appetite and lack of sexual control; hence acceptable methods of fertility control included marital abstinence and containment of male sexuality by reducing the availability of contraceptives, abortion, and prostitution. Twentieth-century demands for reproductive control eventually were based on assumptions that women, like men, are sexual beings entitled to sexual relations without the intent of pregnancy. One could argue that the nineteenth-century efforts, by succeeding in legally prohibiting contraception and abortion for nearly a century to follow, did not help the cause of securing women's reproductive control. Yet the nonlinearity of reproductive control efforts is not quite the point. What is important from the perspective of the continuity of the women's health megamovement is that the theme of reproductive control has been repeatedly "on the agenda" despite different framings in different historical eras.

Finally, the term "megamovement" refers to a series of waves of movement activity over time, not to the number of participants in the movement. Social movements need not be large nor representative of the general population to have a broad social impact (Kingdon 1995; Klandermans 1992; Tarrow 1994). Although the waves of women's health activism tended to be led by predominantly white, middle-class, educated women, this does not negate their status as social movements or their influence on health care institutions.[6] (Nor does it suggest that these activists are not interested in the needs of poor or minority women; in some waves, most notably during the Progressive Era, women's health advocacy was very much focused on gender-based notions of social welfare.) Buechler (1990) argues that white, middle-class women tend to be the leaders of women's rights movements generally because, being relatively privileged by class and race, they are more likely than other women to experience and identify discrimination based on gender. In addition, however, relatively privileged women are more likely to have time available for participation and to have access to resources (e.g., financing, social contacts) needed to mobilize social action and to build an organizational base. In the case of health movements, privileged women also may have greater contact with the health care system and more leverage in the marketplace as consumers of personal health services.

All told, women's health movement waves, as the most conspicuous manifestations of women's health activism, illustrate the remarkable influence that organized groups of women have had on U.S. health care and policy.

THE CULTURAL SIGNIFICANCE OF WOMEN'S HEALTH

Recurring public attention and collective action in women's health reflects both an enduring cultural concern with the health of women and the deeply rooted and evolving cultural relationship between women and health care institutions. Women's health is not only crucial for the survival of the community, but women's traditional roles as healers and as caregivers for their children and other family members uniquely position women as both health care consumers and providers. Paul Starr (1982:22) observes that the transformation of American health care from a household-based to a market-based commodity involved "a shift from women to men as the dominant figures in the management of health and illness." This transformation, along with the dramatic changes in women's social roles during the nineteenth and twentieth centuries, created numerous opportunities for conflict and accommodation between women and health care institutions, and it helps account for the women's health megamovement.

It is commonly asserted that the cultural significance of women's health resides in women's maternal function and their role in cultural continuity, since no society can endure without producing and nurturing new members. For example, Sue Rosser (1994:ix) asserts that "since women are the bearers of both male and female children, the health of the nation depends on the health of its women." The health risks of maternity, to be sure, have long been apparent. Judith Leavitt (1986) shows how early American women's diaries and other documentary evidence indicated a general awareness, despite the absence of reliable statistics, of the dangers of pregnancy and childbirth, with respect to both maternal mortality and disability. In addition, even before the biological mechanisms linking the mother's health with that of her fetus and infant began to be understood in the early 1900s, the survival and health of children were known to depend on the health of the mother. Before the availability of safe substitutes for mother's milk, for example, the death of a mother in childbirth or from childbed fever often resulted in the death of her child (King 1993; Meckel 1990). The disability of the mother because of childbirth injury or repeated childbearing reduced her capacity to produce more children or to care for newborns. Finally, attending women during childbirth and caring for new mothers and infants were traditionally the responsibilities of other women, including midwives, family members, and neighbors. For all of these reasons, the production and survival of children depended upon the health of women.

The importance of women's health for cultural continuity is not, however, sufficient in itself to account for the recurring episodes in women's health activism over the last two centuries. Another critical element has been the ongoing, often conflicted relationship between women and American health care institutions. The emergence of modern health care, beginning in the mid-nineteenth century, involved a renegotiation of women's roles as health care providers within the home and outside the home, as well as a reconceptualization of what constitutes a medical service, particularly with respect to reproductive functions. Furthermore, because women are about half the population and give birth, they have provided a key client base for medical practice. Accordingly, women often have been the target of medical entrepreneurship, and in addition, women with financial resources have been able to use their purchasing power to influence the development of medical practice and the creation of gender-specific health care institutions. Those women who were not able to afford private medical care often were a major target of social and public health reform led by more privileged women. Finally, both the dramatic changes in gender role ideology, including concepts of human sexuality, and the expansion of women's social and economic roles throughout the nineteenth and twentieth centuries, including their increasingly public involvement in social reform activities related to public health, have meant that any accommodation between women and health care institutions would have been inherently unstable. A plausible hypothesis is that the recurring episodes of women's health activism coincided with fundamental changes in women's social roles and self-conceptions that both brought them into conflict with health care institutions and enabled them to mobilize for change.

The renegotiation of women's roles as health care providers and as consumers has been an ongoing and often contentious process. In the American colonies, women provided much of the family's health care, primarily through herbal medicine and midwifery. Childbirth was an exclusively female domain. Women's traditional roles as midwives began to diminish in the late 1700s, when medical men first practiced midwifery and attempted to establish themselves as experts in obstetrical practice and other aspects of women's health. Women were both competitors and potential clients of these new providers in a market characterized by a multiplicity of health care practitioners, few effective medical treatments, and prodigious competition for patients.

Modern American medicine evolved out of a period of intense competition among rival medical paradigms and organizations of alternative medical practitioners throughout the nineteenth century (Rothstein 1992). Women were actively involved in medical matters during this century, both as patients and as practitioners, and the shifting structures in medicine provided opportunities for women's involvement and collective action. As practitioners, women participated in and led various medical "sects" that challenged the aggressive therapies and authority of "regular" medicine (including its childbirth practices) and offered alternative, gentler therapies such as botanics and the "water cure." Despite overt discrimination by the regulars—including exclusion from medical schools, medical societies, and hospital training—women sought training and acceptance as regular physicians, founded women's medical schools, and established women's hospitals both to serve women patients and to provide medical training and employment for women physicians. By the end of the century, women were about 6 percent of U.S. physicians, a peak not to be attained again until the second half of the twentieth century (AMA 1991).

As patients, women have been a key market and economic mainstay of the medical profession. In contrast to the current view that medicine ignores or neglects women, the recruitment of women patients was critical, historically, to physicians' practices, and the development and control of medical treatments for women played a key part in the profession's attempts to establish itself both economically and socially. From colonial times, when male physicians first began to displace lay midwives, throughout the nineteenth century, physicians viewed attending childbirth as a way of building a medical practice, since both the woman and her family would be recruited as patients. When the first medical schools were founded in America, beginning with the Medical College of Philadelphia in 1765, midwifery was the first subject in the curriculum (Wertz and Wertz 1989). Walter Channing, a Boston obstetrician and champion of the use of ether in childbirth in the mid-1800s, regarded midwifery as the basis of physicians' livelihoods (Scholten 1984). In a well-known manual for young physicians published in 1882, D. W. Cathell, a Maryland physician, advised that "No one can succeed without the favorable opinion of the maids and matrons he meets in the sick room. The females of every family have a potent voice in selecting the family physician," and he went on to observe that "obstetrical practice . . . paves the way to permanent family practice" despite its relatively low fees (Cathell 1916:59,65).

As the medical historian W. F. Bynum put it, in the nineteenth century, "more often than not, the abstract patient was referred to as female" (Bynum 1994:211). This may have reflected both the preponderance of women in physicians' patient populations and the tendency of medicine in the second half of the century to pathologize women's biology more so than men's. The dominant late-nineteenth-century theories of women's health, which equated it with reproductive health, have often been perceived as an attempt by the medical profession to oppress women and exclude them from public life, but they also can be interpreted in the context of the profession's attempt to establish its authority and to secure a female client base. The theories focused on the relationship between women's health and their reproductive organs and on the fulfillment of women's maternal function (Smith-Rosenberg and Rosenberg 1984). Invoked by male physicians and others to justify attempts to exclude women from higher education and to limit their activities to the domestic sphere, the theories also provided a medical rationale for physicians' organized campaign for legal prohibition of contraception and abortion during the late 1800s.[7] Both the late-nineteenth-century medical conceptions of women's health and the physicians' campaign against contraception and abortion recently have been interpreted, in part, as attempts to establish the professional expertise of regular physicians, to differentiate them from their competitors on the basis of both technical expertise and social respectability, and to secure their professional authority and economic position (Mohr 1978). The theories also illustrate the importance of the female client base to physicians in private practice.

In addition, a medical specialty focusing on the reproductive health of women, obstetrics-gynecology, formed relatively early within American medicine. Obstetrics developed out of midwifery and expanded its repertoire during the 1920s and 1930s to include prenatal care, in part because of the influence of (and perceived competition from) prenatal care programs established by public health nurses and women social reformers. Gynecological surgery began to develop as a field of expertise in the late 1800s, concurrent with advances in surgical methods generally and with the development after 1867 of antiseptic and aseptic techniques; the repertoire of gynecologists soon included ovariotomy, oophorectomy, hysterectomy, tubal ligation, and a procedure to repair vesicovaginal fistula (a debilitating childbirth injury caused by a tear between the vagina and bladder, resulting in continuous urine leakage). Some physicians began to specialize in gynecological surgery, in the sense that they devoted their practices to it, but there were no formal mechanisms for defining or certifying specialists until the development of specialty boards with the authority to examine and license specialists in the early twentieth century. Gynecologists also became providers of contraceptive services during the 1920s and 1930s, in part because of competition from new lay women–controlled birth control clinics. Obstetrics and gynecology merged in 1930, creating the American Board of Obstetrics and Gynecology, only the third specialty board created (after ophthalmology and otolaryngology). The board limited examination to physicians who treated only women, thus excluding general practitioners and creating its market niche as providers of women's health care.

By the mid-twentieth century, obstetrician-gynecologists had become key providers of well-woman health care and the gatekeepers to fertility-control services, including abortion and contraception. Their role as disseminators of contraception was enhanced when the first oral contraceptive received approval by the Food and Drug Administration (FDA) in 1960. During the Women's Health Movement of the 1960s and 1970s, women activists targeted obstetrician-gynecologists for particular criticism, and they established lay-controlled clinics to provide fertility-control services on women's terms. When women began entering medical schools in increased numbers in the 1970s, obstetrics-gynecology quickly became a popular specialty choice among women residents (Weisman et al. 1980).

In the current health care marketplace, women remain major consumers. They not only use more products and services than men, they are believed to be responsible for most health care–purchasing decisions for themselves and for their families. Marketing statistics, for example, suggest that women make or influence at least two-thirds of all health care–purchasing decisions and that families may become customers of a hospital through an initial experience with maternity care (Dearing et al. 1987). The growth of hospital-sponsored women's health centers in the 1980s and 1990s has been attributed, in part, to hospitals' attempts to capture the women's market. Women also predominate among nonphysician providers of health care and continue to increase their numbers and influence within the medical profession. Currently, about one in five physicians is a woman, and by the year 2020, women will comprise more than one-third of the U.S. medical profession (Council on Graduate Medical Education 1995).

Therefore, while women's health problems may not always have been addressed by mainstream health care institutions in ways that contemporary women would have preferred, women have been far from invisible in American health care. The development of the American medical profession and of health care organizations has involved, among other things, a history of negotiating roles with women consumers, debating women's roles within medicine, recruiting and retaining women patients, providing services exclusively for women (albeit generally reproductive services), expanding and adapting health services to changing conceptions of women's roles and new technologies, and incorporating (some would say "coopting") organizational innovations created by women. The recurring waves of the women's health "megamovement" reflect a cyclical pattern of questioning and renegotiating the relationship between women and American health care institutions, which continues today.

2

The Women's Health
Megamovement

On several occasions throughout U.S. history, various aspects of women's health have become topics of public debate and organized social action, and together these episodes could be said to comprise waves in a women's health "megamovement." The movement waves include the women's health component of the Popular Health Movement, which peaked in the 1830s and 1840s; the late-nineteenth-century women's medical movement and campaigns against contraception and abortion; Progressive Era movements to establish government-funded maternal and child health services and to legalize and disseminate birth control; the Women's Health Movement of the 1960s and 1970s; and the women's health agenda of the early 1990s. In each wave, groups of primarily middle-class women organized to improve the state of all women's health, often by creating institutions to meet specific needs that were not being addressed in contemporary practice. These episodes, furthermore, generally coincided with social movement cycles in which concerns for women's rights were prominent, with dramatic changes in women's social and economic roles and shifts in prevailing gender role ideologies, and with important stages in the development of the American medical profession or of the health care system generally. Each episode also had important consequences for women's health care and policy.

The waves in the women's health megamovement are discussed chrono-
logically. For each wave, consideration is given to prevailing gender role ideology and the status of women, the contemporary state of American health
care institutions, the movement participants, the women's health issues addressed and the strategies used to address them, and the movement's legacies
for health care and policy.[1] Finally, the recurring themes and commonalities
in repertoires across waves are summarized.

THE POPULAR HEALTH MOVEMENT

The first wave occurred as part of the Popular Health Movement, which
peaked in the 1830s and 1840s, when Americans first organized to take control of their health and health care. This movement has been described as one
component of a wave of American reform activity between 1815 and 1860,
abetted by a growing middle class with the commitment and resources to devote to social causes that also included abolitionist, temperance, and women's
rights movements (Walters 1997). Women's active involvement in these social
reform efforts represented their main avenue of political participation, since
all free men at the time were able to vote, but women were not (Skocpol and
Ritter 1995). Although the Popular Health Movement did not focus on
women's health alone, women were prominent among its leaders and adherents, specific issues in women's health were targeted for reform, and women's
special responsibility for the health of their families and communities was
promoted (Morantz 1984).[2]

The Popular Health Movement emerged during a period when American
gender role ideology was undergoing an important transformation. After the
Revolutionary War and coincident with early industrialization, a gender role
ideology had begun to emerge that simultaneously delimited and expanded
women's social roles. This ideology prescribed "separate spheres" of activity
for men and women, in which men were expected to participate in the "public" sphere—to labor in fields or factories to support their families and to participate in electoral politics—and women were expected to participate in the
"private" sphere—to labor in the home, bearing and rearing children. At the
same time, however, gender role conceptions ascribed new prestige to
women's domestic responsibilities. Linda Kerber (1986, 1995) describes "Republican motherhood" as a new role conception in which women were vested
with a civic duty to produce morally virtuous and educated citizens for the
new republic; this ideology combined domestic and political responsibilities

in the sense that women served the state by bearing and socializing children. In the early 1800s, women's roles were further elaborated as part of the ideology of the Second Great Awakening, in which Protestant religious leaders preached both about the possibility of moral "perfectionism" and about women's unique capacity and duty to create the conditions for perfectionism in the home and community. The new concepts of womanhood evolved over the course of the nineteenth century into a more general idealization of women's domestic role, called the "cult of true womanhood" and the "cult of domesticity" (Cott 1977; Welter 1983). Important components of these developing ideals of womanhood were an assumption of the moral superiority of women and a belief in women's sexual "passionlessness." The latter derived originally from religious rather than medical teachings, but some physicians later provided biological explanations for what they perceived as women's lack of sexual appetite (Cott 1984). Ironically, beliefs about women's domestic virtues and moral superiority provided women with a basis for extending their maternal role into the community in the form of a variety of social movements focused on moral reform and social welfare. Women's health became one of the public issues that engaged nineteenth-century women.

The social context out of which the Popular Health Movement emerged also included a highly competitive and turbulent medical marketplace in which gender issues were prominent. The tensions involving gender were related to the nature of women's role in health care in colonial America. In the colonies, when life was mostly rural, most health care had been provided in the home by female family members, and basic health care, often through use of medicinal herbs, was regarded as part of the woman's domestic responsibility. Domestic medicine was practiced on the basis of oral tradition and, after 1700 when books became more widely available, on the basis of a number of popular medical guides (Cassedy 1991). Medical practice in general was undefined and unregulated. Any person, male or female, could use the title "doctor," and those who did so included men who had received formal education in European medical schools (women were excluded from medical schools at the time), a larger group of individuals who had served an apprenticeship with a colonial practitioner, and people with no formal training of any kind. There were no American medical schools until the 1760s and no effective licensing laws. Other medical practitioners in the colonies included clergymen and a variety of folk healers such as midwives, Indian doctors, bonesetters, and herbalists. Since few effective medical treatments were known at the time, the public had little hope that medical providers of any type could cure disease and little basis (other than the personal attributes of providers and the price of services) for distinguishing among the various practitioners.

Health care for women, when administered by non–family members, was provided primarily by lay midwives. These were local women who assisted in childbirth, provided early infant care, and often attended women during the lying-in period following birth. Midwives also provided health care unrelated to childbirth. The diary of Martha Ballard, a midwife practicing in rural Maine from 1785 to 1812, reveals that she treated women and children for rashes, burns, and minor illnesses (Ulrich 1990). Poor or homeless women could obtain maternity care in almshouses or a few charity hospitals, but these settings tended to be both socially stigmatizing and unsafe because of the high risk of infection (Lynaugh 1990).

By the first half of the nineteenth century, health care options were becoming increasingly diverse, and rivalries intensified among competing medical practitioners in a growing market for medical services. "Regular" physicians were men of the middle and upper classes, concentrated in Eastern cities, who had received some type of formal medical training in European or American medical schools and presented themselves to the public as practitioners of mainstream medicine. (There were 42 regular medical schools in America by 1850 [Rothstein 1992], but the first woman student was not admitted until 1847, when Elizabeth Blackwell entered Geneva Medical College in New York State.) These physicians adopted "heroic" treatments—bloodletting, blistering, dosing, and purging—intended to effect dramatic physiological changes in the patient and, it was believed, to rid the body of disease. These treatments were used for many conditions, including problems during pregnancy, childbirth, and puerperal fever, and physicians believed that patients expected aggressive methods (Rothstein 1992). Such treatments, however, were attacked by rival practitioners and by some regulars as ineffective and dangerous.

Male physicians who had been trained in Europe had begun to attend childbirth in the colonies after 1750, but the practice of male birth attendants was not uniformly accepted or initially widely adopted. Physicians competed with midwives for clients on the basis of their superior knowledge of anatomy and their potential for providing shorter labor and safer childbirth through the use of forceps; also, although anesthesia was not yet available, physicians sometimes used opium to alleviate pain during childbirth (Donegan 1984; Scholten 1984; Walsh 1977). The earliest adopters of male birth attendants were urban middle- and upper-class women who could both afford the physicians' higher fees and lend respectability to their practices (Scholten 1984; Wertz and Wertz 1989).

There is considerable scholarly debate about why American women began to accept male birth attendants in the late 1700s, since cultural taboos against male birth attendants were strong, lay midwives were plentiful, and no licensing laws restricted the practice of midwives. In addition, American midwives were not subjected to the same degree of violence or charges of witchcraft as their counterparts in Europe (Ehrenreich and English 1978). Judith Leavitt (1986) argues that it is not surprising that wealthier women of this period were willing to defy cultural taboos and choose male birth attendants of their own social class who promised more comfortable and safer childbirth than that provided by midwives. (Poor women and slave women did not have the option of purchasing the services of alternative birth attendants.) At the time, childbirth was a nearly universal and recurring event in women's lives—fertility estimates for the period suggest more than eight births per woman (Bogdan 1990). Although statistical evidence is not available, documentary evidence reveals that both maternal and infant mortality were high by current standards, and many women suffered permanently debilitating childbirth injuries. For many women, fear of childbirth must have contended with modesty in deciding what type of birth attendant to use.

There is no evidence, however, that physicians provided safer deliveries than lay midwives. In fact, because physicians treated patients for a variety of conditions other than childbirth, they may have been more likely than midwives to transmit puerperal fever (Leavitt 1986; Rothstein 1992). By the early 1800s, furthermore, physicians competing with midwives had to contend not only with the tradition of female birth attendants but also with the contemporary views of woman's moral purity and sexual passionlessness. So strong were cultural taboos against display of the female body that American medical schools—which had begun to teach midwifery in the late 1700s because it was viewed as a skill fundamental to establishing a medical practice—did not include direct observation of childbirth until 1850. Most medical students became physicians without ever witnessing a delivery (Speert 1980). Thus a typical midwife would have been considerably more experienced than the majority of physicians.

The diversity of medical practitioners in the early 1800s also was reflected in the number of apothecaries, bonesetters, and adherents of a variety of medical "sects" advocating prevention, self-care, and gentler treatments than those used by regular physicians. Often the sects were led by lay persons who had developed their own systems of healing. The major sects included Thomsonian botanics, hydropaths, homeopaths, and eclectics. These "irregulars" were attacked by mainstream physicians as "quacks," although the therapeutics of the regular physicians were not generally more effective than those of the irregulars. For their part, sectarians accused regulars of practicing on the basis of "superstition" and of being financially motivated to ignore the causes, and hence the prevention, of disease (Starr 1982; Morantz-Sanchez 1985).

The growth of the sectarians reflected popular dissatisfaction with the harsh therapeutics of regular physicians, as well as the antielitism that characterized the Jacksonian period. Sectarians and their followers opposed attempts by regular physicians to control access to medical knowledge and to establish state licensing laws granting them exclusive privileges; in fact, those states that had established such laws rescinded them during the 1830s (Starr 1982). The sectarians viewed themselves as antielitist, as more reasonably priced than regular physicians, and as providing safer and less debilitating care. They advocated lifestyle changes and self-care, promoted their ideas through popular health manuals, and established schools to train practitioners in their alternative healing systems. Consistent with the democratizing principle, the sects actively recruited women, both as followers and as practitioners, and many of the first generation of women physicians received their training in sectarian institutions (Morantz-Sanchez 1985).

Hydropathy and Thomsonian botanics were particularly popular among women. Hydropathy was based on European methods that were introduced in the United States in the 1840s. Hydropaths used water treatments—ingesting water and various applications of water to the body—for the amelioration of many conditions, and they stressed the importance of healthful habits such as exercise and proper diet. The water-cure establishments they administered were frequented by both women and men, but they offered specific benefits to women. These included respite from domestic responsibilities, female companionship in the residential treatment environment, care by female physicians, and relatively gentle treatments for a variety of women's health problems (Cayleff 1987). Hydropathic training institutes actively recruited women for training, based on the belief that women had unique healing skills and that "no Water-Cure establishment is complete without a qualified female physician" (Cayleff 1987:70). Beginning in 1844, hydropaths also published the widely circulated *Water-Cure Journal*, which included popular articles on a variety of topics related to women's health, such as diet and clothing reform.

Thomsonian botanics also emphasized gentle treatments and the role of women as caregivers. Samuel Thomson was a New England farmer who developed a patented system of botanics to be administered as home treatments and published a popular manual on his system in 1822. His followers were primarily working class, and the sect appealed to women because of its reliance on herbal remedies, because it viewed women as the appropriate caretakers for their families' health, and because of its support for midwives, whom Thomsonians perceived as providing safer, less expensive care than physicians (Ehrenreich and English 1978; Kett 1968; Rothstein 1992). At its peak of popularity, the sect founded infirmaries, associations of practitioners, and medical schools.

Out of this increasingly complex medical milieu, white, middle-class, American women became key participants and leaders in the Popular Health Movement. In essence, this was a social movement to redefine disease as preventable through human action, in contrast to the view that disease was caused by divine intervention; to educate the public—especially women—in healthier lifestyles, hygiene, and self-help; and to wrest control of health care from elitist physicians. Adherents of the movement included lay persons, sectarians, and some regular physicians. The growth of the movement and of the sects was inextricably linked; many participants in the movement were sectarians, and the sects drew on popular sentiments for alternative therapies and self-care. The methods used by the health reformers included public lectures, publication of journals and self-help health manuals, and voluntary self-help associations. Although male health reformers including Sylvester Graham, William Andrus Alcott, and Samuel Thomson are better known today, women were prominent in the movement and in the public arena as lecturers to women and authors of self-help health manuals. For example, Mary Gove Nichols founded water-cure establishments, cofounded the American Hydropathic Institute in New York, lectured women on health topics, and published her lectures on anatomy and physiology in 1842. Harriot K. Hunt, an irregular physician in Boston, lectured during the 1840s on disease prevention. Paulina S. Wright, a follower of Graham, and Lydia Folger Fowler, a regular physician, also were prominent lecturers to women. Women lecturers were particularly important to the movement because some of the material—involving female anatomy and sexual matters—would not have been considered appropriate for mixed-sex assemblages and was even found shocking by some gatherings of women, where frequent fainting spells were reported (Shryock 1966).

Women's health was of particular concern to health reformers because woman was viewed, according to a resolution of the American Physiological Society (founded in Boston in 1837), as "only second to the Deity in the influence she exerts on the physical, the intellectual, and the moral interests of the human race" (Morantz-Sanchez 1985:35). These domestic responsibilities, in turn, required women to be educated in matters of health and to enjoy good health in order to carry out their social responsibilities. Local ladies' physiological societies were voluntary associations formed during the 1840s and 1850s that became important vehicles for disseminating health information to women on personal, family, and community health and for providing a social situation in which women could share experiences and discuss their health concerns.

The Ladies' Physiological Institute of Boston and Vicinity, founded in 1848, illustrates some of the general concerns and strategies of these groups. According to its constitution, the society was formed to educate women about "the laws of life and health, and the means of relieving sickness and suffering," and the expectation was that women would apply this knowledge both in their families and in their communities, consistent with their expanding domestic role (Verbrugge 1979:48). Members included white, nonemployed, married or widowed women of the middle and upper-middle classes, who paid annual dues to attend weekly lectures by invited speakers and group discussions called "conversationals." Women physicians, including Harriot Hunt, were also among the members. The speakers, both male and female, represented the range of medical theories available at the time; they included regular physicians, hydropaths, homeopaths, botanics, mesmerists, and phrenologists. In associations of this type, lectures covered such topics as basic anatomy and physiology, nutrition, exercise, personal hygiene, dress reform (including use of corsetless clothing), the evils of masturbation, natural (drug-free) childbirth, midwifery, and the limitation of family size (Morantz 1984; Verbrugge 1979). Smaller families were promoted as healthier for women and also as consistent with new concepts of child rearing and middle-class lifestyles implicit in the conception of Republican motherhood. The promotion of smaller families, however, did not imply an endorsement of contraceptive methods. Martha Verbrugge (1979) notes, for example, that when Dr. Frederick Hollick, a well-known lecturer and a proponent of contraception, donated some of his books to the Boston Ladies' Physiological Institute's library, the board of directors closely controlled their circulation.

Nevertheless, through the lectures of the physiological societies, fertility control was publicly advocated for the first time in the United States. Furthermore, the way in which the issue was framed—as a means of perfecting, rather than preventing, motherhood—influenced public discourse on the subject for decades to come. The methods of limiting family size that were promoted by the health reformers were sexual restraint and marital abstinence, since these methods were consistent with prevailing views of women's moral purity and sexual passionlessness. Because true women were assumed not to enjoy sexual intercourse and to engage in it only within marriage for the purpose of conceiving a child, the only respectable way to limit family size was to limit marital sexual intercourse. Historians have argued, furthermore, that the public advocacy of family size limitation by this means probably enabled middle-class women to attain greater control over marital sexual relations and frequency of childbearing than had previously been available to them (Cott 1984; Gordon 1990a; Morantz 1984).

Because the U.S. birthrate went into steep decline after 1830, however, some historians and demographers have concluded that contraceptives and abortion must have been in wide use, despite contemporary rhetoric about abstinence and sexual restraint. (For one thing, the menstrual cycle was not yet understood, and popular advice literature often misspecified the woman's fertile period, so that the "rhythm method" would not have been highly effective [Brodie 1994].) Indeed, there is evidence of a booming commercial enterprise in abortifacients and contraceptives of varying degrees of efficacy. Abortion prior to "quickening"—the point in the pregnancy when the woman first feels the fetus move—was not then illegal, and although the first local laws dealing with abortion appeared between 1821 and 1841, they were concerned primarily with regulating the sale of commercial abortifacients that were deemed unsafe, not with limiting the practice of abortion. James Mohr (1978, 1984) shows that abortion had become commercialized as early as the 1840s and was probably increasing in frequency, as evidenced by advertisements for abortifacients (mostly herbal) in newspapers and magazines, by information available in popular health manuals, by the documented practices of several well-known abortionists, and by the appearance of some private women's clinics. Susan Cayleff (1987:157) points out in her study of hydropathy that "the implied availability of abortive techniques" probably was one factor attracting women to water-cure establishments. With regard to contraception, Robert Dale Owen (who had inspired Hollick's work) described coitus interruptus, vaginal sponges, and condoms in a pamphlet first published in 1831 and reissued for several decades thereafter (Brodie 1994). Various commercial douching preparations were being marketed by midcentury. Although the health reformers did not publicly advocate these methods, their arguments for the health and socioeconomic benefits of family size limitation may have unintentionally encouraged their use.

The various social reform movements of the early and mid-1800s, including the Popular Health Movement, are thought to have been in decline by the time of the Civil War (Walters 1997), but the Popular Health Movement left a number of legacies for women's health care. Although the movement was in part a reaction against the methods of heroic medicine and the efforts of regular physicians to establish themselves in the eyes of the state as the only legitimate practitioners of medicine, it may in fact have helped set the stage for regular physicians' more active campaign to dominate medical practice. The movement marked a low point in the prestige of mainstream medicine and probably encouraged regular physicians to organize more aggressively around issues other than licensure. The popularity of the sectarians and the establishment of organizations devoted to their training and practice intensified competition with the regulars, who founded the American Medical Association (AMA) in 1847 and excluded sectarians and women from membership.

In addition, the women's health components of the Popular Health Movement initiated public discourse about the role of women as health care providers, about family size limitation, and about women's health and body concerns generally. The movement is credited with stimulating women to enter the field of medicine by articulating beliefs about women's special capacities as healers and by providing opportunities for training in sectarian institutions (Morantz-Sanchez 1985). Women physicians who were so inspired would become important participants in the next women's health movement wave. The public discussion of family size limitation issues served both to articulate the rights of women to control their participation in sexual intercourse within marriage and to focus attention on the apparently increasing use of commercial products for contraception and abortion. The latter was to become a topic of growing public concern and a pivotal issue for regular physicians and the AMA in their campaign for professionalization throughout the second half of the century. Finally, the Popular Health Movement gave birth to women's self-help health groups, which became part of the cultural repertoire of women's health activism, and to the idea that educating lay women about their bodies and about health matters more generally might improve social conditions within the community.

LATE NINETEENTH-CENTURY MOVEMENTS IN WOMEN'S HEALTH

The second wave of social movement activity in women's health occurred in the decades following the Civil War and consisted of a women's medical movement and an organized campaign against abortion and contraception. During this period, medical theories of women's health were promulgated on the basis of new scientific knowledge of anatomy and physiology and beliefs about biological determinism. Women's health was discussed in various public arenas—including the medical and popular advice literatures, the press, the courts, and government—and it was the focus of actions by the AMA and various social reform groups. Within this context, women physicians attempted to define their distinctive expertise and professional role, and a campaign was undertaken to regulate reproductive practices through legislative means rather than moral suasion alone. Although male regular physicians often have been viewed as the dominant force in this campaign, both women physicians and women social reformers were prominent participants.[3]

After the Civil War, women's changing social and economic roles became particularly conspicuous. Rapid urbanization and new technology (such as the invention of the typewriter) opened new opportunities for women's employment outside the home. The first schools to train professional nurses were founded in the early 1870s and facilitated the growth of hospitals. Women's educational opportunities also were expanded by the founding of several women's colleges, and by 1890, two-thirds of American colleges and universities admitted women, and over one-third of enrolled students were women (Muncy 1991). At the same time, an ideology of "virtuous womanhood" assumed women's moral superiority to men and prescribed that "women's actions had to be consistent with moral sensibility, purity, and maternal affection" (Rothman 1978:14). Appropriate roles for women involved caretaking and nurturing—both in the home, with respect to their children and husbands, and in the community, through charitable works and social reform. Women were increasingly active in the public sphere on behalf of benevolent work and a variety of social reform efforts, including renewed efforts for women's suffrage and "social purity" causes such as temperance, control of prostitution, and suppression of obscenity. Although men also were involved in social reform efforts and participated in some of the same organizations as women, women created and led a number of movement organizations.

This was an era of expanding women's clubs and associations, including literary and "culture" clubs as well as organizations dedicated to charitable work or social reform efforts. Among the latter were the Women's Christian Temperance Union (WCTU), founded in 1873; the Young Women's Christian Association, founded in 1866; and the Florence Crittendon Mission, founded in 1883. The General Federation of Women's Clubs (founded in 1890) coalesced a network of women's groups nationwide. Women social reformers also initiated the American settlement movement in 1889, when Jane Addams and Ellen Gates Starr opened Hull House in Chicago. By 1900, there were more than 100 settlement houses in operation, providing career opportunities for the growing cadre of college-educated women. Thus this episode of women's health activism, like the earlier Popular Health Movement, also coincided with a social movement cycle characterized by women's expanding public role.

The health movements of this period also have to be considered in relation to the state of medicine and, in particular, to regular physicians' continuing efforts to dominate the field. Economic competition between regular and irregular physicians continued in the second half of the nineteenth century. In 1850, there were 40,755 U.S. physicians of all types, and this number more than tripled over the next fifty years (Rothstein 1992). Eclectics, the successors of Thomsonian botanics, and homeopaths were the principal competitors of regular physicians in the second half of the century and had founded their own medical schools. As a means of distinguishing themselves from competitors and improving their technical skills, regular physicians founded specialty societies organized around areas of scientific interest. These included gynecology, which began to develop as a field of expertise in the 1870s, concurrent with advances in surgery generally; these advances were made possible by the availability of anesthesia, the development after 1867 of antiseptic and aseptic techniques, and the growth of hospitals. The specialty societies excluded irregulars as well as less socially prominent regular physicians. Adding to the competitive climate, the new specialists competed with general practitioners for patients.

The number of women physicians also increased steadily after 1850, as women's attainment of higher education rose generally. Seventeen women's medical schools were established, and women began to be admitted to such elite medical schools as Johns Hopkins, which agreed in 1890 to admit women on the same basis as men as a condition of receiving a substantial financial endowment from a group of prominent women including M. Carey Thomas and Mary Garrett. By 1900, there were 7,387 women physicians, nearly 6 percent of the U.S. total, and at least 75 percent of them were regulars (Morantz-Sanchez 1985; Walsh 1977). These women, however, met with hostility from many of their male colleagues, and they were excluded from membership in the AMA and from many local medical societies, hospital positions, and hospital-based training programs.

Simultaneously, women's health was being redefined and debated. Although reliable epidemiological data were not available, it is clear from documentary evidence that many physicians and lay observers throughout the nineteenth century believed that American women were increasingly unhealthy (Smith-Rosenberg and Rosenberg 1984). Catharine Beecher—a noted author, domestic reformer, and frequenter of the water cure—surveyed the health of married women she met on her travels and in "health establish-ments," observing in 1855 that "the *standard of health* among American women is so low that few have a correct idea of *what a healthy woman is*" (Cott 1986:264). Although communicable diseases were major health prob-lems at the time and it was estimated in 1894 that one-quarter of the adult population died from tuberculosis (Rothstein 1992),[4] the discourse about women's health was preoccupied with problems related to the reproductive system and maternity. Physicians reported a high incidence of mental disor-ders, particularly neurasthenia and hysteria, among reproductive-age, pri-marily urban middle- and upper-class women. These conditions were frequently interpreted as a manifestation of women's difficulties fulfilling their maternal and other domestic responsibilities, which, despite the pace of social change, were still generally regarded as women's only accessible roles (Smith-Rosenberg 1985).

The medical community, nevertheless, increasingly sought to explain both social roles and disease on the basis of underlying biological causes. Accord-ing to Morantz-Sanchez (1985:205), "After the Civil War, the spiritual argu-ments developed in the antebellum period gave way to more rigid biological sanctions promoting an increasingly inflexible conception of woman's nature and capacity. Indeed, the last third of the nineteenth century was an era of ex-treme somaticism in which physiological explanations for character, class, race, and gender traits became accepted as a matter of course." Physicians pro-mulgated new theories of women's health based on the assumptions that women and men were biologically different and that women's health was controlled by that aspect of their physiology that differentiated them from men—namely, their reproductive organs. There was some disagreement, however, over whether the uterus or ovaries controlled women's health. A medical professor proclaimed in 1870 that "the Almighty, in creating the fe-male sex, *had taken the uterus and built up a woman around it*" (Wood 1984:223–224). A gynecologist argued in 1878 that "physiologically she is a woman because she owns two ovaries . . . giving her sex and personality. In-stead, therefore, of womb-man, she ought to be called ovary-man" (Speert 1980:48). Furthermore, because women, as one physician put it in 1875, have "a greater multiplicity of organs" than men (Rothman 1978:24) and because the body was presumed to have a finite amount of energy that needed to be conserved, women were thought to be weaker and more prone to nervous dis-ease than men. Their normal biological functions—including menstruation and pregnancy—were defined by medical authorities as potentially debili-tating, and both puberty and menopause were viewed as dangerous transitions in women's lives. Energy had to be conserved to ensure the health of the reproductive organs and the safety of these biological processes.

A theorized linkage between the uterus and the brain was elaborated. (Female hormones were not yet understood.) "Reflex irritation" referred to uterine disease as the cause of mental illness, and an argument was made that the brain-uterus link also meant that mental stimulation could be harmful to a woman's reproductive capacity, particularly at puberty. The brain-uterus link extended to medical views of pregnancy as well. Reflecting a general belief in the heritability of acquired characteristics, a theory of "maternal impression" posited that the activities and mental states of the pregnant woman affected fetal characteristics.

Dominant medical opinion therefore favored limiting women's physical and mental activities, especially their educations, to preserve their reproductive capacity and to protect the health of their gestating and future children. Dr. Edward H. Clarke's widely read and influential book, *Sex in Education: A Fair Chance for Girls* (1873), argued the case against higher education for women largely on the basis that menstruation is a debilitating condition. Similarly, Dr. W. Gill Wylie argued at a meeting of the American Gynecological Society in 1891 that "if a girl is pushed at school or her force is used up by constant contact with older intellectual people from the age of ten to fifteen" she is likely to suffer from menstrual problems, uterine and ovarian problems, sterility, nervous disease, and cancer, among other disorders (Speert 1980:63). Such arguments have been interpreted as a "countermovement" in response to women's quest for higher education after the Civil War (Fish 1990).

Treatments prescribed for women's health problems included bed rest during menstruation and medically supervised "rest cures" consisting of prolonged bed rest devoid of intellectual stimulation. A cult of "female invalidism" appeared among women of the privileged classes, in which it was considered appropriate to be bedridden during menstruation and for various nervous disorders (Drachman 1976; Ehrenreich and English 1973a). Well-known patients who received rest cures included Jane Addams and Charlotte Perkins Gilman. Gilman's experience with the rest cure for treatment of hysteria (promoted by S. Weir Mitchell, a prominent neurologist) was the subject of her 1891 short story "The Yellow Wall-Paper," in which she portrays a physician's wife whose condition worsens under the "cure" (Gilman 1994). Some women, however, may have found the rest cure to be a welcome relief. Smith-Rosenberg (1985) points out that in defining nervous disorders as a medical condition and advocating rest cures, physicians acted as arbiters of women's legitimate withdrawal from maternal and household duties.

In extreme cases, "sexual surgery" was used as treatment for a variety of physical and other conditions. This involved the removal of healthy reproductive organs to treat a condition presumed to be linked with those organs. Battey's operation, named for the American surgeon who developed the procedure in the 1870s, consisted of the removal of normal ovaries for a number of both gynecological and nongynecological indications, including excessive menstrual bleeding, menstrual pain, hysteria, insanity, epilepsy, and sterilization of women with mental illness (Dally 1991; Roy 1990; Speert 1980). The operation lost favor by the end of the century, because of growing medical and public opinion against it.

The thriving patent medicine industry also addressed itself to women as customers, both because of women's traditional role as providers of domestic medicine and because of the new elaboration of women's health problems. At the time, patent medicines were unregulated, and self-dosing was prevalent among women. One of the best known and most enduring products was Lydia E. Pinkham's Vegetable Compound, containing 18% alcohol, which was sold from 1875 to 1925. The nostrum was advertised for a variety of "female complaints" including painful menstruation, vaginal discharge, infertility, and prolapsus uteri. Its marketing appealed explicitly to women's anxieties not only about their health but also about the propriety of male physicians treating women and about the safety of medical treatments. Advertising slogans included "only a woman understands a woman's ills" and "woman can sympathize with woman" (Stage 1979:130–131).

Within this period of heightened public attention to women's health, two health-related movements are discernible. One involved the efforts of women physicians to distinguish themselves as experts in women's health, including, at times, openly challenging prevailing medical theories about women and establishing separate institutions for the provision of women's health care. The other movement consisted of a campaign to prohibit contraception and abortion that was supported by an alliance of male and female physicians, lay social reformers, members of the clergy, and legislators. Each of these movements focused on reproductive health issues, reflecting both the dominant theories of women's health and heightened societal concerns about women's changing social roles.

Some historians have referred to the efforts of women physicians during this period as a "women's medical movement" (Drachman 1976; Morantz-Sanchez 1990; Shryock 1966). The women who entered medicine in the second half of the nineteenth century, some of whom had participated in the Popular Health Movement, clearly sought acceptance within the profession, and one medical historian has described this as a "dramatic test case" for the larger women's rights movement (Shryock 1966:179). In addition, these medical women have been portrayed as participants in the first-wave women's movement who were concerned about the state of women's health and believed they had special abilities to improve it. Scholars debate the extent to which these women physicians were united in a cause to reform medical practice on behalf of women. They assuredly did not all agree on issues pertaining to women's health. Morantz-Sanchez argues that there is little evidence that the women physicians' therapies differed substantially from men's, and she points out that after 1880, women physicians were committed professionals who shared a common medical education with their male colleagues and had been socialized to similar views of gender roles; further, women physicians "revered motherhood in sentimental Victorian fashion" and did not challenge the prevailing view that the objective of good health for women was healthy maternity (Morantz-Sanchez 1985:218). Nevertheless, the women physicians of this period left an impressive body of published work challenging conventional medical wisdom on women's health at a time when they were not universally welcomed within the medical profession and, inasmuch as they portrayed themselves as uniquely qualified to understand and treat women, were likely to have been perceived as competitors by many medical men. They also lectured widely on women's health, including to women's societies, and they established hospitals and dispensaries in a number of cities to provide training for women physicians and to care for women and/or children. These organizations reflected women physicians' claims to special expertise in women's health as well as their exclusion from many hospital training programs and from career opportunities in mainstream organizations.

The most apparent way in which these women physicians differed with the prevailing theories of women's health was in their beliefs that women were not inherently sickly and that it was their duty as physicians to help educate women to be healthy and to prevent invalidism (Drachman 1976; Morantz-Sanchez 1985). In contrast to the dominant medical theories, they constructed an alternative viewpoint stressing women's inherent health, and they emphasized the importance of lifestyle in promoting health. They promulgated these views in their practices (which were often in women's hospitals or women's colleges) and in their medical teaching, public lectures, and both scholarly and popular writings.

Many women physicians viewed menstruation, pregnancy, and menopause as normal functions in healthy women, rather than as naturally debilitating conditions that required rest or other medical treatment. They stressed the importance of exercise, useful work and activity (even during pregnancy), comfortable loose-fitting clothing, and education. They viewed physical and mental inactivity among women of the privileged classes as detrimental to their physical and mental health, not as a cure. If only because their own careers contradicted prevailing medical opinions about women's biological unfitness for mentally taxing work, women physicians were strong advocates of women's higher education. Some also criticized the "reflex irritation" theory of mental illness and the overuse of ovariotomy (Dally 1991; Morantz-Sanchez 1985). Elizabeth Blackwell, for example, opposed the removal of ovaries. Finally, despite their general acceptance of prevailing gender role ideology, they sometimes challenged medical views of female sexuality, they recognized the health risks of too frequent childbearing, and they supported the right of married women to control the timing and frequency of sexual intercourse (Drachman 1976).

Even women physicians who usually are regarded as part of establishment medicine, such as the highly respected and prolific Mary Putnam Jacobi, were often skeptical of contemporary theories of women's health and critical of mainstream medical practice. Jacobi wrote a prize-winning 1876 research paper challenging Clarke's thesis that women require physical and mental rest during menstruation. Based on her findings, which included data from a survey of women, she concluded that "the least ill-health is found among the women who have been most highly educated" (Jacobi 1925:481). She also alluded to physicians' economic motives in medicalizing women's health. Writing on the subject of female invalidism in 1895, she pointed out that "it is in the increased attention paid to women, and especially in their new function as lucrative patients . . . that we find explanation of much ill-health among women" (Jacobi 1925:484).

Morantz-Sanchez (1985) argues that many women physicians in the late 1800s believed that their presence in medicine was justified by their essential difference from men and by their special abilities to deal with the health problems of women and children. Indeed, many women physicians concentrated their practices on the treatment of women and children, and some excelled in gynecological surgery. The dispensaries and hospitals founded by women physicians typically specialized in these fields. Women physicians believed that their special abilities included nurturance, sensitivity to patients' feelings, sympathy, and a fundamental interest in the prevention of disease. In addition, they believed that women patients were more comfortable revealing their feelings, as well as their bodies, to women physicians and that women physicians were more likely than medical men to treat patients as "coworkers" in the health care process (Drachman 1976). As Elizabeth Blackwell put it in 1860: "The meaning of the medical movement amongst women in America is the felt necessity for the education of women in Science . . . for the purpose of occupying positions which men cannot fully occupy" (Morantz-Sanchez 1985:65).

The second health-related movement in the post–Civil War period consisted of an organized campaign against abortion and contraception, which peaked in the 1860s through the 1880s. (Although antiabortion and anticontraception activities are often studied as separate phenomena, they can be understood as representative of the contemporary social purity crusades that were concerned largely with regulating sexual morality.) Regular male physicians are often described as the leaders of this campaign, but they were joined in their efforts by female physicians, elite lay social reformers of both sexes, clubwomen, women's rights activists, members of the Protestant and Catholic clergy, and legislators at the state and federal levels. Most notably, Anthony Comstock, who became an agent of the New York Committee for the Suppression of Vice, was a leading lay crusader against obscenity and a major force in efforts to outlaw contraception and abortion. It is arguable whether either could have been regulated without the active involvement of male physicians and male lay reformers such as Comstock. What is clear, however, is that the movement was not simply an effort by men to disempower women in reproductive matters; movement participants included both men and women, and the target of moral reform was both male and female sexual behavior.

The broad appeal of this movement lay in its ideological consistency with contemporary ideas about virtuous womanhood and with what Linda Gordon (1990a) has called "voluntary motherhood." Voluntary motherhood refers to an elaboration of views on family size limitation that were first advocated publicly during the Popular Health Movement and, by the 1870s, were promoted by a combination of free-love groups, suffragists, women physicians, and middle-class women moral reformers. In essence, these views were an articulation of married women's right to control their fertility to preserve their health and to perfect the practice of motherhood. The ideology of voluntary motherhood did not dispute the centrality of motherhood in women's lives; in fact, it both sentimentalized maternity and, despite the growth of female employment and of women's other public activities, promoted motherhood as women's principal occupation. Beginning in the Popular Health Movement, however, concerns had been raised about the risks of frequent childbearing for women's health, and as we have seen, late nineteenth-century women physicians shared these concerns. Because women assumed both the health risks of childbearing and the responsibilities of child rearing, it was argued that women therefore ought to have the right to determine when to have children and how many to have.

Contemporary understandings of human sexuality, however, held that women had weaker sexual appetites than men and that virtuous women did not engage in sexual intercourse for reasons other than procreation. Contraception (both female and male varieties) was viewed as encouraging the sexual exploitation of women, including prostitution, as well as male promiscuity. Abortion was the act of lapsed women. Accordingly, proponents of voluntary motherhood advocated marital abstinence and the right of wives to refuse their husbands' sexual demands in order to control fertility. The identification of virtuous womanhood with abstinence was evident in the campaigns for legislation prohibiting both abortion and contraception and in popular marital advice manuals. Sheila Rothman (1978:82) points out that women social reformers and women physicians "led a purity crusade that made the suppression of birth control information a major plank in the moral reform agenda." For example, Elizabeth Blackwell, Susan B. Anthony, and Frances Willard of the WCTU were participants in the crusade, which was viewed by some as the moral equivalent of the campaign against slavery (Ginzberg 1990; Rothman 1978).

Male regular physicians also played a prominent role in efforts to suppress abortion and contraception. Physician mobilization had begun through the auspices of the newly formed AMA, of which women were not yet members. In 1859, the AMA passed a resolution condemning abortion, even before quickening, and urging state legislatures to take steps to prohibit both abortion and contraception. Scholars have provided diverse interpretations of male regular physicians' motives in opposing contraception and abortion and of their moralistic rhetoric in condemning these practices. These explanations tend to emphasize three factors: male physicians' negative attitudes toward women's expanding roles, including women's entry into medicine and attempts to establish a gendered niche in medical practice; their alarm over declining fertility among white, native-born women and the future of their own social class; and their continuing interests in differentiating themselves from their competitors and asserting their professional authority. James Mohr (1978) points out, for example, that the Hippocratic Oath, to which the regulars subscribed, was generally interpreted at the time as proscribing abortion; furthermore, the regular male physicians who were most active in the antiabortion campaign also tended to be leaders in the drive to professionalize medicine.

A strong case can be made that regular male physicians stood to gain professionally from asserting their authority in reproductive health. The intensity of economic competition among alternative health practitioners, between male and female physicians, and between physicians and commercially available contraceptive and abortive products has been described by a number of scholars. Regular male physicians were increasingly concerned about competition from irregulars, whom they perceived to be providing abortions for handsome fees (Mohr 1978). Also, despite the opposition of women physicians to abortion, male physicians sometimes accused them of providing abortions (Morantz-Sanchez 1985; Walsh 1977). Abortion clinics operated openly in the cities of New England and the Middle Atlantic states, and a growing commerce in abortive agents in the form of drugs and instruments, many of which were ineffective or dangerous, took place by mail-order catalogues and in drugstores (Brodie 1994; King 1992). Commercially available contraceptives included syringes, various vaginal devices (sponges, diaphragms), and condoms.

All medicine at the time was practiced on a fee-for-service basis, and regular physicians treated primarily middle- and upper-class persons who could afford their services. Furthermore, obstetrics was not yet a full-time specialty in which only a subset of physicians practiced, but was part of the general physician's practice. Childbirth was viewed as a reliable source of income for young physicians establishing their practices and as a means of recruiting family members as patients (Bynam 1994; Donegan 1984; Morantz-Sanchez 1985; Scholten 1984; Wertz and Wertz 1989). However, while physicians' professional livelihoods depended on their ability to attract a steady flow of paying women patients, birth rates had begun a steep decline in the early 1800s, especially among the middle class. The white fertility rate decreased by half between 1800 and 1900 (from 7.04 to 3.56), and by 1900 the average family had only three children (Gordon 1990a). The declining birth rate is likely to have posed a serious threat to the livelihood of regular physicians, who depended on attending deliveries, and to have contributed to their attempts to control the market for women's health care. Shyrock (1966:187) points out, for example, that one reason why male physicians opposed medical women was "for fear of economic competition," particularly for "cutting in on the profits of obstetrics cases."

This interpretation of male regular physicians' behavior, however, attaches little importance to the influence of the lay reformers and medical women who promoted various "social purity" causes. A more subtle explanation is that male physicians' interests were served both by attempting to ensure the female obstetric client base and by allying themselves with the views of prominent social reformers. Although staking out a position opposed to contraception and abortion may have helped to ensure childbearing patients, this is not all it did. Alignment with elite women's conceptions of "virtuous womanhood" provided regular physicians with an element of social respectability and moral authority, which was enhanced by publicly criticizing the abortion practices of other practitioners and the crass commercialism of purveyors of contraceptives and abortifacients.

It might have been otherwise. Regular male physicians might have responded to the apparently accelerating demand for contraception and abortion services by asserting their technical expertise in these matters, much as they had done with midwifery. They might have attempted to control the market in abortifacients, for example, by opposing prevailing abortion techniques on the basis of their ineffectiveness or danger to women, and they could have argued for use of more effective and safer surgical techniques, which were becoming available by the late 1800s and were beginning to be applied to treatment of infertility (Marsh and Ronner 1996; Mohr 1978). This strategy, however, would have required a direct challenge to prevailing gender role ideology and to the elite social purity reformers and women physicians who advocated the principles of voluntary motherhood. The path the regulars did take reflected their acceptance of these views, rather than a desire to change them.

The movement to ban contraception and abortion culminated in a wave of restrictive abortion legislation in the states and in both state and federal legislation designed to restrict the dissemination of abortifacients and contraceptives. The Comstock Act of 1873, in addition to "little Comstock laws" enacted in the states and court cases that upheld or strengthened these laws, essentially classified contraceptive devices and abortifacients as "obscene" and prohibited dissemination of both the products and information about them. By 1885, twenty-four states had passed similar laws, and in seventeen states and the District of Columbia, physicians essentially were under a gag order not to discuss contraception with their patients. After enactment of the Comstock laws, contraceptive devices were advertised under ambiguous names or for purposes other than contraception, to evade the authorities (Brodie 1994). By 1900, abortion was illegal throughout the United States. Simultaneously, however, abortion became defined as a medical service under the jurisdiction of regular physicians. The prohibitions enacted by the states generally gave regular physicians control of abortion by permitting them to authorize and perform medically necessary abortions as "therapeutic exceptions" to preserve the life of the woman; thus, rather than being banned outright, abortion became, legally, a medically controlled procedure (Luker 1984). This result has been taken as evidence by some scholars that regular physicians were more interested in asserting their authority than in eliminating abortion altogether.[5]

A major legacy of the late-nineteenth-century episode of public attention to women's health was the legal regulation—though not total suppression—of contraception and abortion information and services, which remained in force until well into the next century. Kristin Luker (1984) points out that the legal prohibition of abortion probably did not change its practice substantially, because much of medical care still took place in the home; female culture could have sustained access to home remedies; patent medicines and other products were still available (though not advertised openly as abortifacients); and physicians would have had strong incentives to provide abortions demanded by their private patients. The same arguments could be applied to contraceptive practices, although Janet Brodie (1994) argues that both the quantity and quality of health "advice" literature declined in the last two decades of the nineteenth century as a result of the Comstock laws.

There can be little doubt, however, that the restrictive legislation drove fertility-control services underground and resulted in denial of access to contraceptive information and devices and to relatively safe surgical abortions for many women, especially those without the financial resources to consult a private physician. In addition, the stigma associated with these practices attached to the physicians who provided them, which is likely to have reduced the availability of these services even to wealthier women. The status of abortion did not change as a matter of public policy until the states began relaxing abortion restrictions in the 1960s, and U.S. Supreme Court rulings legalized abortion in 1973 *(Roe v. Wade, Doe v. Bolton)*, although it remained a medically controlled procedure. Supreme Court rulings upheld married and unmarried persons' constitutional right to use contraception in 1965 *(Griswold v. Connecticut)* and 1972 *(Eisenstadt v. Baird)*, respectively. All of these rulings came after there was considerable evidence that increasing numbers of women were obtaining abortions (both legally and illegally) and that millions of American women, both married and unmarried, were acquiring medical forms of contraception. Hence the rulings legitimized social practices that were already prevalent.

Other legacies of the late-nineteenth-century episode for women's health were a focus on reproductive issues in women's health care; a social consensus that women's biological functions and life events—including menstruation, pregnancy, childbirth, infertility, and menopause—are appropriate areas for medical supervision; and a presumption, because of the ideology of "voluntary motherhood," that it is women's responsibility to control fertility. Alliances between women physicians and women activists were forged on the issue of fertility control as well as other women's rights issues. The seeds also were sown during this episode for continuing debate about the special skills or contributions of women physicians and about the relative advantages and disadvantages of separate institutions for women's health care. These issues are considered further in chapter 4.

PROGRESSIVE ERA MOVEMENTS IN WOMEN'S HEALTH

The third wave of public attention to women's health consisted of two movements organized largely by educated, middle-class women during the Progressive Era and extending into the 1920s. The Progressive Era was characterized by attempts to solve a variety of social and economic problems through a combination of professional expertise, scientific management methods, and the powers of government. The medical profession, for example, was concerned with upgrading and regulating its educational standards and with establishing and certifying competencies of physicians who claimed the skills of specialists. In the realm of social reform legislation, some efforts were related to women's health. For example, protective labor legislation ostensibly intended to facilitate motherhood and to preserve traditional families (e.g., by regulating hours of work or prohibiting women's night work) was enacted in most states between 1908 and 1920; this legislation was supported by organized labor and women's groups, and it often was justified on the basis of protecting the health of women as actual or potential mothers.[6]

Reform efforts that focused explicitly on women's health care included two movements that did not converge at the time on a shared definition of women's health and, in fact, reflected competing conceptions of women's roles and major health concerns. In one movement, women reformers from the settlement movement, women physicians, and clubwomen—who were organized on an unprecedented scale in U.S. history—raised public awareness of infant and maternal mortality and obtained governmental support for maternal and child health programs. In the other, women activists with ties to leftist politics launched a campaign for the legalization of contraception and established a nationwide network of birth control clinics for women. Both groups of reformers had major long-term impact on medical practice, on women's health care institutions, and on health policy.[7]

These two groups—the maternal and child welfare reformers and the birth control activists—were part of what Nancy Cott (1987:49) describes as "multifaceted" feminism in the 1910s. Women's activism, though generally united on the issue of suffrage, was beginning to express itself on multiple issues that exposed increasing diversity in women's interests and different conceptions of women's social roles. The juxtaposition of the two movements discussed here illustrates differences in gender role ideology among Progressive Era feminists: the maternal and child health reformers focused on women's solidarity on the basis of their maternal role and responsibilities, as traditionally conceived, whereas the birth control advocates promoted a newer view of women as emancipated sexual beings. The birth control movement, in dramatic contrast to the earlier ideal of voluntary motherhood, explicitly separated sexual activity from procreation. These competing views of womanhood could not be reconciled during the 1910s and 1920s, and the two movements generally progressed on separate tracks, without mutual support between their respective leaders (Rothman 1978).

The maternal and child health reformers focused their efforts initially on the health of children. Infant mortality had been discovered as a social problem in the mid-nineteenth century, and social policy to address it evolved through several stages. Solutions at first focused on general environmental reform, such as urban sanitation; then on infant feeding programs, including improving the milk supply; and by the early 1900s, on the education of mothers in infant care and feeding (Meckel 1990). Women social reformers played a key role not only in promoting the education of mothers in infant care, but also in extending social programs to improve the health of mothers. Although many and varied groups were involved in maternal education and child welfare programs, activist women and public health nurses played pivotal roles, and settlement house residents such as Lillian Wald, Florence Kelley, and Jane Addams are often credited both with raising the visibility of the child welfare problem and with initiating events that eventually would culminate in federal programs for maternal and child health (Muncy 1991).

The maternal and child health reformers during the Progressive Era subscribed to what Sheila Rothman calls an ideology of "educated motherhood." This ideology emphasized women's primary responsibility for the health of children and the belief that child health could be improved if women of all socioeconomic classes were provided with expert guidance in the tasks of motherhood (Rothman 1978). Educating pregnant women and mothers in basic hygiene, nutrition, breastfeeding, and other aspects of infant care was part of the reformers' program, as was raising public awareness that environmental conditions also affected child health. Working primarily through local voluntary associations and national women's clubs, and influenced by the ideals and strategies of the settlement movement, these reformers lobbied for a federal agency to promote child welfare (Muncy 1991; Skocpol 1992). They achieved their objective in 1912 when Congress established the Children's Bureau in the Department of Labor.

Julia Lathrop, the Bureau's first director and former Hull House resident, began her tenure by conducting systematic studies of the causes of infant mortality and by promoting birth registration as a source of needed statistics. In a 1916 speech, she claimed to have demonstrated "a close connection between infant mortality and the ill health and death of mothers" (Skocpol 1992:495). It is noteworthy that during this period, public action on behalf of infant mortality predated action on behalf of maternal mortality or maternal health. Richard Meckel (1990) argues that professionals' attention to maternal health grew out of the earlier efforts to reduce infant mortality by educating mothers in basic hygiene and the care and feeding of babies. As these efforts began to attain some success after 1914, neonatal mortality from causes not associated with maternal care became more evident; only then did reform efforts shift to improving prenatal and obstetric care of mothers. Another possibility, of course, is that by then the public efforts were institutionalized in the women-controlled Children's Bureau. In any case, by 1920, mother and child health were linked in the public policy discourse.

Convinced that both maternal and child deaths were largely preventable, in 1917 Lathrop had proposed a federal program to provide matching funds to states for maternal and child health programs, especially in rural areas. Intense lobbying by national women's associations, combined with legislators' fears that newly enfranchised women would not reelect opponents of the Lathrop-inspired bill, led in 1921 to enactment of the Sheppard-Towner Maternity and Infancy Act. This legislation expanded the mission of the Children's Bureau and provided the first federal funding of prenatal care and child health services in the United States. Skocpol (1992:481) refers to the Children's Bureau and the Sheppard-Towner Act as "the joint political achievements of women reformers and widespread associations of married women." Services provided in the Sheppard-Towner programs included home visits by public health nurses, child health clinics, and prenatal care. These programs were established in local communities that requested them, often with the endorsement of the local medical society and with the participation of local physicians. The Sheppard-Towner reformers attempted to forge an alliance with local physicians by assuring them that the new programs were not meant to provide curative medical care and therefore would not compete with physicians' private practices (Rothman 1978). By the time Sheppard-

Towner was allowed to expire in 1929, it had established nearly 3,000 publicly funded prenatal clinics (staffed mainly by public health nurses and women physicians), had provided more than 3 million home visits by nurses, and had set a precedent for federally funded health care services.

On another track, the movement to secure women's access to sex education and contraception was taking shape. Although a number of prominent activists were involved in this movement, Margaret Sanger, a New York public health nurse and socialist, became the dominant figure. She popularized the term "birth control" and began a direct challenge of the Comstock law prohibitions against dissemination of contraception in the 1910s. Sanger believed that women's health depended upon their ability to limit childbearing; she wrote in 1920 that "excessive child bearing is now recognized by the medical profession as one of the most prolific causes of ill health in women" (Rothman 1978:191). Indeed, one estimate in 1913 showed that complications of pregnancy and childbirth were the second leading cause of death in American women ages 15 to 44, after tuberculosis (Meckel 1990), and it was later estimated by the Children's Bureau that 25 percent of maternal deaths were the result of illegal abortions (Loudon 1992). Legalized abortion was not publicly advocated at the time, however. Birth control advocates, including Sanger, believed that availability of contraception would obviate the need for abortion and would therefore reduce maternal mortality from illegal abortions (Gordon 1990a; Lader 1995; McCann 1994).[8]

It is important to recognize that the rhetoric surrounding the birth control movement invoked several themes, and the promotion of women's health was not the only rationale articulated. Sanger also argued for women's right of self-determination as a matter of social justice, and, based on new psychological theories, for women's right to sexual fulfillment. In addition, beginning in the 1920s, eugenics thinking was invoked by many birth control advocates, who saw contraception as a means of improving the population by reducing overbreeding of the lower and immigrant classes and by enabling women of all classes to bear only the number of children their families could support economically. The eugenics argument was not based on a valuation of women's health or self-determination, nor did it challenge maternity as women's primary role. Gordon (1990a) and Petchesky (1990) argue that eugenics thinking contributed to the transformation of the birth control movement, beginning in the 1920s, from a women's rights focus to a more conservative emphasis on family planning, understood as an appeal to responsible motherhood and population control.

Influenced by birth control clinics she had visited in Holland, where they had been invented, Sanger opened a birth control clinic in a poor immigrant neighborhood in Brooklyn in 1916; she and her cofounders were promptly arrested for disseminating birth control information. As a result of the appeal of her conviction, the New York State Appeals Court in 1918 provided an opening wedge for the birth control movement. Although the court upheld Sanger's conviction, it also issued a ruling excepting physicians from the prohibitions regarding dissemination of contraceptive information, as long as the physician was aiding "a married person to cure or prevent disease" (McCann 1994:64). The ruling then went on to define "disease" broadly, without reference to venereal disease, for which physicians in New York State already could legally prescribe condoms. This opened the possibility for provision of contraceptives by physicians to married women for a variety of health-related problems. This decision galvanized Sanger's strategy to form an alliance with the medical profession to establish birth control clinics.

Sanger founded the American Birth Control League (ABCL) in 1921 and proceeded on two fronts. One strategy was to work for both state and federal legislation giving doctors exclusive right to prescribe contraception; this was called "doctors-only" legislation. Simultaneously, Mary Ware Dennett's Voluntary Parenthood League, a rival birth control organization, worked for legislation giving women direct access to birth control information as a matter of free speech. Neither legislative approach was successful. Sanger's additional strategy was to establish a network of women-controlled birth control clinics in which contraception would be provided under the supervision of physicians. Her commitment to clinics stemmed from her belief that pessaries (diaphragms) were the best available contraceptive and that their effectiveness depended on a physical examination, fitting, and counseling session. The legal provision of pessaries, furthermore, required physician involvement in the clinics.

Sanger founded a clinic in New York in 1923 with the dual purposes of providing birth control services to women and collecting data to demonstrate the efficacy of diaphragms, and she hired a woman physician to direct it. The ABCL organized affiliates around the country with the help of local women's clubs, and the clinics that resulted received literature and other technical assistance in exchange for financial contributions to the ABCL. Birth control clinics for married women grew in number during the 1920s, despite the precarious legal climate. By 1930, there were 55 clinics in 23 cities in 12 states (Gordon 1990a), and by 1945, there were more than 800 clinics nationwide (McCann 1994). These clinics were financed privately, mainly by wealthy women and foundations.

Despite the ideological gulf between the maternal and child health reformers and the birth control activists, the women's health services they created had some important similarities. Both the publicly financed maternal and child health services established under Sheppard-Towner and the privately financed birth control clinics represented innovative models of health care founded on the dual principles of prevention and the education of women. The maternal and child health services included preventive examinations of both pregnant women and children and emphasized the importance of educating mothers in child care and in healthful habits during pregnancy. The founders of birth control clinics saw them as preventing unwanted pregnancies, along with their related health risks, and as educating women about their reproductive systems and their health in general. Both the Sheppard-Towner services and the birth control clinics provided care to underserved populations—most notably, rural women in the case of Sheppard-Towner, and women who could not afford private physicians in the case of birth control clinics. Both services also provided career opportunities for women physicians, who were more supportive than medical men of public health and preventive care and who also had limited employment opportunities elsewhere (Chesler 1992; Morantz-Sanchez 1985; Muncy 1991; Rothman 1978). Finally, both types of services eventually came under medical control.

The newly consolidated medical profession was concerned in the first decades of the twentieth century with upgrading educational and specialty standards and with attempting to restrict the number of trained generalist and specialist physicians to reduce competition (Stevens 1971). The profession eventually came to view both the Sheppard-Towner maternal and child health services and the birth control clinics as threats to its autonomy and to the economic position of the emerging specialists. In the case of Sheppard-Towner, by 1927 the AMA (as well as other groups) had organized in opposition to renewal of its funding, and the program expired in 1929. (The Children's Bureau continued, however.) Physicians had come to perceive this publicly funded, lay-managed program as "state medicine" that threatened their authority and competed with their private practices. Since Sheppard-Towner was a universal program that was not targeted to the poor, physicians believed that it served patients who would otherwise pay for their services. This position was consistent with a long tradition of American physicians' opposition to subsidized or charity health care; in the nineteenth century, physicians had opposed public dispensaries on the grounds that patients who could pay for their services "abused" the dispensaries and deprived them of income (Starr 1982). Also, in large part because of the influence of the Sheppard-Towner programs, physicians at the time were beginning to redefine their role to include preventive examinations. The AMA took the position that physicians should incorporate prenatal examinations and well-child care into their practices, and it provided training programs for physicians in the techniques of the preventive examination (Meckel 1990; Rothman 1978).

Obstetricians, in particular, saw a new preventive role as an opportunity. Obstetrics was then becoming a full-time specialty, and competition with midwives, who attended about 50 percent of all U.S. births in 1910, was still intense. Obstetrics also was attempting to upgrade its standards of education and practice; it had been severely criticized in the 1910 Flexner Report on the state of medical education, which noted that "the manikin [used in obstetrics training] is of value only to a limited degree" (Speert 1980:80). By asserting their special expertise in prenatal care, obstetricians could both enhance their prestige and extend their practices to the care of women during pregnancy. Accordingly, obstetricians argued that they were better qualified than public health nurses to provide prenatal care, especially because normal pregnancies could easily become abnormal (Rothman 1978). They defined pregnancy as a medical problem requiring medical solutions, and they expanded their practices to include the medical supervision of pregnant women.

In addition to pregnancy, childbirth itself was defined by obstetricians as a "pathological process" routinely requiring such interventions as forceps and episiotomy, and hospital deliveries were promoted as safer than home deliveries. Simultaneously, hospitals began to apply the principles of scientific management to labor and delivery services by systematizing procedures performed by specialist physicians (obstetricians) and nurses (Leavitt 1986). In the 1920s, many hospitals established new maternity wards or built private wings to accommodate new mothers who could afford to pay for these services. Hospital deliveries also were more efficient for obstetricians, since they did not have to travel to patients' homes, and provided a supply of patients for medical training purposes.

Urban women began to prefer hospital deliveries both because of their continued quest for safer and more comfortable childbirth—as evidenced by the organizations promoting "twilight sleep" in childbirth in the 1910s (described in chapter 1)—and because of a breakdown of the traditional social networks that had supported home births (Leavitt 1986). Due to immigration restrictions, furthermore, there were fewer available midwives after 1919. While less than 5 percent of women delivered in hospitals in 1900 (Wertz and Wertz 1989), from the 1920s onward, hospital births increased rapidly, especially in urban areas, and by 1940, 55 percent of births took place in hospitals

(Leavitt 1986). (This trend did not, however, make childbirth safer; maternal death rates did not decline substantially until after 1935.) Both the medical cooptation of prenatal care and the transformation of childbirth from a home-based to a hospital-based event during this period continued the medicalization of American childbirth begun by physicians in the late 1700s.

In the case of birth control services, medical hegemony was attained more reluctantly. Despite the "doctors-only" legislative attempts and a series of judicial rulings that enabled physicians to prescribe contraceptives to married women, physicians, as we have seen, generally had been hostile to contraception and tended to use a strict interpretation of the legal requirement of providing contraception only to cure or prevent disease. This stance also was consistent with the medical profession's Progressive Era campaign to combat venereal disease. Allan Brandt (1987) argues that new scientific knowledge of the pathology of syphilis and gonorrhea caused physicians to view these diseases as a major threat to the traditional family: husbands who had visited prostitutes were thought to infect their innocent wives and children, and venereal disease was now regarded as a major cause of female infertility. Using 1890 census data, one physician estimated in 1904 that one in seven marriages would be sterile due to venereal infections (Brandt 1987). Accordingly, physicians advocated sexual continence outside of marriage, sex education for both men and women, and prohibition of prostitution. The use of birth control was viewed as encouraging, rather than restraining, sexual activity; hence it was viewed as promoting the spread of venereal disease.

During World War I, however, the anti–venereal disease campaign led to the official promotion of condom use for American soldiers, and this had the unintended consequence of increasing the civilian market for condoms after the war (Gordon 1990a). Although it is not possible to ascertain whether condoms were being used primarily for contraception as opposed to disease prevention, their increasing popularity was seen as reflecting a growing demand for contraceptives generally. Increased demand coincided with a shift in gender role ideology during the 1920s, in which the concept of the "wife-companion" sanctioned the expression of sexuality within marriage, independent of childbearing (Rothman 1978). The Depression also increased demand for contraception, as evidenced by a booming business in "feminine hygiene" products, such as Lysol, claiming contraceptive properties (Palmer and Greenberg 1936; Reed 1984; Gordon 1990a). A public opinion poll conducted in 1937 for the *Ladies' Home Journal* reported that 79 percent of U.S. women believed in birth control (Gordon 1990a).

In light of increasing demand, the combination of private physicians' fears of competition from lay-administered birth control clinics and their concerns about the quality of products being marketed as contraceptives increased their willingness during the 1920s and 1930s to prescribe contraception. A key decision by the U.S. Court of Appeals in 1936 *(United States v. One Package of Japanese Pessaries)*, in a case involving Sanger's clinic, permitted physicians to prescribe contraception for the purpose of saving life or promoting patients' well-being (McCann 1994). Gynecologists, who were basically surgeons at the time, were urged by Robert Latou Dickinson—president of the American Gynecological Society in 1920 and a critic of what he perceived to be Sanger's propagandizing of birth control—to become sexual counselors to their married patients and to provide contraception upon request (Reed 1984). In 1937, largely because of Dickinson's efforts, the AMA endorsed the provision of contraception within medical practice. The *One Package* decision and the AMA endorsement both reflected and contributed to a changing climate of medical opinion on birth control. Similar to the Sheppard-Towner case, this change of climate facilitated private physicians' cooptation of a preventive service that would otherwise have been provided only in clinics controlled by nonphysicians and providing charity care (McCann 1994).

The Progressive Era women's health movements had a number of legacies for women's health and health care. For one, all phases of women's reproductive process—pregnancy prevention, prenatal care, and childbirth—were transformed into medical services. This occurred both as a result of the entrepreneurial interests of medical specialists and because reformers framed their new services within a health care model, employing women physicians and public health nurses as providers and encouraging physicians to adopt preventive care (prenatal care and pregnancy prevention services) in their practices.

Another legacy of the episode was the precedent set by Sheppard-Towner for government funding of maternal and child health services, which has become a defining feature of women's health policy in the United States. The Social Security Act of 1935 in a sense restored the maternal and child health programs of Sheppard-Towner under Title V (Maternal and Child Health), although benefits for these services were associated with public assistance and were not universally provided. Similarly, the Emergency Maternity and Infant Care program (1943-1949) provided obstetrical care, including hospital deliveries, and pediatric care for the dependents of World War II servicemen; benefits were limited, however, to the four lowest pay grades of the armed forces (Marieskind 1980; Meckel 1990). The Medicaid program, established in 1965 to provide health insurance for the poor, specifically targeted, among other groups, pregnant women and mothers of young children. Another consequence of these later measures was a new policy linkage of maternal health care benefits with "welfare."

An important legacy of the birth control movement was the growth of a nationwide family planning service and advocacy network. Sanger's Birth Control Federation of America (which had evolved out of the ABCL) was renamed the Planned Parenthood Federation of America in 1942 and remained "the only national birth-control organization until the abortion-reform movement" of the 1960s (Gordon 1990a:337). Birth control clinics, both private and public, experienced a major spurt of growth in the 1960s and 1970s when public funding for family planning was expanded because of a number of factors: the changing normative climate regarding women's sexuality and reproductive rights; the War on Poverty, in which family planning was viewed as a means of reducing indigence; and the growing national alarm about teenage pregnancy (Nathanson 1991). In 1965, the Office of Economic Opportunity established community agencies to provide family planning for low-income women; in 1968, family planning became a required service under Title V of the Social Security Act on the rationale that child spacing improves both infant and maternal health;[9] in 1970, Title X of the Public Health Service Act provided the first major federal support of family planning services for poor and low-income women without regard to age and marital status; and in 1973, states were required to cover family planning services under the Medicaid program (Burt 1993). The growth of birth control clinics, however, had some unintended consequences that are still problematic. Although they were highly successful at increasing access to contraceptive services, particularly for underserved populations, the clinics generally did not provide comprehensive well-woman services, prenatal care, or, until the appearance of the AIDS epidemic in the 1980s, diagnosis and treatment of sexually transmitted diseases. By separating family planning services from other components of women's health care, the clinics contributed to its fragmentation.

THE WOMEN'S HEALTH MOVEMENT OF THE 1960S AND 1970S

The fourth wave of public attention to women's health was the Women's Health Movement of the 1960s and 1970s.[10] This grassroots movement grew out of a social movement cycle that included the civil rights, women's liberation, and anti–Vietnam War movements, and its beginnings coincided with a number of new health programs in the 1960s—such as the enactment of Medicare and Medicaid and the creation of neighborhood health centers and "free clinics"—that were intended to improve the population's access to health services. The movement also coincided with efforts to protect consumers of health care by ensuring patients' rights in therapeutic decision making and the rights of subjects in medical research. Viewed within the context of 1960–1970s efforts to expand both access to health care and patients' rights, the Women's Health Movement appears as an attempt to define uniquely *women's* issues within this larger domain. It was not, however, totally derived from these contemporary movements. Due to its grassroots origins, criticism of mainstream medicine, and emphasis on educating women and on self-help strategies, it has been compared with the nineteenth-century Popular Health Movement both in terms of ideology and tactics (Marieskind 1975; Starr 1982). The general upheaval around health care issues, however, created opportunities for women's health activism.

Previous descriptions of the Women's Health Movement have emphasized its roots in the second wave of feminism that emerged during the 1960s. Crossing generational lines, this resurgence of feminism included older women reacting to the conditions of their lives during the 1950s and younger women of the post–World War II baby-boom generation. Rothman (1978) points out that a new definition of womanhood characterized this period: the idea of "woman as person," which emphasized women's autonomy and right of self-determination. This was a period of rapid and dramatic changes in women's roles: women's rates of college attendance and labor force participation were at an all-time high, women were delaying marriage and childbearing, fertility rates began a steep decline, divorce rates were rising, and more women were combining motherhood and employment. A "sexual revolution" among college students was described by both social scientists and journalists, with emphasis on an increase in premarital sexual activity among white, middle-class women (Nathanson 1991). In other words, women's roles were increasingly diverse and complex; motherhood was becoming an optional or less central role in many women's lives; and young women were asserting a right to sexual fulfillment.

Borrowing from the civil rights movement "master frame," women began to demand equal rights with men, not, as earlier feminists had argued, because women could make a unique contribution to society by virtue of their moral superiority and maternal role, but rather because women were basically similar to men and were therefore entitled to equal opportunities. The National Organization for Women (NOW) was founded in 1966 to bring about women's full civil rights and social participation. Women's reproductive rights were viewed as fundamental not only to their ability to control their fertility but also to their capacity to exercise their political and economic rights. Full gender equality could not exist unless women could choose whether or not to reproduce. At its 1967 convention, when NOW began a campaign to support legalized abortion, it effectively endorsed women's right to decide to eschew motherhood (Rothman 1978).

The campaign for legalization of abortion is generally regarded as the catalyst of the Women's Health Movement. Although abortion symbolizes the new perspective on women's nonmaternal roles, it was by no means the only issue that concerned women's health activists, nor did the movement end with the 1973 U.S. Supreme Court decisions in *Roe v. Wade* and *Doe v. Bolton* that legalized abortion. Kristin Luker (1984) points out, furthermore, that efforts to legalize abortion predate the Women's Health Movement. The state laws governing abortion practices, as we have seen, were a legacy of the antiabortion fervor of the late 1800s, and most of these laws permitted physicians to perform abortions only as "therapeutic exceptions" to preserve the woman's life. By the 1950s, in part because of the visibility of hospitals' therapeutic abortion boards, which had the authority to approve abortions for medical reasons, both the legal and medical communities had become aware that there was no medical consensus on what appropriate medical indications for abortion were. Physicians, furthermore, were increasingly concerned that they could be prosecuted for interpreting the law too broadly. Both physicians' concerns and public awareness of the implications of restrictive abortion laws were heightened in 1962 by the case of Sherri Finkbine. While pregnant, Finkbine had used a sleeping pill containing thalidomide, a hypnotic drug that causes serious fetal deformities if taken early in pregnancy. When her local hospital refused to provide an abortion despite her physician's support, Finkbine sought care in Sweden, where her abortion of a deformed fetus received sympathetic press coverage in the United States.[11] Another sensitizing event was an epidemic of rubella in the early 1960s, which resulted in threatened sanctions against physicians who were providing abortions to infected women (Joffe 1995).

In response to the campaigns of coalitions of professional associations, population control interest groups, and women's groups, three states (Colorado, North Carolina, and California) reformed their abortion laws in 1967, and by 1970 twelve additional states had either reformed or repealed their restrictive laws (Ruzek 1978). Feminists became an increasingly organized constituency on the abortion issue in the late 1960s, when it became clear that reform of state abortion laws—rather than outright repeal—merely respecified the conditions under which abortions were justifiable (e.g., to preserve the physical or mental health of the woman, in cases of rape or incest, in cases of fetal deformities) and did nothing to challenge the medical profession's role as arbiters of abortion decisions or to make abortion services more widely available (Gordon 1990a; Luker 1984; Petchesky 1990; Ruzek 1978). Women began to claim that abortion was not a matter of medical indications, but a woman's right "on demand" and her decision alone to make.

By 1968, women were demonstrating an increasing willingness to defy the law and to contest the definition of abortion as a medical procedure. In addition to speak-outs (in which women related their abortion stories in public), demonstrations, and consciousness-raising groups, women and men organized both legal and underground information and referral services for women seeking abortions. Referral efforts were assisted by the Clergy Consultation Service on Abortion, a nationwide network of concerned ministers and rabbis (Staggenborg 1991). These activities served two purposes: raising public awareness of the abortion issue and providing direct services to women. Freestanding abortion clinics were established in some areas with the help of sympathetic physicians. Self-help clinics provided "menstrual extractions" using suction devices modeled after the vacuum aspiration equipment used by physicians. In Chicago, a group of women known collectively as "Jane" organized an underground counseling and referral service that evolved into an abortion provider in which some of the members performed abortions themselves; Jane provided an estimated 11,000 low-cost illegal abortions between 1969 and 1973 (Kaplan 1995). These lay-organized abortion services were, of course, a threat to the authority of the medical profession. As late as 1970, the AMA, though acknowledging the trend toward liberalized abortion laws, still argued for medically controlled abortions performed only by licensed physicians in accredited hospitals after consultation with two other physicians (Petchesky 1990). Nevertheless, by the time of the 1973 U.S. Supreme Court decisions, which legalized abortion but preserved medical control of the procedure, it had become clear that the old abortion restrictions were essentially unenforceable. As Rosalind Petchesky (1990:123) puts it, "abortion had to be legalized because the pressure of popular practice on doctors, health facilities, and finally the state had become irresistible."

The abortion issue had provided a focal point for women's concerns about their health care in general and had produced an organizational capacity for disseminating information and mobilizing supporters. The Women's Health Movement eventually addressed a number of issues in addition to abortion, including the quality of the physician-patient relationship; the safety of drugs and devices—notably oral contraceptives, diethylstilbestrol (DES), and intrauterine devices (IUDs); reforms in childbirth practices; and the overuse of surgery, including hysterectomies, cesarean sections, and mastectomies. Although the issues were diverse, the unifying theme was women's shared experience of a lack of control over their bodies and their health care. Unlike reformers in previous episodes of women's health activism, these women did not focus on maternal health or on their health in relation to their actual or potential children. Rather, they viewed their health as essential to their full social participation, and they argued that they had a right to the health care they demanded and the right to make informed decisions about all aspects of their care.

At the core of the movement was a direct challenge to medical authority in matters of women's health. Mary Zimmerman (1987:442) describes the Women's Health Movement as "a challenge to many of the assumptions and practices of mainstream modern medicine." In particular, the medical profession was perceived as treating women in a condescending manner, withholding information, overusing surgery and risky drugs and devices, medicalizing women's reproductive functions, and reinforcing sexual stereotypes by encouraging reproduction over pregnancy prevention. The fact that the profession was male-dominated was seen as part of the problem: in 1970, women were only 7.6 percent of U.S. physicians and 7.2 percent of obstetrician-gynecologists (AMA 1991). Obstetrician-gynecologists were the major focus of women's criticism of the medical profession. These specialists were the gatekeepers to contraception and abortion services and were perceived as responsible for medicalizing women's reproductive functions. Furthermore, obstetrician-gynecologists had begun to play a major role in well-woman care (in addition to maternity care) with increased use of the Papanicolaou (Pap) smear for cervical cancer screening after World War II and with FDA approval of the first oral contraceptive in 1960.

The availability of the oral contraceptive not only affected the relationship between obstetrician-gynecologists and women, it is also an example of women's influence on medical technology. The development of "the pill" had been commissioned in 1951 by Margaret Sanger and Katharine McCormick, heir to the fortune of Cyrus McCormick. At the time, biomedical researchers had been focused on developing hormonal treatments for infertility rather than methods to prevent conception, and pharmaceutical companies were skeptical that there was a market for hormonal contraception (Asbell 1995; Chesler 1992). Most states, furthermore, still had laws (though often unenforced) limiting advertising, sale, or distribution of contraceptives. Mc-

Cormick took Sanger's suggestion to finance development of a contraceptive pill by a private research company in Massachusetts, and by 1963, 2.3 million American women were using the new oral contraceptive (Asbell 1995). By the end of the decade, the pill would be attacked by some women's health activists who would claim that it had been inadequately tested, was unsafe, and was dispensed to women without their informed consent (Seaman 1995).

Women born after World War II entered their reproductive years in the 1960s and depended upon physicians for fertility-control services, including therapeutic abortions and prescriptions for oral contraceptives. This brought them into earlier and more continuous gynecological care than previous generations of women. Leaders of the Women's Health Movement were women who were most likely to have come into contact with obstetrician-gynecologists. They were predominantly white, middle-class, urban, college-educated women in their twenties and thirties who wanted access to fertility-control services (Ruzek 1978). This no doubt accounts for the major emphasis of the movement on the health care needs of middle-class women of reproductive age. Although the movement attempted to address the needs of special groups (especially lesbians, minority women, and poor women) in some of its programs and services, the evidence suggests that relatively few movement participants were poor, rural, or older women.

The Women's Health Movement used two basic strategies to increase women's control over their health care. The first approach was educating women by providing information about their bodies, about medical products and procedures, and about the structure of the health care system. The assumption was that the demystification of health care would enable women to take better care of themselves and to become more discerning health care consumers. The educational methods used included health care conferences and courses organized by women, consciousness-raising groups, and publications. The movement produced a vast literature that included popular health manuals, journalistic exposes of unsafe medical products, and analyses of the nature of the cultural relationship between women and medicine.

The best known health manual emerging from the movement was *Our Bodies, Ourselves,* first issued on newsprint in 1970 by a group of women who had organized a women's health course in Boston; it had sold 250,000 copies by 1973, and by 1996, it had sold nearly four million copies in revised, foreign-language, and special-topic editions (Feinberg 1996). One of the goals of the original edition was "to reach as many women as possible with the tools which will enable them to take greater charge of their own health care and their lives" (Boston Women's Health Book Collective 1984:xiii). Laura Kaplan

(1995) describes how a member of Jane discovered the book in 1971, and the service thereafter gave free copies to all women for whom they provided abortions. The best known example of the movement's revelatory literature was Barbara Seaman's 1969 book *The Doctors' Case against the Pill,* which raised questions about the safety of oral contraceptives and criticized the medical profession and the pharmaceutical industry for failing to disclose the risks to women. The book helped influence the FDA to require informational inserts in packages of oral contraceptives, and it was reissued in a twenty-fifth anniversary edition in 1995 (Seaman 1995). Barbara Ehrenreich and Deirdre English published two pamphlets in 1973 (a,b) that analyzed the gender politics of health care: *Witches, Midwives, and Nurses: A History of Women Healers* and *Complaints and Disorders: The Sexual Politics of Sickness.* These tracts are classic feminist analyses of health care that clearly reflect the ideology of the Women's Health Movement and inspired other gendered analyses of social issues. Both were still in print in the 1990s.

The second strategy used by the Women's Health Movement to increase women's control over their health was the creation of new health care organizations as an alternative to mainstream providers and as a vehicle for bringing "women's culture" back into health care. In addition to the abortion referral networks and clinics already mentioned, the movement also established women-controlled health centers (some were called "self-help clinics") as an alternative to mainstream care. These centers were managed by lay women and offered some combination of health education, referral services, advocacy, and clinical services in a supportive, nonhierarchical environment in which women could be active participants in their care and, in some cases, conduct gynecological self-examinations. Physicians (of either sex) worked in some of the centers on a part-time or consultative basis, sometimes for pay and sometimes as volunteers. The best known examples were the Feminist Women's Health Centers that originated in 1971 in Los Angeles and numbered about 48 by 1976 (Ruzek 1978). Most of the centers established during this period provided mainly contraceptive services and gynecological care, although a few, such as the Somerville Women's Health Project that opened in 1971 near Boston, offered expanded primary care services. Sheryl Ruzek (1978) points out that the centers were threatening to mainstream providers because they increased economic competition (particularly for abortion services) and provided effective models of care delivery using nonphysician personnel. Although this resulted in physicians' attempts to close feminist clinics in some communities, it also induced mainstream providers to adopt some of the centers' innovations.

Typically the centers were run by white, middle-class women, including college students, who often had the dual objectives of extending their feminist politics into the community and providing needed health services to underserved women. Most of the women's health centers attempted to appeal to less affluent women by providing free care, charging low fees, or offering sliding fee scales. Some centers, such as the Somerville Women's Health Project, were located in working-class communities and attempted to involve local women in the center's planning and operations. While many of the centers undoubtedly improved access to health care for local low-income women, few claimed success in expanding women's health activism beyond the middle class.

Another type of alternative health care organization that evolved during this period—the freestanding birth center—grew out of a generalized climate of criticism of the medicalization of childbirth and of impersonal, hospital-managed deliveries. The socially diverse groups generating these criticisms included both feminists, who argued for women's control of childbirth, and traditionalists, who argued for greater involvement of husbands and families in the birthing process (Rothman 1991). "Natural" childbirth, "prepared" childbirth, midwife-assisted birth, home birth, and homelike birth centers were among the innovations supported by these groups. Freestanding birth centers, which were established as nonhospital facilities for "family-centered" childbirth for women at low risk of complications, responded both to consumer demands for alternative birthing options and to the needs of certified nurse-midwives for practice opportunities (Rothman 1991; Wertz and Wertz 1989).

The Women's Health Movement of the 1960s and 1970s had a major impact on the health care establishment. In addition to influencing legislation and judicial decisions pertaining to abortion and contraception, it influenced policy with respect to patients' rights, it increased awareness of medical biases with regard to women, and it provided the means for women to educate themselves about their health and health care. The movement also established alternative service organizations that competed with mainstream providers, and this encouraged many traditional organizations to adopt some of the innovations introduced by women's health activists. Hospital-sponsored birth centers and other childbirth alternatives such as rooming-in, childbirth education classes, patient education and information services, and patient support groups are now familiar services in large part as a result of the movement's innovations.

There are some important additional legacies of the Women's Health

Movement. For one, the Women's Health Movement created a cohort of women concerned about matters of health and health care and a network of organizations to sustain this activism. Three notable examples are the Boston Women's Health Book Collective, which celebrated its 25th birthday in 1996; the National Women's Health Network, which was founded in 1975 in response to the DES and oral contraceptive controversies to monitor health regulatory agencies and was the largest national public-interest organization and information clearinghouse on women's health issues in the 1990s; and the National Association for Repeal of Abortion Laws (NARAL), founded in 1969 (and renamed the National Abortion Rights Action League in 1973 and the National Abortion and Reproductive Rights Action League in 1994), a leading advocacy organization for abortion rights into the 1990s. Minority communities eventually mobilized their own organizations, some with both local and national chapters, including the National Black Women's Health Project (founded in 1981) and the National Latina Health Organization (founded in 1986). Lesbian women and women with disabilities also have formed organizations with health advocacy agendas (Ruzek, Clarke, and Olesen 1997).

The movement also helped motivate women to become physicians at the same time that civil rights legislation made medical schools more hospitable to women. Enactment in 1972 of Title IX of the Civil Rights Act, which prohibited sex discrimination in educational institutions receiving federal financial assistance, effectively eliminated the informal quota system that had limited women's admission to medical schools (Council on Graduate Medical Education 1995; Rhode 1989). Increased interest in medical careers among women may seem contradictory, since the movement severely criticized medical authority and expressed distrust of physicians. However, part of the criticism was that the profession was dominated by men, and part of the solution offered by the movement was women-controlled health services. Participation in the women-controlled health centers may have both demystified medicine for many women and convinced them that women could transform the medical profession. In any case, in 1970, 9 percent of U.S. medical students were women, and by 1980 the percentage had risen to 25 percent (AMA 1991). Furthermore, female medical school graduates after 1975 were, for the first time, more likely than their male counterparts to enter training in obstetrics-gynecology (Weisman et al. 1980), and by 1980, women were 30 percent of residents in obstetrics-gynecology (AMA 1991).

In addition, the movement's success in abortion advocacy set the stage for a movement-countermovement dynamic on the abortion issue that shows little sign of waning. This has occurred in part because abortion has been used cynically by politicians since the 1970s and in part because of the strength of moral commitments on both sides of the issue. As we have seen, furthermore, both antiabortion and abortion rights advocates have roots in earlier women's health movement waves that reflect divergent normative conceptions of women's sexuality and social roles.[12] Even if support for legal abortion remains a majority opinion among the public, in an increasingly pluralistic society, opinions are likely to continue to vary on such issues as the conditions under which abortion should be performed and who should bear the financial cost.

Another legacy of the Women's Health Movement was the promulgation of protectionist policies with regard to women's participation as subjects in medical research. Two controversies involving drug-induced fetal damage— thalidomide-induced birth defects and vaginal cancer discovered in the daughters of women who had taken DES during pregnancy—were widely publicized during the 1960s and 1970s and resonated with women's health activists' criticisms of inadequate testing of drugs consumed by women. In the context of the new abortion politics, in which fetal rights were beginning to be articulated by abortion opponents, these cases also heightened concern about protecting the health of fetuses. In 1977, the FDA issued guidelines recommending that all women of childbearing potential—not just pregnant women—be excluded from early phases of drug trials, except in studies of life-threatening diseases (Mastroianni et al. 1994), and biomedical researchers generally became more cautious about including any women of reproductive age as subjects. Ironically, policy that was framed in the 1970s as protecting women (or, more accurately, fetuses) was reinterpreted in the 1990s as excluding women from potentially beneficial clinical studies (Johnson and Fee 1994). As we shall see, women's health advocates in the 1990s argued for a reversal of protectionist policies in order to benefit the health of all women.

THE WOMEN'S HEALTH AGENDA IN THE 1990S

Women's health once again emerged as a public issue around 1990.[13] While it is debatable whether this wave of women's health activism was part of a social movement cycle—in the sense of a co-occurrence of a family of movements reflecting a broad consensus on the need for social change—it did coincide with a resurgence of public attention to women's issues after a period of relative quiescence during the 1980s. Two key events prompted this resurgence. The first was the 1989 U.S. Supreme Court decision in *Webster v. Re-*

productive Health Services, which upheld the state of Missouri's restrictions on abortion, including a prohibition of use of public facilities for abortions not performed to save the woman's life and a requirement that physicians determine the viability of a fetus believed to be of at least twenty weeks gestational age. The ruling was viewed as a victory for the antiabortion countermovement, and it mobilized supporters of abortion rights, especially women who were too young to have participated in the earlier Women's Health Movement. Substantial increases in contributions and membership were reported by NOW, NARAL, and Planned Parenthood following the ruling (Howes and Allina 1994; Staggenborg 1991). The second focusing event was the October 1991 televised confirmation hearings on the appointment of Judge Clarence Thomas to the U.S. Supreme Court, in which Anita Hill, a law professor who had accused Thomas of sexual harassment, was treated unsympathetically by the all-male, all-white Senate Judiciary Committee. The gender dynamics of the hearings have been credited with activating women, as both candidates and voters, for the 1992 elections and, along with perceptions of a growing "gender gap" in voting patterns during the 1980s, with increasing the salience of women's issues in political campaigns and in Congress (Witt, Paget, and Matthews 1994).

The 1990s episode in women's health also overlapped with a resurgence of efforts to enact national health care reform, which heightened public awareness of health issues generally. The 1991 election of a Democrat, Harris L. Wofford, in a special senatorial election in Pennsylvania on a platform including national health care reform, elevated health reform to national prominence as an issue for the 1992 presidential campaign. According to public opinion polls, public support for health insurance reform reached a forty-year peak in 1992 (Blendon, Brodie, and Benson 1995). The health care reform episode provided the women's health advocacy community with an opportunity to formulate an agenda for women within the context of reform proposals, and it contributed to a decline in legislative activity in health issues when reform failed.

In contrast to the Women's Health Movement of the 1960s and 1970s, which had focused on inequalities of power between women consumers and health care providers and created alternative services outside mainstream institutions, the 1990s episode's unifying theme was the demand for equity for women in access to the benefits of biomedical research and medical treatments. ("Equity" referred to parity between women and men, not to equal access to health care among subgroups of women.) Participants argued that women were entitled to an equitable share of health resources and to health care based on research on *women,* and they sought redress for what they perceived as years of neglect of women's health problems in research and in health care institutions.

They made several key claims. First, they claimed that women's health problems were not studied as frequently as men's were, in part because of the biases of those making research funding decisions[14] and because obstetrics-gynecology was not a major focus in the NIH, the nation's largest funder of biomedical research. Second, they claimed that women had been excluded or underrepresented as subjects in federally funded research, resulting in both information deficits about women's health and barriers to women's access to experimental treatments. Several key cases of exclusion were identified and widely publicized as examples of major investments of public resources that did not produce information that could be generalized to women. Two of the cases were studies of the prevention of heart disease, the leading cause of death in both women and men: the Multiple Risk Factor Intervention Trial (MR FIT Group 1977), a trial of cholesterol-lowering drugs, included 15,000 men and zero women; and the Physicians' Health Study, which tested the effects of aspirin on reducing the risk of myocardial infarction, included 22,071 male physicians and zero women physicians (Steering Committee of the Physicians' Health Study Research Group 1989). The investigators in these two studies defended their exclusion of women on the basis of their perception of heart disease as primarily a problem in middle-aged men and, in the case of the physician study, of a dearth of middle-aged women physicians in 1982 when the study began (Mann 1995). The third case was the Baltimore Longitudinal Study of Aging, which issued a report entitled *Normal Human Aging* that was based on data from an observational study of over 1,000 men and zero women (Shock et al. 1984). Although women were a majority of the elderly population, the study included no women during its first twenty years because, according to the researchers, bathroom facilities for women were not available in the research site when the study began. The title of the monograph, which implicitly equated "normal" with "male," further incensed critics.

Some countered that these studies were not representative of all federally funded research during the same period and that exclusion of women might be scientifically appropriate in some circumstances (Kadar 1994; Mann 1995; Meinert 1995). These arguments, however, did not negate the impact of these studies as powerful symbols used to make a larger political point. The cases were particularly compelling because they were large-scale, expensive studies of conditions affecting both women and men, and the information they provided would be used in treatments for both sexes. Yet they excluded women, and no parallel studies focusing on women were funded simultaneously. Consequently, the cases illustrated a cultural contradiction: apparent gender bias among supposedly objective scientists who should have been aware of the epidemiology of heart disease, of the demography of aging, and of the bio-psychosocial factors that might plausibly produce gender differences in these conditions or in their treatments.

Concern about underrepresentation of women in some studies in which they were included also was raised. Underlying this concern was the assumption that women and men may react differently to treatments or preventive interventions for the same diseases. An insufficient number of women in a study population prevents researchers from conducting statistically valid analyses of gender differences (whether resulting from biological or psychosocial factors) in disease etiology, disease course, or the effectiveness of treatments, particularly drug treatments. Although many in the biomedical community argued that it was not necessary to investigate gender differences in most studies, women's health advocates countered that the current lack of evidence for gender differences could be due to inadequate investigation of these differences in the past.

Third, some participants claimed that women's health research had been too narrowly focused on reproductive health problems and, specifically, on the health of mothers in relation to their fetuses or newborns. Early studies of women and AIDS, for example, had focused on "women as vectors for transmission to men and children" rather than on the disease's impact on women (Rosser 1994:27). This focus also limited research attention to women of reproductive age and neglected the health problems of midlife and older women. Between 1980 and 1990, the number of women in the U.S. population ages 35 to 49 increased by nearly 40 percent (U.S. Bureau of the Census 1995:15), and many of the leaders of the 1990s women's health episode were members of the post–World War II baby-boom generation who were approaching midlife. It was not surprising that these women tended to be interested in menopause and in health problems associated with aging. They argued for a respecification of the definition of "women's health" to recognize women's longer life expectancy than men's and the diversity of women's social roles other than maternity.

Fourth, they claimed that women researchers were underrepresented as directors of studies funded by the federal government. In 1989, for example, women were only 14 percent of principal investigators of research projects sponsored by the NIH (Council on Graduate Medical Education 1995). Finally, they claimed that women were disadvantaged in their health care because of the lack of research, inadequate training of physicians, and fragmentation of services (Auerbach and Figert 1995; Clancy and Massion 1992; Rosser 1994).

The major policy objectives were a reallocation of federal funds to support biomedical research on specific women's health problems; changes in federal policies regarding inclusion of women as research subjects; programs to encourage women to become biomedical investigators; reforms in medical education and postgraduate training, including a proposal for a new medical specialty in women's health; and targeted improvements in health services delivery for women. The episode produced changes in federal policy on including women in trials of new drugs and other clinical studies[15] and in an unprecedented spate of federal legislation and government program initiatives in women's health between 1990 and 1994. Key accomplishments included passage of legislation authorizing major commitments of federal funds for women's health research and preventive services (including programs to extend breast and cervical cancer screening to low-income women), to ensure the quality of mammograms, and to prevent infertility through sexually transmitted disease (STD) screening. Accomplishments also included programmatic changes in the executive branch of government, including new offices and positions dedicated to the coordination of women's health activities. Government attention and action, furthermore, helped legitimize the changing normative climate for women's health care, and it created synergies with initiatives outside of government to promote women's health research, reforms in medical education, and the creation of new services.

The leaders of the 1990s episode were empowered women who had attained positions of influence in government, in the biomedical community, and in women's health advocacy and interest groups, some of which were composed of professional women. The key coalition consisted of women in Congress and their staffs, women in the biomedical community—including NIH officials, academic researchers, and practicing physicians (by 1990, nearly one in five was a woman)—and leaders of women's health organizations who were sophisticated in the promotion of health care issues (through newsletters, professional journals, and the media) and adept at mobilizing human and financial resources. Some of the organizations involved in this episode had originated in the earlier Women's Health Movement, and some were newly organized single- and multi-issue groups. Examples of new single-issue organizations included breast cancer patient advocacy groups, which had begun to appear in local communities in the 1980s and later formed national networks. Examples of new multi-issue groups with professional constituencies included the Society for the Advancement of Women's Health

Research, formed in 1990 by women at NIH (led by Dr. Florence Haseltine, director of the Center for Population Research) and others in the biomedical community to promote research on women's health; and the Jacobs Institute of Women's Health, founded in 1990 with a bequest to the American College of Obstetricians and Gynecologists and the American Association of Obstetricians and Gynecologists Foundation, to study and improve women's health care from a multidisciplinary (biomedical and social sciences) perspective. A major distinction between this movement wave and the 1960–1970s wave was the concerted effort to work through mainstream institutions and to use the power of government to effect changes.

The political climate in which women's health emerged as a public issue for the 1990s was, on the face of it, generally hostile to women's health issues. The abortion politics of the Reagan and Bush administrations had produced a chilling effect on biomedical research related to the development and testing of new contraceptive methods, on studies of sexual behaviors related to prevention of unwanted pregnancies and STDs (including HIV/AIDS), on infertility research, and on research using fetal tissue. Women's health advocates began to perceive that biomedical research on conditions important to women was being seriously compromised. Within the NIH, attempts were being made to expedite the implementation of a 1986 policy, which was to have gone into effect in 1987, urging applicants for NIH research grants and contracts to include women in study populations.[16] At about the same time that concerns were coalescing within the NIH, the Congressional Caucus for Women's Issues was beginning to focus on health issues. The bipartisan caucus, whose members included both women and men, had been founded in 1977 and had focused initially on legal and economic equity for women; in 1989, it began to formulate a legislative agenda on women's health. Members of the caucus and their staffs worked closely with individuals in the NIH and other federal agencies and with representatives of several professional associations and women's health interest groups to begin to formulate an agenda that would have broad appeal. According to Patricia Schroeder and Olympia Snowe (1994:92), "we, as caucus co-chairs, began to look for a new middle ground that could be embraced by congresswomen on both sides of the abortion divide." (The caucus took no official position on abortion rights until 1993.) Accordingly, they defined women's health issues broadly, not only with respect to reproductive issues, and they framed the issues as matters of fairness and objectivity within biomedical science. They developed policy initiatives that, in some cases, provided antiabortion legislators with an opportunity to support women's issues. Abortion politics, therefore, helped create a climate in which legislators became more receptive to a wide range of women's health issues.

In addition, a strategy was crafted that would simultaneously publicize their agenda and bring pressure on the NIH to address women's health issues. Since the NIH was due for reauthorization, a "policy window," in the terminology of John Kingdon (1995), presented itself. In December 1989, the caucus co-chairs joined with Henry A. Waxman, chairman of the Subcommittee on Health and the Environment and a Caucus member, in requesting that the General Accounting Office (GAO) evaluate the success of the 1986 NIH policy encouraging inclusion of women in study populations. The GAO report, which showed, not surprisingly, that NIH had failed to implement its policy (Nadel 1990), was released on 18 June 1990 in a subcommittee hearing that was carefully orchestrated for maximum public impact. Among those attending, representatives of the media outnumbered representatives of the NIH. The newly formed Society for the Advancement of Women's Health Research, whose members included key women's health advocates within the NIH as well as other health professionals, prepared position papers and helped coordinate media contacts. The results of the report, along with details of the studies excluding women that were described earlier, were widely disseminated in the national press, and release of the report is generally acknowledged to have been the event that captured the attention of policymakers and galvanized public opinion on the issue of inequities in women's health research (Auerbach and Figert 1995; Schroeder and Snowe 1994). Participants in the episode refer to the report as "the catalyst," "the hottest issue," "the smoking gun," and "an explosion."

A number of key events occurred in the wake of the GAO report. In July–August 1990, the Women's Health Equity Act (WHEA) was first introduced in the House of Representatives and in the Senate. (It was reintroduced in subsequent sessions in revised versions.) The WHEA was modeled after the Women's Economic Equity Act and included twenty separate bills, some of which had been previously introduced, in three areas: research policy and funding levels, access to health services, and prevention of breast and cervical cancer. The research policy provisions of the WHEA included a proposal to revise NIH's policies to *require* inclusion of women and analyses of gender differences in clinical studies and a proposal to create an NIH office of women's health to coordinate and monitor efforts to improve women's health research. The specific topics targeted for research funding were breast and ovarian cancer, AIDS, osteoporosis, and contraception and infertility. The first victory for the WHEA was the 1990 approval of the Breast and Cervical

Cancer Mortality Prevention Act, which created state grants, to be administered by the Centers for Disease Control, to make screening services more accessible to low-income women.

In anticipation of legislative directives, which they wished to avoid, federal agencies took action in direct response to the GAO report and the introduction of the WHEA. At a meeting in September 1990 that included members of the caucus and officials of the NIH and the Public Health Service, the NIH announced creation of the Office of Research on Women's Health (ORWH), with the mission of establishing an NIH-wide policy for women's health research, coordinating and monitoring NIH women's health research, and developing initiatives to increase the participation of women as subjects in clinical research and as biomedical researchers (Kirschstein 1991). At the same meeting, the Assistant Secretary for Health agreed to prepare an action plan on women's health for each agency of the Public Health Service, and participants agreed to hold a "summit" on women's health to solicit testimony from the research community and from women's health advocates on research needs. (The summit was held in 1991 and produced a broad research agenda on women's health problems throughout the life span, which has been called a "laundry list" [Culliton 1991], but it provided no basis on which to prioritize research needs and no implementation plan [NIH 1992].)

On the same day, the Secretary of Health and Human Services announced his recommendation that Dr. Bernadine Healy, a cardiologist, be appointed as NIH director; in 1991, she became the first woman to hold this post. Healy moved quickly on the women's health agenda by announcing plans in April 1991 for the Women's Health Initiative, which she called a "moonwalk for women" (Schroeder and Snowe 1994:100). The initiative was a massive research project focusing on key health problems of older women: prevention of breast cancer, heart disease, and osteoporotic fractures. Ultimately projected to cost $625 million, the fourteen-year project would be the largest research study ever funded by NIH. The project was to include a three-branch clinical trial assessing the effects of low-fat diet, hormone replacement therapy, and calcium and vitamin D supplementation and including 63,000 postmenopausal women in forty-five clinical centers across the country; an observational study of an additional 100,000 women; and a community prevention study (Rossouw et al. 1995).

Plans for the Women's Health Initiative, however, did not take the pressure off NIH. Several of the key research provisions of the WHEA were included in legislation to reauthorize the NIH, beginning in 1990. These provisions included providing statuatory authority for the NIH office on women's health;

codifying NIH policy requiring inclusion of women in clinical studies; authorizing $225 million for basic research on breast cancer, $75 million for research on ovarian and other reproductive cancers, and $40 million for research on osteoporosis and bone disorders; establishment of contraceptive and infertility research centers; and establishment of a clinical research program in obstetrics and gynecology at the NIH (Auerbach and Figert 1995). Although supported in both houses of Congress, what became known as the "women's health provisions" of the reauthorization bill were opposed by the NIH, which resented what it perceived to be micromanagement of its programs. In particular, funding "earmarked" for specific purposes is generally resisted by the NIH, where the culture values scientific, rather than political, determination of research priorities. Perhaps the most vivid illustration of fault lines in the women's health research agenda occurred in 1992, when Healy openly opposed some of the women's health provisions, including earmarks, thus alienating women's health advocates in Congress. In a letter to the Secretary of Health and Human Services in May 1992, Healy called the women's health provisions in the NIH reauthorization bill "unnecessary"; President Bush used this same term when he vetoed the bill in June 1992.

The 1992 elections brought a Democratic administration, tripled the number of women in the Senate (to six), and increased the number of women in the House of Representatives by two-thirds (to 48 members), contributing to the designation of 1992 as the "Year of the Woman." The political climate for women's health issues became more favorable, not only because of a strengthened base of support in Congress but also because of the Clinton administration's support of reproductive rights and commitment to health care reform. President Clinton appointed women to some key health posts—Donna E. Shalala as Secretary of the Department of Health and Human Services, Jocelyn Elders as Surgeon General, and Hillary Rodham Clinton as coleader of the Task Force on Health Care Reform—and he signed the NIH Revitalization Act, including the women's health provisions, into law in June 1993.

The renewed efforts at national health care reform during the early years of the Clinton administration (1992–94) also affected the women's health agenda. As we have seen, by the time of the 1992 elections, women's health groups were mobilized and were well positioned to frame an agenda for women within the context of the health care reform debate. The key issues at stake for women in the various health care reform plans under consideration were whether or not all women would be covered by health insurance and the content of the basic benefits package that would be provided. However, because health care financing became a highly charged, partisan political issue, the bipartisan Congressional Caucus for Women's Issues had difficulty, at least at first, finding common ground. The caucus did achieve consensus on a statement of principles, based on guidelines issued by the Campaign for Women's Health (1992, 1993), a coalition of over 100 diverse organizations that formed to influence health care reform. (The Campaign for Women's Health is discussed in more detail in chapter 5.) The caucus endorsed the principles of universal access to health insurance (as distinct from universal coverage), a basic benefits package including key preventive and treatment services for women, and primary care availability in diverse settings and by a range of providers (Schroeder and Snowe 1994).

The health care reform debate also forced the abortion issue to the surface. Inclusion of a full range of women's health services, including reproductive health services, in the basic benefits package was a key issue for the dominant coalition of women's health advocates who, as we have seen, viewed women's health as including, but not exclusively defined by, reproductive health. To be an effective proponent of a comprehensive benefits package for women, including a full range of reproductive health services, the caucus adopted an official pro-choice position on abortion in January 1993. Inclusion of abortion benefits, however, was shaping up to be a highly controversial issue both inside and outside Congress. In Congress, some representatives were staking out positions based on abortion coverage (Joffe 1995; Johnson and Broder 1996). The Christian Coalition was against funding of abortions in health care reform proposals generally and opposed the Clinton Health Security Plan for this and other reasons (Skocpol 1996). The Clinton plan included "pregnancy-related services" as covered benefits, with abortion—though not specifically mentioned in the plan—generally understood as meeting the criteria for coverage that were proposed by the Task Force working group on benefits coverage (Bergthold 1995). Abortion rights advocates, however, were concerned that abortion might not ultimately be covered, or might be "compromised away" in the final program. When the effort at national health care reform ultimately failed in 1994, women's health advocates were relieved that the abortion issue had not been the cause.[17]

The failure of national health care reform coincided with another major shift in the political climate, and the elections of 1994 produced a Republican-controlled Congress. In January 1995, the new leadership of the House of Representatives abolished legislative service organizations; consequently, the caucus continued as a congressional member organization without a budget, and its former staff established a private organization, Women's Policy, Inc., to continue the nonpartisan informational services and policy analyses that had been provided previously by the caucus. In the 104th Congress, expectations were not high for new legislative initiatives in women's health, and advocates saw serious threats to women's health care in proposals for restructuring Medicaid and Medicare, for reducing Title X funding for family planning services, for limiting late-term abortions, and for restrictions on federal funding for abortion services. Although many research studies and other projects initiated during the early 1990s continued, the episode's momentum had slowed in Congress by 1995 (Women's Policy, Inc., 1996a).

One of the major legacies of the early 1990s episode—in addition to the biomedical research projects that were funded and initiated—was the level of institutional change initiated within government. New policies governing women's participation as subjects in biomedical research were part of this change. In addition, following the establishment of the NIH Office of Research on Women's Health in 1990, other offices to coordinate women's health research and activities within other federal agencies were established. (There had been some discussion among women's health advocates about proposing a separate center on women's health within NIH, but many viewed this as segregating women's health concerns, rather than as a mechanism to encourage the institutes to integrate women's health issues within their programs; hence the ORWH was proposed instead.) The Office on Women's Health in the Office of the Assistant Secretary for Health, Department of Health and Human Services, was created in 1991 to advance and coordinate a comprehensive women's health agenda across the Public Health Service, and in 1993, President Clinton appointed Susan Blumenthal, a psychiatrist, as the nation's first Deputy Assistant Secretary for Women's Health. Additional offices included the Office for Women's Services in the Substance Abuse and Mental Health Services Administration (established in 1992), the Centers for Disease Control and Prevention's Office of Women's Health (established in 1994), and the FDA Office of Women's Health (established in 1994). Women's health coordinators were appointed in other Public Health Service agencies and in regional offices. The presence of these new offices, despite some budget cuts in 1995, provided an organizational mechanism for keeping women's health issues on the agenda, for monitoring progress over time, and for promoting research and services. It remains to be seen how the role of these offices will evolve and whether they will attain sufficient resources and influence to produce significant change.

Another legacy was the influence of women's organizations and women's health advocacy groups on health policymaking as a result of collaboration between these groups and women in the biomedical community and in government. The case of breast cancer activism provides a vivid example of the influence of women's health advocacy groups. By the early 1990s, breast cancer activists had established national networks of organizations providing education and information, direct services, and political action. The National Breast Cancer Coalition (NBCC) was formed in 1991 to influence national breast cancer policy, and it represented nearly three hundred organizations in all states by 1994 (Love 1995). The combined efforts of the breast cancer groups and the Congressional Caucus for Women's Issues, for which breast cancer had been an early priority, succeeded in attaining increased federal funding allocations for breast cancer research (in the NIH and the Department of Defense) and for programs to extend screening services and to establish and enforce quality standards for mammography. Between 1990 and 1993, funding for breast cancer was increased nearly fivefold. The caucus credits the "clout of the breast cancer lobby" in 1992 with helping obtain an earmark of $210 million in the Department of Defense budget for breast cancer research (Schroeder and Snowe 1994). The breast cancer groups also demanded direct involvement in setting the research agenda, which resulted in unique programs to involve consumers in grant reviews. (The role of the breast cancer organizations is discussed in more detail in chapter 5.)

During the early 1990s, women's health became overtly political, with some potential unintended consequences. The heightened visibility of women's health issues and the apparent growing public support for these concerns provided opportunities for political gain by groups with varied agendas. For example, physicians' associations or other special interest groups could frame an issue as "women's health" to garner support, even if their initiatives or issues were not endorsed by women's groups. Lawmakers (male and female) might be eager to support such issues in an attempt to gain favor with female constituents. Examples of policy initiatives in the 1990s that were promoted largely outside the women's health advocacy community—and sometimes over the objections of women's health groups—included state and federal legislation requiring insurance coverage of minimum hospital stays for women following childbirth and the promulgation of guidelines recommending regular mammography screening for women in their forties. These examples illustrate that women's health advocates do not always control the "women's health agenda."

Another possible unintended consequence of the 1990s episode in women's health activism is noteworthy. Because of the explicit and widely publicized focus on increased investments in biomedical research, including the ongoing NIH-funded Women's Health Initiative and new breast cancer research, the episode may have overemphasized a biomedical model of women's health and promised more than it could ultimately deliver. Those framing the agenda—including many women physicians and researchers—were professional stakeholders in the biomedical research enterprise, with confidence in their scientific expertise. However, one risk of raising consumers' expectations for new treatments is that the research agenda could lose credibility if results are not perceived as definitive, if new treatments are not readily adopted in medical practice or made widely available to women, or if social and environmental factors affecting women's health are not also addressed. Another risk is that consumers might increasingly demand new or experimental treatments in the absence of effectiveness data. Ruzek (1995a,b) has drawn attention to the tendency of some women's health advocacy groups in the early 1990s to advocate new treatment technologies uncritically, such as autologous bone marrow transplants (ABMT) for women with late-stage breast cancer. She attributes this to two factors: the advocacy groups' general distrust of health insurance companies, which are perceived as attempting to deprive women of expensive treatments to control costs; and the politics of national health care reform, which transformed women's health advocacy groups into lobbyists seeking more expansive benefits for their constituencies. In addition, however, the rhetoric of the women's health movement episode in the 1990s, which was under way well before national health care reform efforts began, may have increased women's faith in the capacity of biomedicine to solve their health problems.

CROSSCUTTING THEMES

The U.S. women's health megamovement consists of a series of waves of public attention to women's health and body issues, extending over two centuries, with the waves generally coinciding with social movement cycles and heightened women's rights activism. Furthermore, the episodes occurred at critical junctures in which both women's social roles and health institutions were undergoing important transformations. Opportunities therefore existed within each episode for renegotiation of the meaning of women's health and the relationships between women and health care institutions.

On the face of it, these movement waves addressed diverse health issues reflecting, in part, the changing roles and interests of women in the context of prevailing concerns in the larger society. The movements also used a variety of strategies to influence the nature of health care. However, a number of recurring themes across these movement waves reveal some commonalities in women's health concerns in different historical eras. They include women's attempts to obtain health education and to expand the information base about their health and bodies; women's efforts to participate as formal and informal providers of health care, especially to other women; and women's efforts to control their fertility, including the timing and circumstances of childbearing.

The historical continuity of women's quest for health and body information is apparent across waves and may be rooted in their traditional role as domestic healer as well as in their enduring role as family caregiver. Women have sought to educate each other in health matters in affiliative and self-help groups. The early women physicians were lecturers and health educators of women. Health care institutions established by women in all eras have emphasized education and counseling. Women's demands for information about their health were a major factor in the recent policy initiatives to expand the biomedical research agenda to include more of women's health problems and to increase the participation of women as subjects in clinical studies.

In addition, each wave contended with the dual role of women as consumers and providers of health care. Women had traditionally been health care providers for their families, but as the medical marketplace began to grow and diversify in the early 1800s, women's roles as midwives and domestic healers became a subject of active debate and a point on which competing medical practitioners differed. In the Popular Health Movement, the issue had to do with a conflict between the increasing practice of midwifery by male physicians and the traditional female culture surrounding childbirth, which was supported by most sectarians. By the late-nineteenth-century episode, as more women gained access to medical training, a key issue had to do with articulating roles for women within medicine on the basis of beliefs about the special capacities of women physicians as providers for women patients generally, not only in childbirth. In the Progressive Era, conflicts emerged between private physicians and new services (prenatal care and birth control clinics) established by public health nurses and women social reformers. In the 1960s and 1970s, lay-controlled women's health services were established by women as alternatives to mainstream medical institutions. In the 1990s, the growing cadre of women physicians served as prominent proponents of reforms in medical education and practice and of efforts to expand the biomedical research agenda with regard to women's health.

Finally, each wave articulated a perspective on women's role in reproductive control, and together these waves suggest that fertility control is a fundamental women's health concern that persists across historical eras and is often a key target of organized social change efforts. The recognition that fertility control is integral to women's health and social well-being was apparent during the Popular Health Movement and in each subsequent movement wave. The demand for fertility control has been framed in various ways depending upon the sociohistorical circumstances, including the prevailing gender role ideologies and understandings of human sexuality. Indeed, efforts to improve the status of motherhood and to increase women's control over their fertility were two sides of the same coin. In the waves of the megamovement, fertility-control efforts were apparent in the successive movements for family size limitation, voluntary motherhood, birth control and family planning, and reproductive rights. The successive social change strategies that accompanied these different conceptions of reproductive control included public education and moral suasion on matters of hygiene and marital abstinence; state and federal legislative regulation of contraceptive and abortive agents; efforts to legalize contraception and abortion through legislation and the courts; direct action tactics to provide illegal contraceptives and abortion services; establishment of lay-controlled services; and mainstreaming of fertility-control services. During the twentieth century, the strategies of direct confrontation and establishing alternative services illustrate women's persistence in pursuing reproductive control despite legal prohibitions and the sometimes hostile stance of the medical profession.

The megamovement waves also illustrate a continuity of cultural repertoires in women's activism. The traditions of collective action in women's health include creating organizations at the local level to educate women about their health, to involve women in the health of the community, or to provide social support (e.g., the ladies' physiological societies of the mid-1800s; women's self-help groups in the 1960s and 1970s; breast cancer support groups beginning in the 1970s). They include organizing state and national networks of interest groups for political action in women's health (e.g., associations of women's clubs working in the Progressive Era for federal programs in maternal and child health; coalitions of breast cancer patient advocacy groups in the 1990s lobbying for increased funding for breast cancer research and for a role in setting research agendas.) They also include establishing new organizations for the provision of clinical services and health education to women when desired services were not available from mainstream providers. Health organizations created by women have spanned the nineteenth and twentieth centuries and have included hospitals specializing in the care of women and/or children, prenatal care clinics, birth control clinics, abortion referral services and clinics, and various types of women's

health centers. Some of these organizations were initiated in hostile environ-
ments, including during periods when the services in question were illegal (as
in the case of Progressive Era birth control clinics and pre–*Roe v. Wade* abortion services), so that the women involved were subjected to the risks of legal
sanctions and public criticism. The history of these organizations illustrates
both the tenacity of their inventors and the enduring tension between separatism and assimilation as principles on which to base women's health care.
An apparent lesson from the megamovement waves is that the creation of separate women's health care organizations often has spurred changes in mainstream institutions. (These issues are discussed further in chapter 4.) This
diversity of repertoires in the women's health megamovement, furthermore,
suggests a high level of adaptability and a capacity for mobilization across issues and eras.

The impact of the waves of the women's health megamovement may be
considered at several levels. For individual participants, involvement in various movement activities and organizations might have been empowering in
a number of ways. For example, involvement could have increased women's
knowledge about health and access to health-producing resources; it could
have resulted in gaining new social and political skills transferable to other issues or areas of life; and it could have created a new collective identity among
women. It is particularly noteworthy that women participated in movement
activities at some personal risk in all waves. These risks included social stig-
matization for speaking in public or verbalizing unpopular or taboo topics
such as reproductive control; public criticism from elite groups such as the organized medical profession or the church; and arrest and imprisonment for
illegal acts such as providing contraceptives and abortions. The experience of
taking such risks could have been both personally and politically empowering to many women. With regard to movement impact on health care institutions and public policy, the waves of the megamovement transformed
medical practice in specific ways (e.g., by motivating obstetricians to incorporate prenatal care into their practices), created new health care organizations
(e.g., birth control clinics) that often influenced mainstream providers, and
set precedents for regulation (e.g., legal restrictions on abortion) or public
funding (e.g., the Sheppard-Towner Act) of specific health services. Depending on one's ideological perspective, of course, not all of these changes would
be viewed as positive or as broadening women's social and economic opportunities. However, the waves influenced women's political culture and thereby
created the basis for future waves of health activism. In particular, the varied
repertoires of collective action and networks of activist groups have provided

access to policymaking and the organizational resources for ongoing women's health advocacy.

This discussion has presented a more complex picture than the usual consideration of women's health movements as distinct entities focused on a single service or issue. In addition, it has attempted to highlight the ways in which women who have organized for collective action have sought to control their health and build health care institutions that are more responsive to their needs. Because women, traditionally, were providers of domestic medicine and key clients of various health care practitioners contending for their patronage, they have been uniquely culturally positioned as both providers and consumers of health care services. Moreover, the American tradition of women's organization and advocacy for social reform extended frequently into matters pertaining to personal and public health. Women have therefore been particularly important agents for change in health care institutions. That the waves of women's health activism have continued into the 1990s suggests the relevance of women's health movements for current health care policymaking.

3

Patterns of Health Care Use

IN ARGUING for an expanded biomedical research agenda in women's health and for gender equity in access to the benefits of health care, women's health advocates in the early 1990s challenged prevailing notions about women's health care. Their claims that women were disadvantaged in their health care, however, were difficult to reconcile with the evidence that women have longer average life expectancy than men, have lower age-adjusted mortality than men, and consume more health services than men throughout most of the life span. Thus women would appear to have greater access to care than men and to benefit from that care. Yet women's higher overall use of services does not necessarily mean that women receive better care than men or similar care for the same conditions. Nor does it mean that women generally enjoy better overall health status than men throughout life or that all subgroups of women—defined by age, race/ethnicity, or socioeconomic level—have equal access to health care. And, during periods of change, it does not mean that shifting practices or policies have equal impact on women and men.

Gender differences in health care patterns are, at least in part, the consequence of sociohistorical factors and of health care institutions that structure basic health care differently for women and men. Some gender differences may be appropriate, and some may reflect inequities. Health care delivery organizations, furthermore, are constantly changing and affecting the health care patterns of both women and men. What is the evidence for gender inequities in the current health care environment, and what are the prospects for change?

GENDER DIFFERENCES IN HEALTH

Most discussions of health care use begin with a consideration of individuals' needs for care, as reflected in their current health status or risks to health. The standard indicators of health in the U.S. population reveal a number of differences in health status between women and men, but they cannot be easily interpreted as favoring one sex or the other. Nor are the reasons for these differences fully understood. A brief summary of gender differences will help place contemporary concerns about women's health care in context and will help illustrate why gender differences in health care use are not a matter of epidemiology alone, but also one of social and historical factors.

There is no "gold standard" for assessing health status or for comparing the health of women and men. Typical indicators of health in populations include average life expectancy at birth, mortality patterns, and morbidity patterns. (Use of health services is also sometimes used as an indicator of health status, but this is problematic because individuals may use health care for reasons other than illness, such as disease prevention, and greater use of services does not necessarily predict improved health.) Morbidity is measured in several ways, including incidence and prevalence of specific conditions assessed through physician reports or health care organization statistics; self-reported symptoms, illness episodes, disabilities, and days lost from work or other major activities because of illness or disability; and self-assessments of overall health status or quality of life. Methods that rely on self-reports, such as community-based epidemiological surveys, may be subject to bias if women and men perceive and report symptoms differently or if the measurement instruments are biased. Methods that rely on utilization statistics, such as office visits to physicians or hospital discharge data, reflect only those persons who obtain care and may be biased if one gender seeks care more often than the other or if there are systematic differences in how women's and men's visits or diagnoses are recorded.

American women live longer than men and have lower mortality than men at all ages. However, women appear to experience more disease and disability than men throughout most of the life span. It is not clear, however, how much of women's apparent excess morbidity is due to health differences that result from either innate or acquired risks, learned illness behaviors, or health care system factors. The causes of observed differences in health between women and men have, in fact, been the subject of much inquiry by social scientists, who have drawn attention to the importance of considering social and cultural factors, as well as biomedical factors, as determinants of health. In particular, the apparent contradiction of women's lower mortality but higher morbidity has generated a considerable body of research during the last twenty years (Walsh, Sorensen, and Leonard 1995). These issues are likely to continue to be debated for some time.

With regard to life expectancy, women in the United States now live an average of nearly seven years longer than men: in 1994, the average life expectancy at birth was 79 years for females and 72.3 years for males (NCHS 1996a). The difference in average life expectancy favoring females has increased from two years in 1900 (when average life expectancy at birth was 48.3 years for females and 46.3 for males) and reflects trends in other developed countries. Worldwide, females now have longer average life expectancy at birth, with the exception of a few countries in southern Asia (United Nations 1995). Women's advantage in average life expectancy is larger in developed countries than in developing countries, and it is thought to have emerged in industrial nations beginning in the late 1800s as a result of changes in gender-linked risks to health at different ages. This included a gradual decline in maternal mortality.[1]

Men in the United States currently have higher mortality rates than women at all ages. The sex differential in mortality, favoring women, increased steadily from the early 1900s to about 1970, when it began to stabilize (Verbrugge 1990; Waldron 1995; Wingard 1984). Currently, the leading causes of death in the United States are the same for both sexes: heart disease and cancer. In 1993, deaths from heart disease and cancer accounted for 56 percent of deaths of women and 55 percent of deaths of men (NCHS 1996a). Lung cancer was the leading cause of cancer deaths for both white and black women, followed by breast and colorectal cancers. Since 1970, the age-adjusted death rate from lung cancer has been rising steadily in women, reflecting women's increased cigarette smoking after World War II, while the death rate from other cancers has been fairly stable. Breast cancer death rates have been declining since the late 1980s, except among black women, for whom the breast cancer death rate increased 16 percent between 1980 and 1992 (NCHS 1995).

In 1993, black women were 28 percent more likely than white women to die from breast cancer (NCHS 1996a).

Cerebrovascular diseases (stroke) were the third leading cause of death in women in 1992. However, in men, the third leading cause of death was not disease-related: for white men, the third leading cause of death was unintentional injuries, including motor vehicle accidents; for black men, the third leading cause of death was homicide and legal intervention. For white women in 1993, the fourth leading cause of death was chronic obstructive pulmonary diseases, followed by unintentional injuries; for black women, the fourth leading cause of death was diabetes mellitus, followed by unintentional injuries. In 1993, HIV/AIDS was the fourth leading cause of death among U.S. women ages 25 to 44 and the leading cause of death among black women in this age group; the incidence of AIDS was increasing more rapidly among women than among men (CDC 1995a; NCHS 1996a).

Although U.S. women live longer than men, they report more disease and disability than men and more time lost from regular activities because of disease and disability, throughout most of the life span. Studies of self-assessed overall health status uniformly find that women perceive themselves to be less healthy than men, but the gender difference generally is small and disappears among the elderly. For example, in the 1994 National Health Interview Survey, the percentages of women and men rating their health as "fair" or "poor" were 8 percent of women and 6 percent of men ages 25 to 44; 18 percent of women and 15 percent of men ages 45 to 64; and 28 percent of both women and men ages 65 and over (Adams and Marano 1995).

As to specific conditions, women report higher rates than men of most acute and some chronic conditions. Among acute conditions (i.e., those ordinarily lasting less than three months), women ages 18 to 44 in 1994 reported, for example, higher rates than men of respiratory conditions, infective and parasitic diseases, digestive system conditions, acute urinary conditions, and headaches, and men ages 18 to 44 reported higher rates than women of wounds and lacerations and of fractures and dislocations. Women generally reported receiving medical attention more often than men for the same acute conditions, and women ages 18 to 44 reported more restricted-activity days, more bed days, and more work-loss days associated with acute conditions than did men of the same ages; however, among persons ages 18 to 44, men reported more restricted-activity days, bed days, and work-loss days associated with injuries (Adams and Marano 1995).

Among chronic conditions, in 1994 women reported, for example, higher rates of arthritis, migraine headaches, dermatitis, and bladder disorders, and men reported higher rates of ischemic heart disease, visual and hearing impairments, deformity or orthopedic impairment, and gout (Adams and Marano 1995). The percentage of women reporting that they were limited in the "amount or kind of major activity" because of chronic conditions is higher than the percentage of men in nearly all age groups. The greatest gender difference occurs among persons ages 75 and over: 10 percent of men and 17 percent of women reported limitations in 1994 (NCHS 1996a).

Women report more general disability than men in all age groups. Disability in noninstitutionalized persons often is measured by assessing the individual's ability to perform activities of daily living (ADLs)—including self-maintenance activities such as bathing, dressing, eating, and so on—and instrumental activities of daily living (IADLs)—including housework, meal preparation, shopping, and so on. These disabilities increase with age, and the gender differences are particularly pronounced in persons ages 75 and over (NCHS 1996a). Women, however, are more likely than men to be IADL-disabled at all ages, and this finding could result in part from the fact that IADLs are gender-linked activities: that is, given prevailing gender roles, they are less likely to be performed by men, whether or not they are disabled.

Data from the 1980s Epidemiological Catchment Area study of mental health problems revealed that women had significantly higher rates than men of major depressive episodes, anxiety disorders, somatization disorder, and eating disorders, whereas men had higher rates of alcohol and drug abuse and antisocial personality (Glied and Kofman 1995). The gender difference in the rates of depression, furthermore, persists in different race/ethnicity groups and by level of income, education, and occupation (Horton 1995). The 1992 National Comorbidity Survey found that women were more likely than men to have an affective disorder or an anxiety disorder in their lifetime, whereas men were more likely to have a substance use disorder or antisocial personality disorder (Kessler et al. 1994). Depression in women occurs predominantly during their childbearing and child-rearing years, often during pregnancy or the postpartum period (Weissman and Olfson 1995).

Women's health researchers recently have compiled data on acute and chronic conditions that are unique to women, are more prevalent in women, or that affect women and men differently (Collins et al. 1994; Fogel and Woods 1995; Horton 1995; NIH 1992). Aside from conditions that are unique to one sex (such as cancers of the reproductive organs), there are a number of conditions that are more prevalent in either males or females. For example, autoimmune diseases, such as lupus erythematosus and rheumatoid arthritis, are more common in women than in men. And because women live longer

than men, they are more susceptible to late-onset conditions such as osteoporosis, fractures attributable to osteoporosis, and Alzheimer's disease. In
part because of their longer life expectancy, women are thought to be more
likely than men to experience more than one chronic condition simultaneously and to spend more years in a frail elderly condition (NIH 1992).

Women are more likely than men to be victims of domestic violence and
sexual abuse, and health consequences to women of these experiences are just
beginning to be understood (Commonwealth Fund Commission on Women's
Health 1996a). Women ages 18 to 64 who reported in a 1993 survey that they
had experienced childhood sexual abuse or spouse abuse were twice as likely
as nonabused women to rate their current health as "fair" or "poor" and were
significantly more likely to report gynecological diagnoses, a sexually transmitted disease (STD), or a diagnosis of depression or anxiety within the past
five years. Women who had been victims of rape within the past five years
were significantly more likely than other women to report a disability, gynecological diagnosis, urinary tract infection, STD, or diagnosis of depression
or anxiety in the past five years (Plichta 1996). Holmes and colleagues (1996)
recently estimated that there may be over 32,000 rape-related pregnancies in
the United States annually among women ages 18 and over, and most of these
pregnancies are associated with domestic and family violence.

In addition, there are a number of diseases for which etiology, disease pres-
entation, or disease course differ for women and men. For example, some
STDs are asymptomatic in women and therefore may be detected and treated
later than in men; consequently women are more likely than men to suffer
long-term effects of these diseases, including pelvic inflammatory disease, reproductive problems, and infertility. AIDS manifests differently in women
than in men, and the 1993 Centers for Disease Control's expanded definition
of AIDS recognized such female symptoms as persistent vaginal yeast infections and invasive cervical cancer (Donovan 1993). Heart disease typically occurs about ten years later in women than in men, in part because of the
protective effect of estrogen in premenopausal women; furthermore, the first
sign of heart disease in men is often a heart attack, whereas the first sign in
women is often angina (Collins et al. 1994).

The interpretation of standard indicators of gender differences in health is
not, therefore, straightforward. That women live longer than men does not
necessarily mean that they are biologically more robust or that they enjoy better health status than men at all stages of life. That women report more illness
than men, and more limitations of major activities because of illness, does not
necessarily mean that they are more susceptible than men to all health prob-

lems. Furthermore, lumping all women together can be misleading because there are clear gradients in some health indicators by socioeconomic level (e.g., the percentage of persons reporting fair or poor health status is inversely correlated with family income) and differences among women by race/ethnicity (e.g., the percentage of black adults reporting fair or poor health is nearly twice as high as the percentage of white adults of comparable age). The complexity of the epidemiological data provides fertile ground for multiple interpretations and debate about gender effects on health status and on gender-based needs for health care.

GENDER DIFFERENCES IN USE OF HEALTH CARE

A ubiquitous finding in health services research is that adult women consume more outpatient and inpatient health services than do adult men.[2] Given the known sex differences in incidence and prevalence rates of many conditions, it is, of course, difficult to make accurate adjustments for comparing utilization rates between women and men. Nevertheless, after accounting for the medicalization of pregnancy and childbirth, which generates health care system use by most women, women consume more health care than men of comparable age. The gender differences, however, are relatively small among the elderly (particularly among those ages 75 and over).

A few examples will illustrate the pattern for outpatient care. Women are more likely than men to report having a usual source of health care, typically defined as a particular place that individuals usually go when sick or in need of advice about their health. In the 1987 National Medical Expenditure Survey, 83 percent of women ages 18 and over reported having a usual source of care, compared with 73 percent of men ages 18 and over (Collins et al. 1994). The usual sources of health care reported were overwhelmingly (86%) physicians' offices (including group practices, physician clinics, and health maintenance organizations [HMOs]). Among those without a usual source of care, women and men differed in their reasons: men were more likely than women to report that they seldom or never get sick, and women were more likely than men to report that they use multiple health care sources (Cornelius, Beauregard, and Cohen 1991).

Women interact with the health care system more frequently than do men, for both prevention and treatment. In 1994, 84 percent of females (all ages) reported having made a physician "contact" within the last year, compared with 74 percent of males. (A "contact" is defined in the National Health Interview Survey as a consultation with a physician by telephone or in person for examination, diagnosis, treatment, or advice.) Among persons of reproductive age (ages 15 to 44)[3] in 1994, 82 percent of women and 64 percent of men reported a physician contact of some kind in the last year; this was the largest gender difference for any age group, and there was no gender difference for persons ages 75 and over (NCHS 1996a). The higher rate of physician contacts among women generally persists for all adult age groups and by poverty status and self-assessed health status; the major exception is that among nonpoor persons (i.e., those with incomes 200 percent or more of the poverty threshold) ages 65 and over, there is no gender difference in number of physician contacts (NCHS 1996a).

Visits, as opposed to physician contacts, are a more specific indicator of use of health services. In 1994, women were 51 percent of the U.S. population and 52 percent of the population ages 18 and over, but they made 60 percent of all visits to physicians' offices and 61 percent of all visits to outpatient departments in nonfederal hospitals; among persons ages 15 and over, women made 63 percent of physician office visits and 64 percent of hospital outpatient department visits (Schappert 1996; Lipkind 1996). Women and men were equally likely to make visits to hospital emergency departments (Stussman 1996). With regard to use of outpatient physician services, women are consistently found to have higher rates of utilization, whether measured through household surveys or through patient records. For visits to physician's offices not located in hospitals, to nonhospital clinics, and to HMOs, females (all ages) made 5.2 visits per person in 1993, compared with 3.8 by males (Benson and Marano 1994). According to the 1993 National Ambulatory Medical Care Survey, females (all ages) made 3.3 visits per person per year to physicians' offices, compared with 2.3 by males (Woodwell and Schappert 1995). Six percent of women's visits were for routine prenatal examinations. In 1994, females (all ages) made 30.5 visits per 100 persons per year to hospital outpatient departments for nonurgent care, compared with 20.4 visits by males (Lipkind 1996). The gender difference in visits was greatest among persons of reproductive age.

All of these findings are consistent with women's establishing higher rates of health care use during the so-called reproductive years both for routine preventive care as well as for family planning services. During these years, women frequently access the health care system to obtain forms of medical contraception, and prevailing medical recommendations call for regular pelvic examinations and Pap smears for sexually active women (U.S. Preventive Services Task Force 1996). Obstetrician-gynecologists most often provide these services, and in 1992, visits to obstetrician-gynecologists accounted for 30 percent of all visits to physicians' offices made by women ages 15 to 44, but only 9 percent of visits made by women ages 45 to 64 (NCHS 1995). (It is not yet known whether the post–World War II baby-boom generation of women, who established their health care utilization patterns during the 1960s and 1970s and may have been more reliant upon obstetrician-gynecologists for preventive care than earlier cohorts, will continue to visit obstetrician-gynecologists for regular care beyond the reproductive years.) In addition to visits to physicians' offices, some women use family planning clinics (including public health department clinics, hospital-based clinics, and freestanding clinics) for contraceptive services. According to the 1988 National Survey of Family Growth, about 7 million women ages 15 to 44 made one or more family planning clinic visits in the last year, and clinics were more likely to be used by adolescent, low-income, and black women (Mosher and Pratt 1990).

Outpatient care for mental health problems can occur in the offices of psychiatrists, psychologists, social workers, or others; in outpatient clinics or health centers; and in community mental health centers. Women accounted for 59 percent of office visits to psychiatrists in 1989-90, and women ages 65 and over made significantly more visits than men of comparable age (Schappert 1993a). In addition, 54 percent of the visits made by women, compared with 44 percent of visits made by men, included medication therapy. In general, women received more psychotropic drug prescriptions than did men, and the reasons for the gender difference are not fully understood (Glied and Kofman 1995).

The use of nontraditional or "alternative" therapies—sometimes called "complementary medicine"—is receiving increased attention by researchers, since their popularity is thought to be increasing. There is no standard definition of these therapies, however. They have been defined, alternatively, as therapies that are not taught in U.S. medical schools, are not provided by mainstream physicians, or are not reimbursed by health insurance plans.[4] A national survey of 1,539 persons ages 18 and over conducted in 1990 found no significant gender difference in the use of nontraditional therapies in the last year (Eisenberg et al. 1993). The survey measured sixteen therapies and found that 34 percent of respondents had used at least one in the last year; the most commonly reported were relaxation techniques (13% of respondents), chiropractic services (10%), and massage therapy (7%). The highest frequency of use was found among nonblack persons ages 25 to 49 who were highly educated and had higher incomes. Such individuals would be more likely to be able to pay for these services out of pocket.

For inpatient care in 1993, females accounted for 60 percent of all short-stay nonfederal hospital discharges, including deliveries, and for 72 percent of all discharges among persons ages 15 to 44 (Graves 1995). When deliveries, which accounted for 22 percent of all hospital discharges among women in 1993, are excluded, women accounted for 53 percent of hospital discharges and for 58 percent of discharges among persons ages 18 to 44 (Benson and Marano 1994; Graves 1995). In 1993, 7 percent of females (all ages) and 6 percent of males reported at least one short-stay hospital episode, excluding deliveries, in the previous year; among persons ages 18 to 44, 5 percent of women and 4 percent of men reported at least one episode, excluding deliveries (Benson and Marano 1994). However, in psychiatric hospitals and other mental health organizations providing inpatient care, women accounted for only 42 percent of all admissions in 1990; this was attributable, in part, to men's predominance among those admitted to public facilities, including state and county hospitals and VA medical centers, for such serious conditions as schizophrenia and alcohol and drug-related disorders (Glied and Kofman 1995).

Women receive more in-hospital surgical procedures than men, and most of the gender difference is accounted for by childbirth-related procedures, surgery on the reproductive organs, and diagnostic dilation and curettage of the uterus. The most common inpatient surgical procedures for women in 1993 were procedures to assist delivery, cesarean section (23% of all births), repair of current obstetrical laceration, and hysterectomy (NCHS 1996a). An estimated 1.5 million surgical abortions were performed in 1992, of which only 7 percent were performed in hospitals; 89 percent were performed in clinics, and 4 percent in physicians' offices (Henshaw and Van Vort 1994).

Because women live longer than men and are more likely to survive their spouses, and because they are more likely than men to be functionally disabled at older ages, they are the major users of long-term care, including nursing homes (Horton 1995; Moon 1994; Rowland and Davis 1994). In 1989, women were 72 percent of persons residing in nursing homes in the United States, and they were more likely than men to have stays of two years or longer (Moon 1994). Among persons who reach the age of 65, 45 percent of women use nursing home care at least once before death, compared with 28 percent of men (Murtaugh, Kemper, and Spillman 1990). Among older persons who are not institutionalized, women are more likely than men to live alone; in consequence, women are more likely than men to use formal (paid) home health care services, and men are more likely than women to be cared for by family members (Horton 1995). Women and men also receive somewhat different services from home health agencies, reflecting gender differences both in functional incapacities and in gender roles. For example, more elderly women than elderly men received help doing light housework in 1993 (Dey 1996).

Thus, for most indicators, women consume more health care services than men. Little attention has been directed, however, to understanding whether the aggregate gender difference in consumption is appropriate, let alone whether it results in better health outcomes for women.

GENDER DIFFERENCES IN CONDITION-SPECIFIC SERVICES

Greater overall use of services by women does not necessarily equate with more appropriate care received or with better outcomes. For conditions on which women and men may be compared, some studies suggest that women may be diagnosed later, receive less aggressive treatment (which sometimes may be more appropriate treatment), or experience more adverse effects of treatment than men. Most noteworthy are studies of access among patients with kidney disease to dialysis and transplantation; of diagnosis of lung cancer by sputum cytology; and of diagnosis and treatment of heart disease (Council on Ethical and Judicial Affairs of the AMA 1991). The reasons for the observed gender differences in care received are not well understood, however. These differences might be due to physicians' gender biases or delays in referral or treatments for women, to an inadequate knowledge base for the treatment of women with these conditions, to gender differences in patients' preferences for treatments, or to a combination of factors. In the case of heart disease, the observed gender differences in diagnosis and treatment could be related both to the research emphasis on male subjects, as discussed in chapter 2, and to the consequent perception of the disease as primarily affecting men.

Several studies provide evidence of a possible referral bias in the diagnosis and treatment of women with coronary artery disease. For example, studies have found that women are less likely than men to be referred for cardiac catheterization following exercise radionuclide study (Tobin et al. 1987) and that women hospitalized for coronary heart disease are less likely to undergo angiography or revascularization (Ayanian and Epstein 1991). A study of post–myocardial infarction patients found that although women reported greater functional disability from angina, they were less likely to undergo catheterization or bypass surgery (Steingart et al. 1991). Krumholz et al. (1992) found no gender difference in rates of coronary angiography among patients who had recently had a myocardial infarction, although among patients who underwent catheterization, men and women were equally likely to receive angioplasty, but men were more likely than women to receive coronary bypass surgery. Another study found that among patients at low risk for cardiac death, women were less likely to be referred for bypass surgery, which actually may be a more appropriate treatment pattern (Bickell et al. 1992). In other words, rather than women being undertreated, men may be too aggressively treated.

Other studies have investigated the relationship between gender and survival following myocardial infarction (MI) and found that women are more likely to die than men. Two studies found that women experiencing MI were older and more often had a history of hypertension and/or congestive heart failure, risk factors that explained the mortality difference (Fiebach, Viscoli, and Horwitz 1990; Maynard et al. 1992). Another study found higher in-hospital and one-year mortality rates for women after controlling for major risk factors such as age and congestive heart failure, and diabetic women were at even higher risk of death (Greenland et al. 1991). Weaver and colleagues (1996) found that women enrolled in an international clinical trial of thrombolytic treatments in over 40,000 patients with acute MI were at greater risk than men for both fatal and nonfatal complications, after adjusting for baseline status. Less aggressive treatment of women earlier in the disease course might account for these findings.

Some researchers find that women undergoing coronary artery bypass surgery suffer a higher rate of perioperative mortality than men, which some authors have attributed to women's smaller size, including smaller diameter of the coronary arteries (Fisher et al. 1982; Loop et al. 1983; Hannan et al. 1992b). The development of cardiac surgery techniques and postoperative management on male patients may account for this phenomenon. Khan et al. (1990) found that higher in-hospital mortality from bypass surgery among women was explained by preoperative functional class and age differences between women and men referred for surgery; however, the findings suggested the possibility of a referral bias in which women were referred for treatment later in the course of their disease when their prognosis was poorer. Women also experience greater procedural mortality from percutaneous transluminal coronary angioplasty (Eysmann and Douglas 1992; Hannan et al. 1992a; Kelsey et al. 1993), although the reasons are unclear.

Investigators also have explored possible gender differences in screening or treatment for HIV infection or AIDS, because of concerns about the biomedical community's delays in acknowledging and studying these conditions in women. Faden, Kass, and McGraw (1996), for example, point out gender biases in the early Centers for Disease Control case definition of AIDS and in research studies of HIV and AIDS, which, they argue, resulted in medical harm to women. Studies of gender differences in treatment and survival after infection with HIV or AIDS diagnosis have produced mixed results, however. Although one study found no gender difference in AIDS mortality (Ellerbrock et al. 1991), another found that women had a significantly shorter median survival time following AIDS diagnosis than men: 11.1 versus 14.6 months, respectively (Lemp et al. 1992). The latter study found no gender difference in survival when only those receiving zidovudine (AZT) were analyzed. Hellinger (1993) examined the use of AZT and health care services by HIV-infected persons and found that while asymptomatic women were 20 percent less likely than asymptomatic men to receive AZT, there were no gender differences in AZT use for symptomatic patients or patients with AIDS. Also, although women with AIDS tended to make more outpatient visits, they were 5 percent less likely than men with AIDS to be hospitalized and 20 percent less likely than male intravenous drug users with AIDS to be hospitalized. A subsequent study found that among non–drug users with AIDS, men were twice as likely to receive AZT and *Pneumocystis carinii* pneumonia (PCP) prophylaxis, although survival was similar for women and men (Turner et al. 1994). Among drug users, no difference in access to AZT or PCP prophylaxis was found, but survival was slightly better for women. For both drug users and non-drug users, men tended to receive AZT earlier in the course of their illness, but this was associated with a *higher* risk of death. In addition to drug therapy differences, women made more ambulatory care visits (which was associated with longer survival) and were equally likely to see an AIDS specialty provider.

Thus, there is some evidence that women with heart disease and HIV or AIDS may receive less appropriate care than men with the same conditions, and there is some evidence that men might be too aggressively treated. Because gender differences in treatment of conditions that women and men have in common have not been extensively studied, it is difficult to draw overall conclusions about gender differences in the quantity or quality of care for the same conditions.

EXPLANATIONS FOR GENDER DIFFERENCES IN HEALTH CARE

Alternative explanations for women's generally greater use of health services have been proposed, based on quite different assumptions about how the use of health care is determined. They focus, respectively, on gender differences in the need for care, on gender differences in health-seeking behavior, and on health care system factors that differentiate treatment for women and men.

These explanations are not mutually exclusive, and each contributes to an understanding of gender differences in utilization patterns. One of the key points argued here, however, is that health care system factors play a larger role than is usually acknowledged.

Most frequently, women's higher utilization of services is viewed as a function of their greater objective "need" for care. Pregnancy is assumed to generate a set of needs for care (including preconception, prenatal, delivery, and postpartum services), and pregnancy-prevention also entails a cluster of medically mediated services. Apart from pregnancy-related care, it is argued, women's higher utilization results from their poorer health status—their generally higher rates of morbidity and disability—compared with men. Use of health care based on need is assumed to result from a rational decision process in which the individual identifies a need for care and accesses the health care system for treatment or preventive services. (Problems in accessing care, or the possibilities of overtreatment of women—or of undertreatment of men—are not explicitly considered when a "need" framework is used.) Many researchers currently believe that "need" is the best explanation for gender differences in health care use. Lois Verbrugge (1989), for example, concludes that morbidity is the strongest determinant of health care and that it accounts most strongly for gender differences in utilization of services.

The "health-seeking behavior" explanation, in contrast, interprets women's higher utilization of health services largely as a function of learned behavior patterns. According to this view, women use more services than men because they have been socialized to acknowledge and articulate bodily signs and symptoms; to perceive a greater need for care, including preventive care; or to seek the help of others, including health care providers and informal sources of care, more readily than men (Hibbard and Pope 1986; Mechanic 1978). The socialization of women to health-seeking behavior may be, in part, a legacy of nineteenth-century views of women as inherently sickly because of their reproductive organs, but it is also likely to reflect the cultural expectation that women assume caregiving responsibilities on behalf of their children and other family members. Because of this gender-based role expectation, women would be expected to seek health information more actively, to have a lower threshold than men for seeking formal care, and to be more tenacious than men in overcoming barriers to access.

Research support for these hypotheses is mixed. Hing, Kovar, and Rice (1983:16) conclude from analyses of national data sets that "females perceive more symptoms and, perhaps as a consequence, they visit doctors more often than males do." Cafferata and Meyers (1990) suggest that women's higher rates of psychotropic drug prescriptions can be explained by their greater tendency to define themselves as ill. Wilensky and Cafferata (1983) report that women are more likely than men to use physician services for chronic conditions. However, Verbrugge (1985) argues that while women are more attentive than men to bodily discomforts and therefore more likely to interpret minor health problems as illness, for major health problems—such as life-threatening chronic diseases or severe acute conditions—women and men do not differ substantially in their likelihood of seeking care. Waldron (1995) reports that for most types of cancer and ischemic heart disease, women delay as long or longer than men before seeking care.

Explanations focusing on the health care system have been least well articulated. In this perspective, women's higher health care utilization is viewed, at least in part, as a function of the gendered nature of health care institutions. The health care delivery system might contribute to women's higher utilization rates for regular and preventive care through such mechanisms as aggressive marketing of health services and pharmaceutical products to women; the medicalization of women's biological processes such as menstruation and menopause; the medical control of pregnancy prevention services; physicians' biases about women's health care needs or availability for preventive care or follow-up treatment; funding mechanisms supporting specific women's services; or inefficiencies in the provision of well-woman care because of the fragmentation of services. Moreover, if women make more preventive visits, they also would be exposed to more opportunities for symptom reporting, testing and diagnoses, false-positive test results, and iatrogenic conditions, all of which may contribute to greater subsequent utilization. Finally, if medical biases or an inadequate research base contribute to later diagnoses or inappropriate treatments for women for some diseases, such as heart disease, this could also contribute to greater subsequent utilization.

Despite these alternative explanations for women's greater use of health services, the dominant model of health care utilization developed by health services researchers does not explicitly address gender issues. The "behavioral model of health services use" was originally formulated by Ronald Andersen and Lu Ann Aday in the 1960s (Aday 1993a; Aday and Andersen 1974; Andersen 1995), when a major concern in health policy was increasing access to medical services among traditionally underserved groups such as the poor and the elderly. Consequently, the original model focused on individuals' and families' decisions to use formal medical care (usually outpatient care) and sought to identify the variables—particularly the mutable variables that might be amenable to policy intervention—that facilitated or impeded use of care.

Utilization of medical care was conceptualized as a function of characteristics of individuals at risk (including "predisposing," "enabling," and "need" variables) and of the health care delivery system (including availability and organization of services). "Predisposing" variables included sociodemographics (such as sex), social role obligations, and attitudes and beliefs about health care (such as beliefs in the efficacy of care). "Enabling" variables were conceived as factors that enhance access to the health care system. They included the resources available to individuals, such as health insurance coverage and discretionary income, as well as community variables such as the proximity of health services, their organizational characteristics, and the availability of public transportation. The presence of enabling resources was termed "potential access." "Need" variables included both self-assessed (perceived) need for health care and "evaluated" need, that is, need assessed through professional judgment. Research applying this model has generally found that "need" variables are the strongest predictors of utilization.

Inequities in access to health care would be presumed to exist if individuals with the same level of need do not receive the same level of care, or if non-need variables, such as race/ethnicity or income level, were the strongest determinants of utilization (Aday, Andersen, and Fleming 1980). Equitable access, according to Andersen, occurs "when demographic and need variables account for most of the variance in utilization" (Andersen 1995:4). By demographic variables, Andersen means age and sex, which "represent biological imperatives suggesting the likelihood that people will need health services" (Andersen 1995:2). These variables are also regarded as immutable from a policy standpoint (Aday 1993a).

In the behavioral model of health services use, therefore, sex has been treated as a biological variable predisposing persons to use services. In this logic, controlling for sex reduces unexplained variation in utilization, and any residual effect of sex on utilization, after other variables are controlled, is attributed to biology. The implicit assumption has been that women need more services than men because of their reproductive function. Controlling for sex, however, is not the same thing as examining the effects of gender. Researchers generally have not questioned the structure of health care institutions with regard to reproductive services or the medical definition of what constitutes a reproductive health service. Nor have they considered how gender roles or statuses might interact with the "need" for health care or with health care system variables. The main effects of sex and enabling factors are considered in the model, but interactions between sex and such non-need variables as health insurance coverage, level of discretionary income, or availability of services also might produce inequities in health care use. The latter variables are mutable from a policy standpoint.

Another interesting aspect to the theoretical treatment of sex in the behavioral model of health services utilization is that it reflects a more general confusion about the gendered nature of health care. On the one hand, health services researchers have tended to accept women's use of both outpatient and inpatient services related to pregnancy (i.e., prenatal care visits and childbirth services) as "needed" services, and in comparisons of women's and men's utilization, they attempt to remove the effects of these services in statistical analyses. (See, for example, a study by Cleary, Mechanic, and Greenley [1982] of outpatient medical care use in a rural area of Wisconsin, in which childbirth-related services were excluded to examine sex differences in use of outpatient medical care.) On the other hand, gender-specific services not related to pregnancy (e.g., family planning visits by either sex, visits for services related to the diagnosis or treatment of problems of the reproductive system of either sex) are not statistically controlled. Thus the logic of removing from comparisons any services that one sex would not need is not consistently applied.

Despite its assumption of biological essentialism, the behavioral model of health services utilization helps identify a number of indicators of "potential access" to health care that are highly relevant to gender. The relationship of gender to health insurance is discussed in the next section.

GENDER AND FINANCIAL ACCESS TO HEALTH CARE

National concern over rising health care costs and the debate in the early 1990s over national health care reform focused attention on financial access to health care, particularly through health insurance coverage, and on declining "potential access" to care in the U.S. population. Between 1980 and 1994, the age-adjusted percentage of nonelderly (under age 65) persons without health insurance of any kind increased from 12.5 percent to 17.8 percent, and in 1994, 40 million people were uninsured (NCHS 1995; NCHS 1996a). The Council on the Economic Impact of Health System Change projects that the number of uninsured could reach 66.8 million by 2002, in part because of the decline in employer-based health insurance (Rovner 1996). Financial access to health care therefore has been declining.

A large body of research shows that having health insurance, either public or private, increases the likelihood that both women and men have a usual source of care and made a physician visit during the last year; that cost sharing reduces use of care, especially preventive services and mental health services; and, among women, that having insurance increases the use of early prenatal care, clinical preventive services, and mental health services (Brown et al. 1995; Davis 1995; Glied and Kofman 1995; Muller 1990; Reisinger 1995, 1996; Weissman and Epstein 1994; Wyn, Brown, and Yu 1996). The question of whether women and men have equivalent access to health insurance is quite complicated, however. Currently, Americans' access to health insurance depends upon their employment status, family status, age, and economic resources. This is because most private health insurance, since World War II, is secured either through employment (or the employment of a family member) or through private purchase, and public insurance depends in part on means-tested eligibility and family status (in the case of Medicaid) or on age (in the case of Medicare). Clearly, if women and men are differently distributed on these social categories, then they will have differential access to health insurance. Once insured, furthermore, benefits may vary for women and men with respect to the services covered or the level of copayments. The wide variation in private health insurance options, particularly with the increasing diversity of managed care plans, makes comparison of benefits by gender quite complicated.

When both private and public sources of health insurance are considered, women are slightly more likely than men to have insurance coverage at any point in time.[5] For example, in 1992, an estimated 13 percent of women ages 18 and over were uninsured, compared with 18 percent of men (Reisinger 1995). Among adults of reproductive age (ages 15 to 44) in 1993, an estimated 19 percent of women and 22 percent of men were uninsured (Women's Research and Education Institute 1994a). The gender gap disappears among the elderly, since virtually all persons ages 65 and over are insured under the Medicare program.

Women and men differ in the types of health insurance coverage they have, however. Most nonelderly Americans have private health insurance through their employment or are dependents on a family member's employer-based insurance. In 1993, 62 percent of women and 63 percent of men ages 18 to 64 had employment-based health insurance; among women, white women were more likely than women who were members of racial and ethnic minorities to have employment-based insurance (Wyn and Brown 1996). However, because women are less likely than men to be employed full-time in jobs that provide health insurance benefits and because women change jobs more frequently than men, women in the population overall are less likely than men to have private health insurance through their own jobs or unions (Jecker 1994; Muller 1990). Among persons ages 18 to 64 in 1993, 38 percent of women had private health insurance through their own jobs, compared with 53 percent of men, and 24 percent of women had coverage through a family member's job, compared with 10 percent of men; 10 percent of both women and men had privately purchased policies (Wyn and Brown 1996). One study of full-time workers in 1993 found that married women were more likely than married men to decline coverage through their own employer to be insured on the spouse's policy (Buchmueller 1996). Dependence upon a spouse's health insurance places women at risk of becoming uninsured in the event of marital dissolution, widowhood, changes in the spouse's employment status, or changes in the employer's coverage of dependents. The percentage of nonelderly Americans covered by employment-based health insurance has been declining since the mid-1970s, and dependent coverage may become more difficult to obtain if employers continue to seek ways to reduce health insurance costs.

Women are more dependent than men on publicly funded health insurance programs, particularly Medicaid. In 1991, 31 percent of females and 24 percent of males of all ages had some type of public health insurance for all or part of the year: females were more likely than males to be enrolled in Medicaid (12% vs. 9%, respectively) and in Medicare (15% vs. 11%), but females and males were about equally likely to be covered by the Civilian Health and Medical Programs of the Uniformed Services (CHAMPUS), the Department of Veterans Affairs, or other military programs (about 4% of both women and men) (Costello and Stone 1994). Among the nonelderly (persons ages 18 to 64) in 1993, 9 percent of women and 4 percent of men were enrolled in Medicaid; among nonelderly women, African American and Latina women were more likely than other women to be Medicaid enrollees (Wyn and Brown 1996). Major restructuring of Medicaid or Medicare (e.g., by funding Medicaid through block grants to the states) therefore could disproportionately affect the health care of women.

Since 1965, the Medicaid program has been the nation's major public program for providing health and long-term care coverage to low-income persons. Medicaid is a means-tested entitlement program covering specific groups, and although the program is administered by the states, federal guidelines require states to provide certain benefits for specific groups. In the 1980s, Congress mandated expanded coverage for pregnant women and young children. In part as a result of these expansions, Medicaid enrollment rose by more than 50 percent between 1988 and 1994, and in 1994, children and adults in low-income families comprised 73 percent of Medicaid beneficiaries (Kaiser Commission on the Future of Medicaid 1995). Females accounted for 70 percent of Medicaid beneficiaries under age 64 (Davis 1995). Among persons of reproductive age (ages 18 to 44) in 1992, 11 percent of women were covered by Medicaid, compared with 5 percent of men (Reisinger 1995). Medicaid paid for nearly one-third of all U.S. births in 1991 (Singh, Benson, and Frost 1994), and in 1993, 29 percent of pregnant women had Medicaid coverage (Holahan, Winterbotton, and Rajan 1995), and Medicaid paid for more than 45 percent of births in ten states (National Governors' Association 1995). Also, between 1984 and 1991, Medicaid expenditures for family planning services used by enrollees rose 41 percent, so that Medicaid became a major payer for these services nationwide (Ku 1993).

The limited and evolving nature of the Medicaid program has important implications for women. For one thing, coverage is limited to persons meeting specific eligibility requirements based on income and other categorical criteria, so that not all needy women qualify. In 1994, for example, Medicaid covered only 55 percent of poor Americans (Kaiser Commission on the Future of Medicaid 1995). A poor, nonelderly woman who was neither pregnant, the mother of dependent children, nor disabled would not have been eligible for Medicaid (Collins et al. 1994). Analyses conducted for the Commonwealth Fund of women ages 19 to 64 with family incomes below 200 percent of the poverty level from 1990 to 1992 found that 31 percent of these women had no health insurance of any kind (Short 1996). Also, changes in Medicaid eligibility status, for example, because of changes in the family's income level, may jeopardize the continuity of the woman's health care: 63 percent of women disenrolling from Medicaid become uninsured (Short 1996). The Medicaid expansions between 1984 and 1990—which extended coverage to pregnant women whose family incomes were below 133 percent of the federal poverty level—were intended in part to increase women's access to early prenatal care and hence to improve birth outcomes (Alpha Center 1995; Coughlin, Ku, and Holahan 1994). The expansions, however, linked benefits for women to pregnancy and included provision of prenatal care and maternity services; benefits for women ended 60 days after delivery unless the woman was eligible for cash benefits or assistance under Aid to Families with Dependent Children (AFDC) (Collins et al. 1994).[6] The Medicaid program does not provide a mechanism for integrating pregnancy-related care with other health care services for women or for continuity in women's health care after delivery. Finally, both the implementation of mandated Medicaid benefits and the provision of non-mandated benefits vary across states, resulting in nonuniform coverage. States vary, for example, in their coverage of abortion services for Medicaid enrollees: in 1995, only 16 states and the District of Columbia provided Medicaid coverage of abortions under most circumstances (NARAL 1996).

Medicare was enacted in 1965 under the Social Security Act as a health insurance program for the elderly. Although Medicare covers virtually all adults ages 65 and over, because of their longer life expectancies and lower incomes than men after age 65, women may be regarded as more dependent than men on Medicare and more susceptible to increases in premiums or to changes in benefits. (In 1995, women were 56% of U.S. residents ages 65 to 74, 61% of persons ages 75 to 84, and 72% of persons ages 85 and over [U.S. Bureau of the Census 1995].) In 1992, women were 57 percent of Medicare enrollees (Reisinger 1995). One analysis of the Medicare benefit structure found that coverage is less adequate for chronic diseases that are more prevalent in women than in men, such as arthritis and depression (Sofaer and Abel 1990).

Because of the limitations of Medicare coverage, such as cost-sharing requirements and lack of coverage for prescription drugs and long-term care, most Medicare recipients purchase private supplemental insurance or receive such insurance from a former employer. In 1994, women ages 65 and over were equally likely as men of comparable age to have private supplemental coverage (75% of women vs. 76% of men) but twice as likely as men to supplement Medicare with Medicaid (7% vs. 3%, respectively) (NCHS 1996a). In other words, women are less likely than men to be able to afford private supplemental insurance, including long-term care protection. The importance of supplemental insurance to women has been shown in studies of clinical preventive services obtained; women ages 65 and over who have private supplemental insurance have been found to be more likely than women with only Medicare coverage to receive Pap smears, clinical breast examinations, and mammography (Blustein 1995; Makuc, Freid, and Parsons 1994).

The adequacy of private health insurance coverage for women also is an important issue. Private health insurance policies vary in their coverage of specific women's health services. For example, a 1993 study by The Alan Guttmacher Institute (1994) of private-sector health insurance coverage of reproductive health services found that obstetrical care was routinely covered in all types of plans; however, health insurance policies varied in the extent of coverage, and some policies restricted benefits for pregnancy as a preexisting condition (Muller 1990; Women's Research and Education Institute 1994a).[7] There also was wide variation among insurance plans in coverage of cancer screening (Pap smears and mammography), reversible contraception, and abortion (Alan Guttmacher Institute 1994). Managed care plans of various kinds typically provided more extensive coverage than indemnity insurance plans for routine gynecological care, reversible contraceptive services (including oral contraceptives), and infertility services. (A growing proportion of both privately and publicly insured persons are enrolled in managed care, which is discussed below in this chapter.) Among managed care plans, however, there was variation in services covered, the level of copayments for specific services, and in the allowable interval for screening services such as Pap smears or mammography (Bernstein, Dial, and Smith 1995; Bernstein 1996). Private health insurance plans also vary in coverage of mental health services. In general, coverage of mental health services is more limited than that for physical illness, and higher cost sharing is characteristic for these services (Glied and Kofman 1995). For women with comorbidities, who require longer-term treatment, such limited coverage could be a major barrier to care.

The adequacy of health insurance coverage for women of reproductive age recently was assessed by the Women's Research and Education Institute (1994a) in a study of out-of-pocket expenditures for reproductive and preventive services. Using data from the 1987 National Medical Expenditure Survey, the study found that many health plans failed to adequately cover these services, and as a result, women ages 15 to 44 had out-of-pocket expenses for health care that were 68 percent higher than those of men in the same age group. The gaps in coverage identified in the study included exclusion or inadequate coverage of pregnancy-related services in some individual and group policies; failure of some states to mandate insurance coverage for mammography, infertility treatment, or Pap smears; and failure of some HMO plans to cover oral contraceptives or drugs related to fertility treatments. According to these analyses, women of childbearing age paid 56 percent of the cost of contraceptives in 1993 out of pocket.

Overall, then, nonelderly women are slightly more likely than nonelderly men to have health insurance at any point in time, largely because of their greater reliance on the Medicaid program. Women also spend more out of pocket for basic health care than men do, particularly for such gender-specific services as contraception. Moreover, because women are less likely than men to be insured through their own employment and more likely than men to rely on public insurance, they are more vulnerable to the limitations on dependent coverage in employer-based insurance plans and to the politics of Medicaid and Medicare. Women therefore have much at stake in debates about the future of publicly funded health insurance programs and in health insurance reforms.

GENDER AND NONFINANCIAL BARRIERS TO ACCESS

In addition to lack of health insurance or inadequate health insurance, other factors may constitute barriers to access to care, even for individuals who have insurance. These nonfinancial barriers are not likely to be removed by health care reform efforts that focus only on insurance coverage. Factors such as the availability of services within reasonable proximity of the individual's residence, the availability of transportation and child care, physical features to accommodate the disabled, and organizational characteristics (such as reasonable hours of operation, comprehensive on-site services, and efficient referral mechanisms) are all important facilitators of access to care. Such barriers have been said to produce "rationing by hassling" because individuals may give up before obtaining care (Leigh 1995:191). Informational barriers may exist if individuals are not aware of the availability or location of services. In addition, cultural diversity may necessitate translator services, outreach programs, or other culturally sensitive services to promote access for specific subpopulations (Millman 1993).

Some of these nonfinancial barriers may differentially affect women and men, and the cumulative effect of barriers may be greater for one gender than the other. Few studies have investigated this possibility, however. In a 1989 survey in Michigan, women reported significantly more access problems, both financial and nonfinancial, than men, and the most common problems reported in the sample overall were having to wait one week or more for a nonroutine physician visit, inadequate insurance coverage or inability to pay for services, physicians not accepting patients, and services located more than thirty minutes away (Bashshur, Homan, and Smith 1994). Some barriers, such as absence of child care, are likely to be particularly burdensome to women. For example, access to inpatient services, such as residential alcohol and substance abuse treatment programs, may be impaired if services do not consider patients' parenting responsibilities (Glied and Kofman 1995).

One of the most critical gender-linked nonfinancial barriers to access is the lack of availability of specific women's health services in some communities. For example, the geographic maldistribution of providers of obstetrical services, including prenatal care, was documented in the 1980s and linked, in part, to the unwillingness of about 30 percent of obstetricians to accept Medicaid patients; their reasons had to do primarily with low Medicaid reimbursement rates, delays in reimbursement, and concerns about medical malpractice liability (Brown 1988; Horton 1995). A 1989 study found that one-fourth of all U.S. counties had no prenatal care clinic for poor women (Singh, Forrest, and Torres 1989). Although they have not eliminated availability problems, the recent Medicaid expansions appear to have had positive effects on physician participation in Medicaid-reimbursed maternity services in some states and on private hospitals' provision of obstetrical services (Alpha Center 1995).

Fertility-control services provide other examples of availability problems. The unmet need for these services is presumed to be great. For one thing, most pregnancies in the United States are unintended—that is, unwanted or mistimed—according to the reports of women in national surveys (Forrest 1994).[8] In 1990, 44 percent of all U.S. births were the result of unintended pregnancy, and this percentage had been increasing since 1982 (Brown and Eisenberg 1995), reflecting both an increase in the proportion of unintended pregnancies and a decline in the use of abortion to resolve those pregnancies. Some fertility-control services, including abortion, are controversial or subject to legal restrictions, so that providers may opt not to offer them. In addition, some religiously controlled health care organizations place restrictions on delivery of specific services (e.g., abortion, emergency contraception, sterilization). The recent increase in affiliations between religious and nonsectarian organizations serving diverse populations has raised questions about the continued availability of fertility-control services in some communities served by these providers (ACLU 1995; Delbanco and Smith 1995; Family Planning Advocates of New York State 1996).

The case of abortion availability has received the most attention. Access to surgical abortion services is thought to have declined in recent years because of a number of factors, including the continued politicization of abortion and increased legal restrictions on service provision; the increasing incidence of antiabortion protests, particularly at freestanding clinics, where over 90 percent of abortions are performed; the geographic maldistribution of services; and, due to a decline in the number of residency programs in obstetrics-gynecology that provided abortion training, a reduction in the availability of trained providers (Forrest and Henshaw 1993; Henshaw 1995; Joffe 1995; MacKay and MacKay 1995; NARAL 1996; Radford and Shaw 1993). Henshaw and Van Vort (1994) reported that in 1992, 84 percent of U.S. counties had no known abortion provider of any type (physician, clinic, or hospital), and 30 percent of women of reproductive age resided in those counties. The number of hospitals providing abortions decreased by 18 percent between 1988 and 1992, and only 7 percent of abortions were performed in hospitals in 1992 (Henshaw and Van Vort 1994). While the number of nonhospital facilities providing abortions did not change substantially, 24 percent of women having abortions in nonhospital settings in 1992 traveled at least fifty miles from home to obtain the procedure because of the unavailability of a local provider (Henshaw 1995). Geographic distance from the provider is important because the woman incurs increased costs associated with travel and because the risk of complications is greater if the procedure is delayed to later gestational stages. In addition, some states' legal restrictions on abortion, such as mandated waiting periods or counseling that require the woman to make more than one visit, increase the travel burden and risks associated with delay.

Physicians' ability and willingness to provide abortion services also is an issue. In 1995, 43 states had laws stipulating that only physicians may perform abortions, and 46 states had laws that permitted physicians, health care facilities, or both to refuse to participate in abortion for reasons of conscience (NARAL 1996). Despite their specialization in women's reproductive health, most obstetrician-gynecologists do not provide surgical abortions. A 1995 survey by the Henry J. Kaiser Family Foundation found that one-third of obstetrician-gynecologists performed surgical abortions, a decline from 42 percent in 1983 (Kaiser Family Foundation 1995a). One contributing factor was that medical training in abortion procedures was not widespread. In 1991–92, only 12 percent of the 268 residency programs in obstetrics-gynecology provided routine training in first-trimester abortion, and 30 percent of programs offered no abortion training (MacKay and MacKay 1995). Effective January 1, 1996, the Accreditation Council for Graduate Medical Education (ACGME) required that residency programs in obstetrics-gynecology provide training in abortion or in managing the complications of abortion, but it is not yet known how this policy will affect abortion availability.[9]

The availability of nonsurgical abortion methods could increase access to abortion services. Nonsurgical methods—including oral contraceptives used as "morning after" pills, mifepristone (RU 486), and methotrexate in combination with misoprostol—can be provided in the privacy of physicians' offices, thus increasing the number of providers potentially available for abortion services. On the other hand, the availability of these methods is not likely to eliminate the need for surgical abortion as an alternative for those who prefer it, as a backup procedure, or for late-term abortions.

In sum, nonfinancial barriers to health care can be considerable, and they also have a clear gender component. An important implication of these observations is that financial access alone cannot guarantee women's ability to obtain health care services when and where they are needed.

GENDER EQUITY OF ACCESS?

Given all of these factors, can women and men be said to have equitable access to health care? There is little consensus on the meaning of "equitable access" to health care in general, let alone in relation to gender. We have seen that assessing equity of access in terms of need for care is difficult, and there are a number of gender differences in the financial and nonfinancial determinants of health care use. Gender equity of access also can be considered in terms of normative standards of fairness.

Considerations of equity of access from an ethical perspective typically are based on conceptions of distributive justice, namely, defining fair allocation of the benefits and burdens (including the financial costs) of health care among members of society. Within the distributive justice frame, there are different principles on which allocations of health care may be justified. For example, allocations may be based on utilitarian notions of maximizing the public health; on libertarian notions of free market enterprise and individuals' ability to purchase services; on communitarian notions of moral traditions; or on egalitarian notions of health care as a means of ensuring individuals' fair equality of opportunity. Most considerations of distribution principles assume that personal health care—although it is not the only determinant of health status—is a social good, like education, that helps provide individuals with the opportunity to participate fully in society and to pursue their personal objectives.[10] Although health care often is assumed to be a good to be maximized, some critics of women's health care, in particular, have questioned the premise that "more care" equates with "appropriate care." They point out the iatrogenic effects, increased dependency on providers, and other burdens to women that can be associated with higher levels of health care consumption (Sherwin 1996).

Beauchamp and Childress (1994:350) suggest that American society is evolving from a traditional view that access to health care should be based on ability to pay—either directly or through health insurance—toward a consensus that "all citizens should be able to secure equitable access to health care, including insurance coverage without temporal gaps and unjust exclusionary clauses." The definition of equitable access, however, is a contested issue that inevitably raises the question "access to what?" and involves the application of normative standards to definitions of what constitutes appropriate health care. Equitable access might be defined, for example, as equal access across social groups (e.g., defined by age, race/ethnicity, socioeconomic level, or gender) to preventive and curative health care services on the basis of all objectively determined needs or subjectively determined wants. (How needs would be objectively determined is, of course, another issue that is open to debate and multiple approaches.) Alternatively, equitable access might be defined as provision of needed health services without differential burdens across social groups; burdens that make accessing care more difficult for some social groups might include longer travel or waiting times, higher out-of-pocket costs for care, or information deficits. Or again, equitable access might be defined as a right among all persons, regardless of social category, to a basic standard of care, sometimes called a "decent basic minimum" (Daniels 1985). In the current policy climate, furthermore, considerations of equitable access coexist with efforts to balance health care costs and quality of care. Accordingly, the need to produce efficiencies in the care delivery process and to provide services with demonstrated efficacy or effectiveness (i.e., improved outcomes for patients) is increasingly important in discussions of access and of normative definitions of basic health care (Millman 1993; Sharpe and Faden 1996; Weissman and Epstein 1994). These issues, further-more, are relevant to both national health care policy and, in the private sec-tor, the design of benefits in health insurance plans.

It is immediately apparent that claims can be made that gender-specific is-sues are relevant in any consideration of equitable access. It can be argued, for example, that women have different health care needs than men throughout the life span, because of their different reproductive systems, acquired risks, or longer life expectancies. It can be argued that gender roles inevitably cre-ate inequalities in the burdens of seeking care because, for example, women have fewer financial resources than men and greater family caregiving re-sponsibilities. It can be argued that the very fact of women's higher utilization rates may constitute a burden, if, for example, these higher rates are due to fragmentation of the service delivery system for women, if they do not result in improved outcomes for women, or if they result in higher financial costs to women. It can be argued that the operational definition of the "decent min-imum" must be gender specific and include services that only one sex needs (for women, prenatal care, childbirth services, medical contraception, abor-tion, breast cancer screening, etc.).

Norman Daniels's attempt to conceptualize the "decent minimum" pro-vides an illustration of how the gendered nature of health care can be ob-scured in equity considerations. Daniels does not explicitly address gender issues, but he uses some gender-specific examples in his discussion of health care needs. Relying on a biomedical conception of disease, he regards health care needs as "those things we need in order to maintain, restore, or provide functional equivalents (where possible) to normal species functioning" (Daniels 1985:32). Assuming that the distinction between disease and the ab-sence of disease may be readily determined using a normative biomedical standard, he asserts that infertility may be regarded as a disease, but that "unwanted pregnancy" is not a disease; he accepts treatment of infertility as a basic health care need but regards the medical treatment of unwanted pregnancy (like cosmetic surgery) as meeting other social goals than the cure of disease. He therefore implicitly equates fertility enhancement, but not fertility curtailment, with normal species functioning. There are, of course, alternative conceptualizations available. For example, an unintended pregnancy, like infertility, could be regarded as a disability. Or again, women's needs to control their fertility could be regarded as normal species functioning or as health maintenance. Contraception and pregnancy termination services also may be regarded as health care needs because they are socially constructed as medical problems and are controlled by the medical community; that is, women generally do not have access to these services except through formal health care services. The basic point is that any attempt to conceptualize a "decent minimum" of health care or a basic benefits package has to contend with questions of gender-based needs and gendered health services.

Thus while gender equity of access to health care and in treatment within the health care system seems an appropriate goal, it requires an understanding of gender-based needs, gender-based obstacles to care, and the gendered nature of basic health services. The institutional context within which health care is defined and delivered is highly relevant to any consideration of gender equity.

FRAGMENTATION IN WOMEN'S HEALTH CARE

Recently, women's health advocates concerned with how women's health care is delivered have drawn attention to the ways in which women's basic care is "fragmented."[11] Specifically, they refer to the separation of the reproductive and nonreproductive components of basic well-woman care, without provisions for coordinated care of the whole woman. Clancy and Massion (1992) describe the state of American women's health care as "a patchwork quilt with gaps." In recent decades, there has been a tendency in U.S. health care to separate organizationally, or to fail to coordinate, reproductive health services and other components of women's basic care, and within reproductive services, there has been a tendency to separate financing and delivery of maternity care (including prenatal care) from fertility-control and screening services (Brown 1988; Muller 1990). The consequences of fragmentation are thought to include inefficiencies in the delivery of care to women; higher costs to the woman, her insurer, and society at large; undue access burdens on women; risks to women of both gaps and redundancies in services; and increased iatrogenic effects. In addition, since no provider has been trained in, or is accountable for, care of the whole woman, important health problems—such as the health consequences of sexual abuse or domestic violence—have been neglected both in research and in clinical practice.

These consequences, furthermore, are relevant for all women, regardless of life stage or reproductive status. Women's "reproductive health care" has no standard definition and is often assumed to be relevant only to women of so-called reproductive age, to refer only to fertility-control services, or to be a code word for abortion. Broadly defined, however, it refers to services related to the female reproductive system at any stage of life. These services include pregnancy-related care (including preconception counseling and risk assessment, prenatal care, labor and delivery, and postnatal services); contraceptive and sterilization services; abortion services; infertility diagnosis and treatment; diagnosis and treatment of STDs; medical and surgical care of the reproductive system; and gender-specific clinical preventive services, such as Pap smears and breast cancer screening. All women have female reproductive systems, but not all women are in need of pregnancy-related services. (Approximately 15% of U.S. women do not bear children in their lifetimes [NCHS 1996a].) Therefore, to the extent that the provision of preventive and other services are linked with pregnancy-related care, women who are not at risk of pregnancy may not receive them. Consequently, the concerns about fragmentation of services do not apply only to women of reproductive age, to pregnant women, or to heterosexually active women.

Fragmentation of women's health services arose as a result of three socio-historical phenomena: medical specialization, the organizational and programmatic separation of reproductive and nonreproductive services, and the politicization of some reproductive services. Medical specialization contributed to fragmentation as a result of the early formation of the specialty of obstetrics-gynecology and the growing role of this specialty in the provision of well-woman care (as described in chapter 1). This contrasts with Western European countries and Canada, where most well-woman care is provided by family practitioners (who represent a larger proportion of the physician work force than in the United States) and obstetrician-gynecologists are regarded as specialists to whom referrals are made (Starfield 1992). In the United States, the female reproductive system has been the province of obstetrics-gynecology and not typically within the repertoire of other physicians who may treat women for nonreproductive conditions. Women's health care therefore has been organized around the practices of medical specialties, not around the multifaceted needs of patients.

Interestingly, in ongoing efforts to define "primary care" medicine, the problem of integrating women's basic health services has rarely been addressed. Since the 1960s, the term "primary care" has been used both to distinguish the training, competencies, and practices of generalist and specialist physicians and to define a particular health care function, regardless of the type of provider. Primary care has also been defined in terms of structure and process features, such as the point of first contact between the patient and the health care system, continuity of care (longitudinality), comprehensiveness, and coordination of services across practitioners and visits (Starfield 1992). The Institute of Medicine Committee on the Future of Primary Care recently presented a definition of primary care as "the provision of integrated, accessible, health care services by clinicians who are accountable for addressing a large majority of personal health care needs, developing a sustained partnership with patients, and practicing in the context of family and community" (Donaldson et al. 1996:1). By "integrated" services, this definition means comprehensive care at any stage of life, coordinated services and information, and continuity of care over time by one provider or a team of providers. These concepts were formulated in gender-neutral terms, however, and the operationalization of primary care for women was not discussed.

There is no standard definition of primary care, and there is debate about its features, the type(s) of provider who should serve as the first-contact coordinator of care for individuals, and the types of organizational arrangements that facilitate effective primary care. Furthermore, with the growth of managed care and the increasing use of "gatekeepers" in these plans, different professional groups have sought to be designated as "primary care providers" in managed care plans. Most notably, obstetrician-gynecologists have promoted their specialty's role in the overall health care of women and have attempted to position themselves for recognition as primary care providers to women throughout the life span. In a 1991 survey of fellows of the American College of Obstetricians and Gynecologists, 48 percent of respondents identified themselves as primary care providers (Leader and Perales 1995). In some states, the specialty has advocated legislation designating them as primary care providers or requiring managed care plans and other insurers to provide women with direct access to obstetrician-gynecologists (ACOG 1993; Johns 1994).[12]

By the mid-1990s, conceptions of primary care for women were beginning to be formulated. A 1993 conference, "Women's Health and Primary Care," convened by George Washington University questioned the "gender-neutral" approach to primary care and stressed the importance of integration of reproductive health services into primary care for women (Weiss and Soloway

1994). Proposals for a new medical specialty in women's health (Johnson 1992; Rosser 1994) and for expanded medical training in women's health in medical schools, in residency training, or in fellowship programs were promulgated (Clancy and Massion 1992; Dan 1994). These proposals specified some content and process features of primary care for women, often emphasizing the need to integrate services and the importance of a multidisciplinary team approach including a variety of medical specialties as well as nonphysician providers (e.g., nurse practitioners, certified nurse-midwives, psychologists). The theme of integrating and coordinating services that typically are provided by various medical specialties also appeared in new medical textbooks on the primary care of women (Carlson and Eisenstat 1995; Lemcke et al. 1995; Seltzer and Pearse 1995). Organizational strategies for integrating women's health care in multidisciplinary settings were highlighted in the 1993 Conference on Women's Health Centers convened by the Jacobs Institute of Women's Health (Schaps et al. 1993). Thus it was only in the 1990s that the perverse effects of medical specialization on the primary care of women began to be recognized and addressed within the professional community.

The second phenomenon contributing to fragmentation of women's basic health care has been the establishment of organizations to provide specialized reproductive health services outside of mainstream health care institutions. This occurred, as we saw in chapter 2, largely in conjunction with twentieth-century waves in the women's health megamovement. Separate organizations for provision of prenatal care, family planning, and abortion services were created originally to promote and disseminate new services, especially to rural, poor, or low-income women. These organizations served the additional important function of legitimizing some new and initially controversial services. While the services for which separate organizations were created often became integrated into the practices of mainstream providers with whom the new organizations competed for patients, persistence as separate organizational forms was facilitated by a variety of public policies and funding streams—such as Title X of the Public Health Service Act for family planning services and Title V of the Social Security Act for prenatal care clinics—designed to extend access to underserved groups. Although they provided only limited services, some of these separate women's health organizations became "safety-net" providers for underserved subpopulations of women, and, indeed, low-income, minority, and adolescent women were major clients who often relied on these organizations as their usual source of health care.

What is less well recognized is the high likelihood that a typical woman will use one of these organizations at some point during her lifetime. For example, according to the 1988 National Survey of Family Growth, 58 percent of women ages 15 to 44 reported using a family planning clinic, such as a Planned Parenthood clinic or a public health department clinic, for their first family planning visit (Mosher and Pratt 1990). The use of organizations receiving public funds for specialized reproductive health services may be some women's first or only contact with the health care system, may provide a component of care for women who obtain other services elsewhere, and may be part of the health care careers of a substantial proportion of U.S. women.

The third contributing factor to fragmentation is the politicization of some reproductive services, which creates barriers to access for these services. The most prominent examples are abortion and, for adolescents, contraceptive and STD prevention services. These services have become the topics of sustained public debate characterized by strongly held moral viewpoints as well as diverse opinions about the role of government as a provider of services. Politicization has several consequences for women's health care. One consequence, of course, is that the use of public funds for these services is contested and precarious, as has been the case with controversies surrounding funding levels for Title X and the use of public funds to support abortion services. In addition, some women may not seek controversial services for fear of exposure and embarrassment. Alternatively, women may intentionally seek the services outside their usual source of care to maintain their privacy; for women insured as a dependent on a family member's insurance policy, for example, seeking care from another provider, even if it means paying out of pocket, avoids disclosure to the policyholder. Politicization also creates incentives for mainstream providers to avoid the controversial services, so that women who are patients of these providers are compelled to obtain the services elsewhere. Indeed, confrontational tactics have been used by antiabortion protesters as a deliberate strategy to discourage physicians from providing the service. Surgical abortions, as we have seen, are provided largely in clinical settings where women may seek care without coordination by their regular provider. This poses a potential risk to health in the event of a complication or the need for follow-up care.

The medical and organizational fragmentation of health care has a number of implications for women of all socioeconomic levels. For one, women may receive basic health care from several types of providers concurrently and in a variety of health care organizations, both public and private. Although the use of more than one type of provider might result in more comprehensive services, it also introduces the potential problems of lack of coordination of care, redundancies in services received, higher risks of iatrogenic conditions, and higher costs to the woman or her insurer. On the other hand, some women might rely on one provider or on a specialized service site, such as a family planning clinic, that does not provide comprehensive services. Depending on the provider's service mix, women who rely on one regular physician or on one site might be at increased risk of not receiving key preventive tests or other needed services. Fragmentation therefore could be regarded as a structural barrier to women's ability to obtain health services appropriate to their needs.

Therefore, although women are more likely to report having a regular source of care and consume more overall health services than men, they rely on a more complex array of providers, and they may not in all cases have access to comprehensive, coordinated primary care services. Fragmentation of basic health care services for women suggests that their utilization patterns will be diverse, may vary across life stages (particularly as need for specific reproductive services changes), may include multiple concurrent sources of care, may result in gaps or redundancies in services if care is not coordinated, and may be highly sensitive to political processes affecting public financing of health services and programs. The diversity of health care options for women also suggests that they are likely to vary in their beliefs about which types of providers are appropriate for their needs and in their preferences for specific practitioners or health care organizations.

This discussion is not to suggest that the solution to fragmentation is a "one-size-fits-all" model of health care for women. Rather, it draws attention to the need to understand the implications of variation in women's patterns of health care in order to design appropriate delivery systems.

WOMEN'S SOURCES OF REGULAR HEALTH CARE

Surprisingly little is known about how U.S. women seek health care. The ongoing national surveys, for example, typically do not measure the types of physicians and other providers used for basic care or the combinations of providers or organizational settings used.

Available research suggests that three types of physicians provide most primary health care services to women—family or general practitioners (who treat both male and female adults and children), general internists (who treat both male and female adults), and obstetrician-gynecologists (who treat adult women). Estimates of the relative contributions of these specialties to women's primary care vary, however. Using data from the National Ambulatory Medical Care Survey, Barbara Bartman and Kevin Weiss (1993) estimated that 60 percent of all nonobstetric visits to office-based physicians in 1989 and 1990 by women ages 15 to 64 years of age were to family or general practitioners, internists, and gynecologists; among these specialties, 55 percent of visits were to family or general practitioners, 21 percent were to internists, and 24 percent were to gynecologists. Also using the 1989–90 National Ambulatory Medical Care Survey, Leader and Perales (1995) analyzed visits for "general medical examinations" (defined as annual or routine checkups, excluding gynecologic and prenatal examinations) made by women ages 15 and over to these three types of physicians: they estimated that 27 percent of these visits were to family or general practitioners, 13 percent were to internists, and 60 percent were to obstetrician-gynecologists. The most common reason for visits to office-based obstetrician-gynecologists in 1989–90 was routine prenatal examinations (33% of all visits) (Rosenblatt et al. 1995; Schappert 1993b).

Data from the 1987 National Medical Expenditure Survey, analyzed by Leader and Perales (1995), show that among women ages 15 and over who made an ambulatory medical visit (excluding hospital outpatient and emergency room visits) in that year, nearly half (48%) made a visit for a general medical checkup. Among women who made at least one general medical visit that year, 28 percent visited a general or family practitioner only, 21 percent visited an obstetrician-gynecologist only, 6 percent visited an obstetrician-gynecologist and some other physician, and 46 percent visited only other types of physicians. Among women who saw an obstetrician-gynecologist, the most common reason for making a visit was a general checkup (reported by 53% of women), followed by diagnosis or treatment (33%), and pregnancy-related care (23%).

Estimates of the extent to which women rely on obstetrician-gynecologists for their regular health care vary widely and depend, in part, on the wording of survey questions. For example, in the 1987 National Medical Expenditure Survey, 49 percent of women ages 18 and over identified a family or general practitioner as their usual physician, 10 percent an internist, and only 5 percent an obstetrician-gynecologist (Bartman, Moy, and Clancy 1994). In a 1993 telephone survey conducted by Gallup for the American College of Obstetricians and Gynecologists (Gallup 1993; Horton, Murphy, and Hale 1994), 72 percent of a national sample of 1,005 women ages 18 to 65 reported having a physical examination by an obstetrician-gynecologist within the past two years, and of these, 54 percent considered their obstetrician-gynecologist to be their "primary physician"; thus about 39 percent of women surveyed might rely on an obstetrician-gynecologist as their primary physician. (The term "primary physician" was not defined for the respondent.) When asked what type of doctor they would choose "if you could only go to one doctor for your health care needs," one in five women named an obstetrician-gynecologist; among women ages 18 to 39, one in four named an obstetrician-gynecologist. The majority of women in all age groups named a family practitioner. In a 1994 telephone survey conducted by the Gallup Organization for the American Medical Association, 1,519 persons ages 18 and over were asked, "Do you have a personal doctor you usually go to when you are sick?" Eighty-three percent of women responded that they had a personal doctor, of whom only 6 percent identified the doctor as an obstetrician-gynecologist (AMA 1994a). Although many women may see an obstetrician-gynecologist regularly, they may not perceive this physician as the one they would consult if they were ill.

The first national survey that attempted to identify the specialties of physicians women use for regular health care and to measure women's concurrent use of more than one type of physician for regular care was the 1993 Survey of Women's Health conducted by Louis Harris and Associates for the Commonwealth Fund (Falik and Collins 1996; Weisman 1996). (See Appendix for a description of the survey methods.) This survey included a series of questions about the types of providers used by women ages 18 and over, including whether they have a usual source of care (and what type),[13] whether they have a regular physician, the specialty of their regular physician, whether or not they see an additional physician "for female-related problems" (if the named regular physician was not an obstetrician-gynecologist), and the specialty of the additional physician.

Table 3.1 shows the types of physicians used by women, based on a composite of questions about their regular physicians.[14] (Three percent of women surveyed are not included in these analyses because they could not identify the specialties of their physicians.) The largest group of women (39%) reported using either a family or general practitioner or an internist for regular care, without seeing an obstetrician or gynecologist in addition. Sixteen percent of women reported that they saw an obstetrician-gynecologist for regular care. One-third of women reported that they saw both types of physicians for regular care: a family or general practitioner or internist *and* an obstetrician-gynecologist.[15] Three percent of women saw only other specialists, and 10 percent of women had no regular physician of any kind. (The women who had no regular physician were more likely than other women to report that their usual source of care was a hospital emergency room: 16% of women without a regular physician relied on an emergency room as their usual source of care, compared with 3% of women who had a regular physician.)

Table 3.1
Types of Physicians Used by Women for Regular Care and Number of
Physicians Seen and Visits Made in Last Year
(N = 2,447 Women Ages 18 and Over)

Type of Regular Physician(s)	Percent (N)		Physicians Seen in Last Year (Mean, S.D.)[a]		Visits in Last Year (Mean, S.D.)[b]	
Family/general practitioner or internist[c]	39	(953)	1.81	(1.41)	5.02	(7.04)
Obstetrician-gynecologist[d]	16	(386)	2.08	(1.55)	5.36	(6.88)
Family/general practitioner or internist *and* obstetrician-gynecologist[e]	33	(800)	2.39	(1.52)	5.84	(6.92)
Other specialist[f]	3	(67)	2.09	(1.42)	7.28	(8.41)
No regular physician	10	(241)	1.64	(1.82)	3.02	(4.16)

[a] Kruskal-Wallis analysis of variance is significant ($p < .001$). In tests for multiple comparisons, the mean number of physicians seen by women whose regular physicians include both an obstetrician-gynecologist and another primary care provider is significantly different ($p < .05$) from all other categories, except for other specialists.

[b] Kruskal-Wallis analysis of variance is significant ($p < .001$). In tests for multiple comparisons, the mean number of visits for women with no regular physician is significantly less ($p < .05$) than all other categories.

[c] The regular physician is either a family/general practitioner or an internist, and no obstetrician-gynecologist is seen in addition.

[d] The regular physician is an obstetrician-gynecologist (84% of these cases), or an obstetrician-gynecologist is seen in combination with physicians other than general/gamily practitioners or internists.

[e] The regular physician is either a family/general practitioner or internist, and an obstetrician-gynecologist is also seen for "female-related problems."

[f] The regular physician is an "other specialist" and no obstetrician-gynecologist is seen. "Other specialists" include cardiologists, rheumatologists, chiropractors, etc. Cardiologists were named most frequently (N = 19); all others were named by 10 or fewer respondents.

The types of physicians women used for regular care, furthermore, were influenced by a number of factors. We conducted multivariate analyses examining the use of different physician specialties as a function of the types of variables specified in the behavioral model of health services use: predisposing, enabling, and need variables. The predisposing variables available in the survey included age, education, race/ethnicity, marital status, and children in the household; enabling variables included type of health insurance, employment status, household income, and geographic location (region of the country and size of community); and need variables included number of chronic conditions in the last five years (from a list including hypertension, cardiovascular disease, cancer, arthritis, diabetes, lung disease, osteoporosis, severe menstrual problems, and endometriosis), a diagnosis of depression or anxiety in the last five years, and disability or impairment that interferes with social functioning. Women also may select particular types of physicians for their regular health care based upon beliefs about what type of physician is most appropriate, perceptions of needed services, or other attitudes or personal preferences. For example, women who see two types of physicians for regular care may prefer to see a specialist in women's reproductive health for routine gynecological care. The survey, however, did not include measures of such beliefs or preferences as predisposing factors.

The analyses showed that women whose regular physician was a family or general practitioner or an internist and who did not also see an obstetrician-gynecologist tended to be beyond the reproductive years (ages 45 and over), to have no post–high school education, and to reside in rural areas or the north central or western regions of the country. Women whose regular physician was an obstetrician-gynecologist and who did not see another primary care physician tended to be in the peak reproductive years (ages 18 to 34), to have post–high school education, to be African American, and to reside in urban areas. Women who saw two types of physicians for regular care tended to be relatively affluent and to reside in geographic areas where specialists are more likely to be available: they were more highly educated (at least high school graduates), white, married or living with a partner, privately insured or members of a private HMO, urban, and residents of the Northeast.[16] Women using two types of physicians also tended to report more chronic conditions during the last five years. Women with no regular physician tended to be unmarried, to have no health insurance, and to have fewer chronic conditions. (Women whose regular physicians were "other specialists" could not be characterized because of their small number.)

Table 3.2 shows the types of physicians women used for regular care by age and health insurance status and is intended to illustrate that the types of physicians used are not a simple function of either variable. For example, the pattern of using two physicians—both an obstetrician-gynecologist and another primary care provider—characterizes substantial proportions of women in all age categories under the age of 65, regardless of health insurance status. Thus the pattern of using two types of physicians is not unique to the peak reproductive years or to women with a particular type of health insurance. In all age groups under age 65, however, women with private health insurance, including enrollment in private HMOs, were more likely than other women to see both types of physicians. Reliance on a family or general practitioner or an internist for regular care, without an obstetrician-gynecologist, increased with age and characterized at least two-thirds of women ages 65 and over. Among women ages 65 and over, having any supplemental insurance in

Table 3.2
Types of Regular Physicians by Age and Health Insurance[a] (%)

	Type of Regular Physician(s)					
	Family/General Practitioner or Internist	Obstetrician-Gynecologist	Both	Other Specialist	None	(N)
Women ages 18–34[b]						
Private insurance	24	28	37	2	8	(376)
Private HMO	28	20	40	1	10	(153)
Medicaid	35	26	20	3	16	(69)
None	22	23	23	2	29	(96)
Women ages 35–44[c]						
Private insurance	26	23	42	1	8	(348)
Private HMO	38	12	45	2	3	(128)
Medicaid	42	15	31	8	4	(26)
None	30	14	24	5	27	(59)
Women ages 45–64[d]						
Private insurance	43	11	37	2	7	(468)
Private HMO	38	12	46	1	3	(121)
Medicare	47	20	22	4	8	(51)
None	48	5	21	5	22	(63)
Women ages 65 and over[e]						
Medicare plus supplemental	66	5	18	6	6	(332)
Medicare only	70	0	7	8	14	(71)

[a] Cross-tabulations of physician type by type of insurance are significant ($p < .05$) by the chi square test.

[b] Excluded: 20 women who were Medicare beneficiaries.

[c] Excluded: 17 women who were Medicare beneficiaries.

[d] Excluded: 16 women who were Medicaid beneficiaries. The Medicare category includes 14 women with supplemental insurance of some kind.

[e] Excluded: 22 women who had only non-Medicare coverage.

addition to Medicare increased the likelihood of seeing an obstetrician-gynecologist, either as the regular physician or in combination with another primary care provider.

TYPES OF PHYSICIANS AND SERVICES RECEIVED

The types of regular physicians seen, in turn, were associated with services received. Table 3.1 shows that women using two types of physicians for regular care visited an average of 2.39 different physicians in the last year, significantly more than all other women except those relying on "other specialists" for their regular care, and made an average of 5.84 visits in the last year. (Overall, 93% of women made at least one physician visit in the last year, and women with no regular physician were significantly less likely than all other women to have made a visit.) Multiple linear regression analyses were conducted in which the number of visits in the last year was regressed on the same set of predisposing, enabling, and need variables previously described. Controlling for all of these variables, indicators of need, particularly the number of chronic conditions, were most strongly associated with the number of visits. However, women seeing two types of physicians made significantly more visits, independent of need, than women seeing only a family or general practitioner or an internist for regular care: women seeing two types of physicians made nearly 25 percent more visits in the last year than women seeing only a family or general practitioner or an internist (Weisman, Cassard, and Plichta 1995).

The types of physicians women use for their regular health care also would be expected to be related to their receipt of clinical preventive services.[17] (Physician gender also has been explored in relation to women's receipt of preventive services; this is discussed in chapter 4.) Research has demonstrated variation by specialty in the provision of preventive services to women. Obstetrician-gynecologists generally are less likely than family or general practitioners or internists to provide such clinical preventive services as blood cholesterol screening, stool guaiac tests, and adult immunizations such as influenza vaccines and tetanus boosters. Conversely, the major adult primary care providers (general internists and family or general practitioners) are not trained as reproductive health specialists and are less likely than obstetrician-gynecologists to provide pelvic examinations, Pap smears, family planning services, physical breast examinations, and mammography (Bartman and Weiss 1993; Horton, Cruess and Pearse 1993; Leader and Perales 1995; Lurie et al. 1993; Weisman et al. 1989). For example, using data from the 1989–90 National Ambulatory Medical Care Survey, Leader and Perales (1995) found that pelvic examinations were provided in 95 percent of general medical examinations of women ages 15 and older conducted by obstetrician-gynecologists, compared with only 45 percent of examinations by family or general practitioners and 54 percent of examinations by internists. Clinical breast examinations were provided in 88 percent of general medical examinations conducted by obstetrician-gynecologists, in 50 percent of examinations by family or general practitioners, and in 54 percent by internists. Cholesterol tests were provided in 13 percent of examinations by obstetrician-gynecologists, in 22 percent of examinations by family or general practitioners, and in 50 percent by internists. The recommendations made to patients by physicians are thought to be key determinants of whether or not patients receive preventive services.[18] Consequently, a logical hypothesis is that women who use both an obstetrician-gynecologist and another primary care physician for regular care will receive a wider array of preventive services than women who have only one regular physician or no regular physician.

The 1993 Survey of Women's Health measured women's receipt of five clinical preventive screening services that generally are recommended for most women on a periodic basis (although recommended intervals vary by age group): blood pressure reading, blood cholesterol test, Pap smear, clinical breast examination, and mammography. Regardless of the time interval examined (one-, two-, or three-year intervals), women who used both an obstetrician-gynecologist and another primary care provider for regular care received significantly more of these services than other women. For example, women seeing both types of physicians received an average of 4.2 of 5 preventive services within the last three years, compared with 3.7 services among women seeing only another primary care provider. The significant effect of seeing two physicians on preventive services held when number of visits was controlled: a higher number of physician visits often is regarded as increasing the woman's "opportunities" for screening, but these analyses show an independent effect on screening of physician specialty. Analyses also were conducted of receipt of specific services within time intervals for which there was some professional consensus for specific age groups at the time of the survey (e.g., mammography every two years for women ages 50 and over) and controlling for the set of predisposing, enabling, and need variables previously described. These analyses consistently found significantly higher odds of receiving the service among women seeing both types of physicians, compared with all other women except those relying on an obstetrician-gynecologist alone (Weisman, Cassard, and Plichta 1995). However, since the number of women who relied on an obstetrician-gynecologist alone was smaller than the number of women relying on a family practitioner or internist alone, the findings suggest that substantial proportions of women in all age categories were at risk of not receiving key preventive services within recommended intervals.

Women, therefore, have quite varied patterns of physician use. The types of physicians women use for regular health care depend on a number of factors, including age, socioeconomic status, geographic location, and health insurance status. Furthermore, utilization (measured as the number of physician visits and preventive services received within specific time intervals) varies by types of physicians seen, independent of other factors such as age, health insurance, and need. The data examined here do not permit conclusions about what the appropriate level of utilization might be, but they do demonstrate at least one way in which the health care system contributes to variation in women's utilization patterns.

The implications of these results are relevant both for medical training and for the design of health care delivery systems. The basic problem is not that multiple types of physicians are involved in the provision of women's primary care, but that both medical specialization and health care delivery systems create barriers to women's receipt of comprehensive primary care in an efficient, coordinated way. One argument that could be made based on these findings about women's utilization patterns is that there is a need for improved training of physicians in women's health or for a new type of provider (a physician specialist or an advanced practice nurse) who would be trained in women's health and would integrate the components of women's primary care. Another strategic approach to integrating women's basic health care is the creation of organizational models designed for this purpose. One option—the multidisciplinary comprehensive primary care women's health center—is discussed in the next chapter. Another possibility is that managed care organizations, which ostensibly emphasize primary and preventive care and seek efficiencies in care delivery, might chart new territory in defining and implementing primary care for women.

THE IMPLICATIONS OF MANAGED CARE FOR WOMEN'S HEALTH

The growth of managed care is likely to change profoundly the ways in which both women and men obtain basic health care, and there are both promises and problems for women enrolled in managed care. A key promise is that at least some types of managed care plans may conceptualize women's primary care in new ways and provide an opportunity to reduce fragmentation. To the extent that managed care organizations provide incentives to providers to keep women well and to deliver basic care more efficiently, care might be better coordinated than in fee-for-service insurance plans. For example, if the reproductive and nonreproductive components of primary care were integrated under the supervision of a primary care provider or team of providers, well-woman care—including clinical prevention services and health promotion counseling—might be provided in fewer visits per patient. Or again, if managed care organizations develop information systems and proactive methods (such as patient education and reminders) to encourage preventive care, then early detection and treatment of cancer and heart disease could be improved.

Among the concerns that have been raised about women's health in managed care are that plans might place restrictions on women's choice of providers, particularly their access to specialists, or might deny care for treatable conditions or access to experimental treatments. These concerns implicitly compare managed care with private indemnity insurance, on the assumption that care provided in fee-for-service arrangements is more appropriate than care provided in managed care plans. This is a questionable assumption, of course, because fee-for-service insurance provides incentives for overtreatment, a problem addressed by women's health advocates since the 1960s. Another concern is that the volatility of the managed care market and of employers' health insurance options may produce plan switching that interrupts the continuity of care and disrupts relationships with regular providers for many women. Because enrollment in managed care plans is growing rapidly and the plans themselves are increasingly diverse, the implications of managed care have only begun to be investigated, and consumers' concerns have been based largely on anecdotal evidence. It is too early to tell, for example, what types of managed care plans will provide new models of integrated primary care for women and which will tend merely to replicate the fragmented patterns of care that characterize women's health care generally.

The term "managed care" covers a wide range of continually evolving health care plans and no longer applies only to the original prepaid health plans known as HMOs. Managed care encompasses a variety of organizational arrangements that combine health care delivery, financing of health services, and utilization controls within a network of providers who have some type of contractual relationship with the plan to provide care to enrolled populations and, in some cases, assume financial risk for the provision of services. Included are relatively tightly structured group- and staff-model HMOs that may be housed in one physical location; more loosely structured network and independent practice association (IPA) HMOs; and newer managed care models such as preferred provider organizations (PPOs), in which enrollees receive care from a network of approved providers, and hybrid point-of-service (POS) plans, which combine features of an HMO with options for services outside the network. Managed care organizations increasingly describe themselves as "mixed model," since they may incorporate group or staff components with IPA or network components. Finally, managed care organizations may be either for-profit or not-for-profit entities, although for-profit plans have increased in number since the mid-1980s (Davis, Collins, and Morris 1994); in 1994, 69 percent of HMOs were for-profit entities (GHAA 1995).

The percentage of Americans enrolled in managed care plans of various kinds increased rapidly between 1985 and 1995. In 1985, 19 million persons were enrolled in HMOs, compared with 58.2 million in 1995; and an additional 91 million were enrolled in PPOs in 1995 (American Association of Health Plans 1996). Together, these plans therefore enrolled approximately 57 percent of the 1995 U.S. resident population. In 1995, 69 percent of employees of midsized and large companies were enrolled in HMOs, PPOs, or POS plans, an increase of 23 percent since 1992 (KPMG 1995). Both Medicaid and Medicare beneficiaries were increasingly being enrolled in managed care plans as well. In 1990, fewer than 3 percent of these beneficiaries were in managed care, but by 1995, nearly one-third of Medicaid beneficiaries (11.6 million persons, predominantly poor children and their parents) and 10 percent of Medicare beneficiaries (3.7 million persons) were enrolled in some type of managed care (Kaiser Family Foundation 1995b; Rowland and Hanson 1996). These percentages were expected to increase rapidly.

Women were about 53 percent of all HMO enrollees in 1993, and women ages 15 to 44 were slightly overrepresented among enrollees compared with their percentage of the U.S. population (Gabel et al. 1994). This could reflect a number of factors, including the tendency for HMOs to enroll younger and healthier populations; the growth of Medicaid managed care; and a tendency for employees to switch from traditional fee-for-service insurance to HMOs in anticipation of childbirth, due to the benefits structures in HMOs (Robinson, Gardner, and Luft 1993). Women in this age group also accounted for 67 percent of all prepaid health plan visits to office-based physicians in 1991 (Woodwell 1995).

Some managed care plans use primary care providers as "gatekeepers" to coordinate an enrolled individual's use of services, including authorizing referrals to specialists and following up on referral services (Weiner and de Lissovoy 1993). In theory, these plans would be expected to conceptualize what is meant by "primary care" for women, with respect to the range of services that ought to be provided, the type(s) of providers who ought to deliver care, and the types of information systems and other mechanisms needed to monitor and coordinate across episodes of care and among providers. Furthermore, because of the financial incentives (e.g., through capitation) to keep enrollees healthy and to reduce use of high-cost hospital services, women enrolled in these plans would be expected to receive more age-appropriate clinical preventive services, earlier prenatal care, more effective pregnancy prevention services, and fewer unnecessary high-technology treatments than women with conventional fee-for-service health insurance. Research has shown that HMO enrollees tend to receive more preventive services, examinations, and health promotion interventions than persons with private indemnity insurance (Miller and Luft 1994). However, noncapitated plans would not necessarily have incentives to provide regular preventive screening services, and plans with high patient turnover might not invest in prevention for patients who are likely to disenroll.

Several studies have investigated the relationship between managed care and women's receipt of preventive services. A review of studies of the effects of Medicaid managed care plans on women's receipt of preventive services found mixed results, with some studies finding higher rates of preventive services received among those in managed care, and some studies finding no differences (Collins and Simon 1996; Rowland et al. 1995). Similarly, studies of the effects of Medicaid managed care on use of prenatal care have been inconclusive (Alpha Center 1995). Findings for private HMO enrollees also are mixed. For example, using data from the 1992 National Health Interview Survey, Makuc and colleagues found greater use of Pap tests and mammograms among women ages 50 and over who were enrolled in HMOs than among women with fee-for-service private health insurance; however, there were no significant differences between HMOs and fee-for-service insurance among women ages 40 to 49 (Makuc, Freid, and Parsons 1994). Using data from the 1993 Survey of Women's Health, we constructed an index of clinical preventive services received within the last three years and found that enrollment in a private HMO had a significant positive effect on the total number of services women received, compared with private indemnity insurance, after controlling for a set of predisposing, enabling, and need variables and for types of physicians seen for regular care. In examining receipt of specific preventive services, however, a significant effect of HMO enrollment, compared with private indemnity insurance, was found only for Pap smears (Weisman, Cassard, and Plichta 1995).

One possibility is that as HMOs become more diverse, as they enroll less selected populations, and as all providers become more prevention conscious, differences between managed care and fee-for-service insurance plans in the provision of clinical preventive services will decrease. At least one study using national data sets supports this. Weinick and Beauregard (1997) found that privately insured nonelderly women enrolled in HMOs in 1987 were more likely than women with fee-for-service insurance to have received Pap smears, breast examinations, and mammograms; by 1992, however, this HMO advantage had disappeared for privately insured women.

A key research question is how different types of managed care arrangements—including the newer types of plans—compare with each other in providing clinical preventive services and comprehensive primary care to women. The managed care industry does not have a standard definition of primary care or, as yet, the technology to measure the comprehensiveness and effectiveness of primary care services. Some managed care organizations have developed innovative programs and information systems to improve delivery of clinical preventive services to women, but evaluation of these programs has not been extensive. Driven, in part, by the need to demonstrate performance on the measures included in the Health Plan Employer Data and Information Set (HEDIS), which provides the basis of health plan report cards for purchasers and consumers (National Committee for Quality Assurance 1995), plans have focused on improving delivery of early prenatal care and provision of Pap smears and mammography screening. Programs to provide comprehensive preventive screening to women (rather than a specific preventive service) are less common.

With regard to benefits, studies have found variation across plans in routine coverage of some services as well as variation in the level of copayments and, in the case of clinical preventive services, in the allowable interval between tests. Levels of copayments are important because research has found that higher cost-sharing is associated with decreased use of services, particularly among low-income populations (Weissman and Epstein 1994). As noted earlier, a 1993 survey of private health insurers conducted by the Alan Guttmacher Institute (1994) found that HMOs provided routine coverage of Pap tests, mammography, reversible contraception (including prescriptions for oral contraceptives), and infertility treatment more often than conventional indemnity plans, PPOs, and POS plans. However, the study found variation across types of health plans in coverage of reproductive health services. For example, 49 percent of conventional indemnity plans offered by large employers (100 or more employees) routinely covered annual gynecological examinations, compared with 64 percent of PPOs, 88 percent of POS networks, and 99 percent of HMOs. HMOs were found to be more likely than indemnity health insurance plans, PPOs, and POS networks to have billing and claims processing procedures that allow dependents, such as adolescents, to obtain reproductive health services confidentially, without notification of the policyholder.

The 1994 HMO survey by Group Health Association of America and the Henry J. Kaiser Family Foundation found that coverage of reversible contraception and abortion varied by HMO type. The older types of HMOs, group- and staff-model HMOs, were sometimes more likely than the newer IPA and network models to cover specific services, which could suggest a trend toward less coverage; examples included Norplant insertions and removals, diaphragm prescriptions, and abortions (Bernstein, Dial, and Smith 1995). With regard to cost-sharing, comparisons across plans are complicated by the amount of the premium paid by the policyholder (as opposed to the employer), deductibles and coinsurance provisions, and copayments. HMOs generally have no deductibles or coinsurance provisions, but they typically have copayments (averaging $7.00 in 1994) associated with primary care visits (Bernstein 1996). In 1994, between 67 and 75 percent of HMOs had copayments for office visits to a primary care provider, and although most had copayments for reproductive health services, copayments in addition to those for the office visit were often waived. In all, 83 percent of HMOs required some copayments for oral contraceptives, 75 percent for Pap tests, 74 percent for diaphragm fittings, 71 percent for Depo-Provera injections, and 46 percent for tubal ligation (a surgical procedure). For reversible contraceptive services, staff-model HMOs were less likely than other HMOs to require copayments (Bernstein 1996).

Women's health advocates and others have raised questions about women's access to specialists within managed care plans. One concern has been that plans might erect barriers to access to obstetrician-gynecologists by failing to designate them as primary care providers for women or by limiting referrals (Johns 1994), and as noted earlier, some states have enacted legislation to ensure access. (A related concern is the suspected exclusion of community-based providers, such as Planned Parenthood clinics or Feminist Women's Health Centers, from some managed care networks; the participation of such providers in managed care is discussed in chapter 4.) There are some data on variation among managed care plans with respect to how providers for women's primary care are designated. A 1994 survey of HMOs sponsored by Group Health Association of America and the Henry J. Kaiser Family Foundation investigated the types of primary providers for women in different types of HMOs including staff- and group-model, network, and IPA HMOs (Bernstein, Dial, and Smith 1995; Bernstein 1996). Among all types of HMOs, 47 percent allowed women to select an obstetrician-gynecologist as their primary provider, and 70 percent allowed them to self-refer to an obstetrician-gynecologist. In nearly all HMOs of all types, however, family or general practitioners routinely provided pelvic examinations, Pap smears, and breast examinations. Network and IPA-model HMOs were more likely than staff and group-model HMOs to require a new referral for each visit to an obstetrician-gynecologist and to limit the number of self-referrals to one per year. Since network and IPA HMOs are newer models and constituted a majority of

HMO plans in 1995 (HIAA 1996), these results may signal a trend toward increased control of use of obstetrician-gynecologists' services.

Another issue that drew considerable public attention in the 1990s was the imposition of 24-hour limits on hospital stays for mothers and newborns after uncomplicated childbirth, known as "drive-through deliveries." Concerns about shorter lengths-of-stay reflected a general fear that the financial incentives of managed care will operate to reduce enrollees' access to hospital-based or other high-technology services, compared with indemnity insurance. In fact, hospital length-of-stay for both vaginal and cesarean-section deliveries had been declining since 1970 (Centers for Disease Control and Prevention 1995b) because of efforts to control costs, and managed care was not entirely responsible for this trend. Although research evidence on the health impact of length-of-stay for either mothers or newborns was not available, the medical community led efforts for legislation, at the state and national levels, to require insurers to cover minimum postpartum stays consistent with professional guidelines and to provide home visits or other follow-up care after discharge from the hospital.[19] By the time national legislation was approved in the Newborns' and Mothers' Health Protection Act of 1996, more than half of the states had either enacted legislation or had legislation pending (Women's Policy, Inc. 1996b). Lawmakers could scarcely oppose this legislation—despite lobbying against it by employers' groups, the managed care and insurance industries, and providers of alternative birthing services—for fear of being perceived as "antimotherhood." The potential downsides of legislative standard-setting for the medical treatment of childbirth, however, include discouraging innovations in the use of home care or other alternatives to hospital-based childbirth services and higher health insurance costs.

The growth of managed care is fraught with implications for women's health. Two issues that resulted in early, precedent-setting legislative regulation of managed care plans and other insurers—access to obstetrician-gynecologists and coverage of minimal hospital stays following childbirth—pertained to women's health care. Growing public concerns about managed care, combined with the great variability across managed care plans in policies and practices, suggest the need for research that compares various types of managed care arrangements with regard to women's utilization rates, out-of-pocket costs, satisfaction levels, quality of care, and retention. As managed care evolves, the relevant question is no longer how managed care plans compare with indemnity insurance, but how various types of managed care arrangements compare with each other and which models are the most effective providers of women's health care.

CONCLUSION

This chapter began with the observation that women's health advocates in the early 1990s were concerned about gender inequities in health care. Considerations of gender equity, however, have to contend with gender differences in needs and services. It is difficult to compare health care utilization patterns and to draw conclusions about appropriate levels of use or equity of access because there are gender differences in incidence and prevalence of conditions that women and men have in common, because some health conditions are gender specific, and because there are sociocultural factors influencing use of health care. Although women in general consume more health services than men, there are some important gender-based financial and nonfinancial barriers to care. For example, while women are more likely than men to have health insurance at any point in time, they are more dependent than men on public insurance, they experience some important limitations in coverage, they pay out of pocket for more of their care, and they may have difficulty obtaining specific services because of availability problems. Furthermore, health care services are highly gendered. Women and men use a different array of health care providers and organizations, and for a variety of sociohistorical reasons, the primary care sector for women is complex and fragmented. Some women therefore receive less than optimal services, and some use more than one provider for basic care and may make excess visits or receive redundant services as a result. Although the growth of managed care holds some promises for integrating well-woman services, for improving prevention, and for reducing inefficiencies in care delivery, the increasing diversity of these plans and trends in regulation make it difficult to project what types of managed care organizations will tend to replicate fragmented care for women and what types will develop more women-centered models of care.

4

Women and Health Care Delivery: Providers and Organizations

ONE OF THE recurring themes and unresolved issues in the women's health megamovement has been the question of whether women's health care generally, or some components of it, ought to be delivered in separate organizations for women or by women providers. The creation of separate women's health organizations, as we have seen, has been a strategy employed by activists in all movement waves. Although most formal health care services currently are provided in mixed-gender settings, and most women receive medical care from physicians who are men, gender as a characteristic of health organizations and of health care providers is a continuing topic of interest and controversy. An important feature of American health care is the persistence and increasing diversity of separate organizations providing services designed for women. In addition, an ongoing debate focuses on women's preferences for, or the therapeutic benefits of, women providers. What is the evidence that either women providers or women's organizations provide solutions to women's health care problems? How are these issues affecting the health care marketplace?

PROVIDER GENDER ISSUES

Provider gender has been a controversial issue throughout the history of American health care. When medical men began to practice midwifery in the late eighteenth century, the moral propriety of mixed-gender health care for women was publicly debated. The first generation of American women physicians in the late nineteenth century attempted to justify their role in the profession, particularly in obstetrics and gynecology, partly on the basis of propriety and partly on the basis of their presumed special expertise in the treatment of women patients. They believed that they were better qualified than men to care for women because of their greater sensitivity to, and sympathy with, women's health concerns generally, and they believed that women patients would feel more comfortable disclosing their health problems to women physicians (Drachman 1976; Morantz-Sanchez 1985). Most male physicians of the period, however, had general practices that included both women and men as patients, and they depended upon childbearing women as a means of establishing their practices. Medical men therefore were not generally supportive of the claims to special expertise made by women physicians, and they did not relinquish the practice of women's health care. Not until the 1970s, when women began to enter the profession (and a wider array of specialties) in greater numbers, was there a resurgence of interest in whether gender-congruent care might be characterized by different patterns of communication, different levels of attention to gender-specific services or psychosocial issues, or better outcomes of care. The hypotheses about the possible benefits of gender-congruent health care for women were reminiscent of the arguments made by women physicians a century earlier.

Since the 1970s, women have dramatically increased their presence in the medical profession, particularly in the specialties most likely to provide primary care. The number of women physicians increased nearly sixfold between 1970 and 1995, and in 1995, 21 percent of U.S. physicians were women, compared with 8 percent in 1970 (AMA 1997). The percentage of women physicians will continue to grow, since women were 38 percent of U.S. medical school graduates between 1992 and 1994 and 40 percent of all medical students in 1993. By the year 2010, the number of women physicians is projected to be nearly 200,000, or 29 percent of all physicians, and by the year 2020, women are projected to be more than one-third of active physicians (Council on Graduate Medical Education 1995). Furthermore, between 1990 and 1995, the number of women practicing in the three specialties providing most primary care services to women—family practice, internal medicine, and obstetrics-gynecology—increased 69 percent, 44 percent, and 49 percent, respectively. In 1995, women were 21 percent of family or general practitioners, 24 percent of internists, and 30 percent of obstetrician-gynecologists, and women were 42 percent of residents in family practice, 34 percent of residents in internal medicine, and 58 percent of residents in obstetrics-gynecology (AMA 1997). In consequence, women in the general population have increasing opportunities to receive basic health care from women physicians.[1]

In addition, the increasing proportion of women in medicine sometimes is expected to bring about changes in medical practice as more women physicians rise to positions of authority in academic institutions and health care delivery organizations. The Council on Graduate Medical Education (1995), for example, has provided a number of recommendations for increasing the number of women in medicine and for ensuring their advancement into high-level positions. There is no assurance, however, that this strategy will, in itself, lead to increased attention to gender issues within the profession or to improvements in women's health care. The work of Rosabeth Moss Kanter (1977) in American corporations provides reason to expect that as the proportion of women in medicine reaches parity with men, the behavior of women and men will become less differentiated. This might, as advocates hope, result from women altering the culture of medicine for all physicians, but it might also result from the uniform socialization of women and men to the prevailing culture of medicine or from the similar exposure of women and men to the incentives of the medical workplace. In other words, an increasing number of women physicians and their ascendance to positions of influence does not guarantee, but could facilitate, changes in the culture or practice of medicine.

Medicine is not the only health care profession that provides some elements of primary care and includes women practitioners.[2] Advanced practice nurses (particularly nurse practitioners and certified nurse-midwives) and physician assistants also provide some basic health services. Although the relative contribution of these groups to primary care has not been a major one, some policy analysts believe that changes in the U.S. health care system may produce increased roles for these professionals in community-based health care settings. In particular, there may be increased financial incentives for health plans to substitute less costly nonphysician services for some medical services and to increase the use of collaborative practices involving physician and nonphysician providers. Recent data reveal that nonphysician personnel provide some primary care and a substantial proportion of outpatient obstetrics-gynecology visits in staff and group-model HMOs (Dial et al. 1995; Weiner 1994). Some managed care plans, particularly staff- and group-model

HMOs, permit enrollees to select a nurse practitioner as the primary care provider for general care (Bernstein, Dial, and Smith 1995). (Furthermore, as we shall see shortly, both nurse practitioners and certified nurse-midwives play important roles in some types of women's health care organizations.) Because nurse practitioners and certified nurse-midwives are overwhelmingly female—96 percent of all employed registered nurses in 1992 were women (Moses 1994)—an increased role for these occupational groups in the provision of adult primary care would increase women's opportunities to receive gender-congruent health care. The confounding of occupational groups and gender, however, means that it is difficult to assess the effects of gender-congruent care within these groups.

Nurse practitioners, originating in the 1960s, are registered nurses with masters degrees who often provide primary care services to adults or children. According to the 1992 National Sample Survey of Registered Nurses (Moses 1994), there were over 42,000 active nurse practitioners in the United States in 1992, about half of whom held job titles as nurse practitioners. The practices of nurse practitioners vary across states and are governed by state nurse practice acts. Nurse practitioners have prescribing privileges in 48 states, although some states require some form of physician supervision, and in some states nurse practitioners may be reimbursed by third-party payers (Leppa 1995; Lynaugh 1994; Mundinger 1994). The Pew Health Professions Commission (1995) recently recommended expansion of the number of training programs for nurse practitioners to increase the available supply.

Certified nurse-midwives, who are registered nurses with additional training in obstetrical care, are legally permitted to practice midwifery in all states and the District of Columbia and have been acknowledged to provide cost-effective quality care for low-risk pregnant women (U.S. Congress Office of Technology Assessment 1986; Brown and Grimes 1993). The American College of Nurse-Midwives reported 5,060 members in 1994 (Walsh and Boggess 1996). According to Gabay and Wolfe (1995), there were about 4,000 practicing nurse-midwives in 1994, and 92 percent provided gynecological care as well as maternity services. Certified nurse-midwives attended about 4.4 percent of all hospital births in 1992, an eightfold increase since 1975. Of the non-hospital births they attended, 64 percent took place in freestanding birth centers, 33 percent took place in homes, and 26 percent took place in clinics, doctors' offices, or other places. Nurse-midwives had some degree of prescriptive authority in 41 jurisdictions in 1995 and could receive private insurance reimbursement in 31 states (American College of Nurse-Midwives 1995).

Physician assistants constitute a third occupational group that may provide basic health care services. These personnel typically have completed two-year training programs at the college level and work under the supervision of physicians. Over 32,000 physician assistants have been trained, and the American Academy of Physician Assistants estimates that about half practice in primary care specialties (Donaldson et al. 1996). In 1990, only about one-third of practicing physician assistants were women, but this percentage will likely increase because women comprised a majority of physician assistants in training by 1990 (Muller 1994).

RESEARCH ON PHYSICIAN GENDER EFFECTS

Despite growing interest in gender-congruent health care for women and increased opportunities to study health care provided by women, relatively little research has addressed the topic directly. Three areas of research may be identified: studies of variations in physicians' practice patterns by gender, studies of gender effects on communication patterns within medical visits, and studies of gender differences in physicians' provision of preventive services to women.

Some of the early research on gender differences in practice patterns was motivated by concerns about the potential impact of an increasing number of women physicians on the productivity of the medical profession and on estimates of physician supply.[3] One consistent finding from this body of work was that women physicians, compared with men, tended to see fewer patients per unit of time and to spend more time per patient visit. For example, data from the National Ambulatory Medical Care Survey showed that on average, women physicians spent more time in face-to-face contact with each patient than did men, and they spent more time with patients who were women than with patients who were men (Cypress 1980). In addition, according to 1980–81 data, women obstetrician-gynecologists had an average of 49 patient visits per week, with visits averaging 17.1 minutes; this compared with 69.5 visits per week to men, with visits averaging 13.8 minutes (Cypress 1984). Although it was hypothesized that longer visits were due to more time spent communicating with patients and therefore might indicate that women physicians do a better job, these studies could not investigate the content of visits.

The type of practice arrangement also is likely to affect length of visit. For example, in a 1984 survey of a national sample of obstetrician-gynecologists who had been in practice for an average of about three years, there were small but significant gender differences in the number of patients seen per hour in both partnership and multispecialty group practices, with women seeing fewer patients than men; however, there were no physician gender differences in solo or institutional (salaried) practices (Weisman et al. 1986b). Bertakis and colleagues (1995) found no significant gender difference in the length of visits among residents in family practice and internal medicine in a primary care center. It is not known whether the gender difference in visit length persists in managed care plans, in which administrative controls would be expected to reduce variation in visit length generally. However, one recent study in a California HMO found no significant gender difference in the number of patients seen per hour by family practitioners and pediatricians (Eyler, Gorenflo, and Musser 1996). Pressures to improve efficiency in care delivery are likely to reduce both the average amount of time physicians spend communicating with patients overall and the gender difference in visit length.

The relationship between gender (both physician and patient gender) and the quantity and quality of communication during observed medical encounters also has been investigated. Dimensions of communication that have been studied include the quantity of information exchanged between physician and patient (e.g., the amount of symptom reporting by patients, the amount of information provided by physicians); the affective tone of the communication (e.g., verbal statements of empathy, nonverbal communication such as voice tone and body language); and the negotiative quality of the interaction (e.g., joint decision making). Because studies have differed with respect to both their populations and methods of observation, conclusions with regard to gender effects on communication are difficult to draw.

In literature reviews conducted in the 1980s, some evidence was found from both survey research and observed medical encounters that gender-congruent provider-patient interactions might be characterized by more effective communication and stronger rapport than mixed-gender interactions; further, there might be specific conditions under which gender-congruent health care could result in better communication, including treatment of gender-specific conditions or conditions of a highly sensitive or sexual nature (Weisman and Teitelbaum 1985, 1989). Roter and Hall (1994) recently concluded that the bulk of the research evidence suggests that women primary care physicians are better communicators than men because they communicate more feelings and emotions; they are more informative; they elicit more patient disclosure; they facilitate more patient participation; they are more empathetic; and they are more attentive listeners. Women patients in particular may benefit from encounters with women physicians because of longer visits, more positive affect, and a more equal distribution of talk in woman-to-woman encounters. The studies of observed medical encounters, however, have not linked gender differences in physicians' communication styles with services received or with patient outcomes, and evidence regarding the impact of physicians' communication styles on patients' levels of satisfaction with care received is mixed. For example, Hall and colleagues (1994) did not find that patients were more satisfied with women physicians, despite their superior communication style, whereas Bertakis and colleagues (1995) found that the patients of female residents were more satisfied with their visits than were the patients of male residents.

In efforts to understand the impact of a growing proportion of women physicians for women's health, researchers have investigated gender differences in the provision of specific women's services. Some investigators have hypothesized that as more women enter the surgical specialties, they might contribute to lowering the rate of overused procedures, such as hysterectomies, or increase the availability of controversial procedures, such as abortion. The evidence is inconclusive, however. A North Carolina study, for example, found that men gynecologists performed 60 percent more hysterectomies than women (Bickell et al. 1994), whereas an Arizona study found that women physicians (specialty not specified) performed significantly more hysterectomies than men (Geller, Burns, and Brailer 1996). With regard to abortion performance, a 1984 national study of 1,420 obstetrician-gynecologists in practice, on average, about three years (and therefore gender-matched on training and experience) found that women were significantly more likely than men to provide abortions: 50 percent of women, compared with 43 percent of men (Weisman et al. 1986a). On the other hand, a 1995 survey of 307 obstetrician-gynecologists (age unspecified) found no significant difference in abortion provision by gender (Kaiser Family Foundation 1995a).

Research also has addressed the effect of physician gender on women's receipt of clinical preventive screening services. The implicit hypothesis in much of this work is that women physicians, compared with men, will take a more holistic view of women's health and therefore will be more likely both to provide screening and preventive services and to motivate their women patients to receive these services regularly over time. Because there is variation among professional groups' guidelines with respect to the appropriate intervals between screenings and the age groups that should be targeted for specific preventive services, some patients may be confused, and the physician's ability to communicate recommendations may be a critical factor in the patient's receipt of screening.[4]

Several recent studies have provided evidence that women receive more clinical preventive services when they see women physicians. For example, in a study of general internists' ambulatory care practices, Hall and colleagues

(1990) found that the patients of female staff physicians were more likely than the patients of men to receive Pap tests and clinical breast examinations, according to performance criteria established for review of patient records. Franks and Clancy (1993), using data from the 1987 National Medical Expenditure Survey, found that women whose usual physician (specialty unspecified) was a woman were more likely to have had a Pap test in the last three years and to have ever had a mammogram; however, physician gender was not associated with breast examinations or blood pressure checks. In a study analyzing claims data for patients enrolled in a Minnesota IPA health plan, Lurie and colleagues (1993) reported a physician gender effect among family practitioners and internists, but not among obstetrician-gynecologists: the patients of women family practitioners and internists were more likely to receive Pap tests and mammograms during the year than the patients of men in these specialties. Kreuter and colleagues (1995) studied patients of family practitioners in North Carolina and found that women seeing a woman physician were significantly more likely than those seeing men to receive Pap tests within a six-month follow-up period, that younger women (ages 35 to 39) seeing a woman physician were more likely to receive mammography, and that both women and men seeing a woman physician were more likely than those seeing a man to receive cholesterol tests. They concluded that women family practitioners screen more aggressively than men, and they raised the possibility that women physicians may conduct unnecessary screening. In an experimental trial of expanded Medicare benefits for preventive services, German and colleagues (1995) found that women patients of women physicians (specialty unspecified) were more likely than the women patients of men physicians to make a free comprehensive preventive visit that included a breast examination, pelvic examination, and Pap smear, in addition to other preventive services. Finally, in a study of screening for colorectal cancer, female residents in internal medicine performed more rectal examinations and fecal occult blood tests on female patients than did male residents, and male residents performed more rectal examinations on male patients than did female residents (Borum 1996).

These studies suggest alternative explanations for the findings that gender-congruent care may enhance screening for women. One possible explanation is that communication is more effective in gender-congruent physician-patient pairs. That is, women physicians, compared with men, might provide better information about screening to their women patients, including alleviating confusion about conflicting professional guidelines for screening, or they might be more persuasive in motivating patients to obtain screening.

Alternatively, and independent of the quality of communication, women physicians might feel more comfortable than men providing certain screening services to women, particularly those involving pelvic, rectal, or breast examinations. Or, women physicians may simply be more aggressive screeners because they are more convinced of the value of preventive care. Or again, women patients might seek out women physicians because they desire preventive services and are more comfortable receiving gender-specific preventive services and follow-up from a woman.

The ability to distinguish among these alternative explanations, which is problematic based on current data, is important for the formulation of policy. For example, if women physicians, compared with men, were found to provide better explanations to patients about the need for preventive services, or better follow-up and reminders for routine screening, then a possible policy recommendation would be to train men in communication and patient follow-up skills. If, alternatively, men practicing family or general practice or general internal medicine were found to be less likely than women in the same specialties to provide clinical preventive services for women, then there might be a need to retrain or certify physicians as primary care providers for women. Or again, if variation in screening were found to be the result primarily of patients' preferences for women physicians for these services, then there might be a rationale for health plans and practices to increase the availability of women physicians, nurse practitioners, or certified nurse-midwives to provide the option of gender-congruent care for women.

Most of the studies of women's receipt of preventive services have been limited in the variables that could be examined. For example, of the six studies just described, three were limited to a single medical specialty (general internal medicine or family practice), two could not control for physician specialty (despite known variations in primary care physicians' patterns of screening associated with specialty, as discussed in chapter 3), and none could control for women's use of more than one physician for regular health care (that is, they could not account for the additional screening opportunities provided by having a second physician).

EVIDENCE OF PHYSICIAN GENDER EFFECTS
IN THE 1993 SURVEY OF WOMEN'S HEALTH

The Commonwealth Fund's 1993 Survey of Women's Health provides an opportunity to investigate the relationship between physician gender and several variables: women's satisfaction with care received from their regular physician, women's assessments of the quality of communication with their regular physician, women's physician gender preferences, and women's receipt of key clinical preventive services. (See Appendix for a description of the survey methods.) Satisfaction with care received was measured in three questions that asked women to rate their current regular physicians (on a four-point scale, ranging from "excellent" to "poor") on the quality of overall care provided, knowledge and competence to treat illnesses, and caring about the woman and her health; no significant differences were found on these items by physician gender. The quality of communication with the regular physician was measured in eight items assessing the amount of time the physician spent with the patient; the physician's effort spent in soliciting symptoms and problems, answering questions, making sure the patient understands information given, caring, and listening to the patient; and the woman's comfort level in talking with the physician. Again, no significant differences were found on these items by physician gender.[5]

There was a strong association, however, between having a regular physician who is a woman and preferring a woman physician. Overall, 18 percent of women in the survey had regular physicians who were women, and among these, 40 percent reported that they preferred a female physician, 4 percent preferred a male physician, and 56 percent had no gender preference. Among women whose regular physicians were men, these percentages were 8 percent, 14 percent, and 78 percent, respectively. This pattern was the same in all age groups of women (despite the tendency of women ages 65 and over to be more likely than women under age 65 to prefer male physicians) and controlling for the specialty of the regular physician.[6] It cannot be determined from these cross-sectional data whether women who saw women physicians preferred them because they had positive experiences with them, or whether they had chosen them because of a preference for gender-congruent care. Since women currently seeing women physicians did not report higher levels of satisfaction with care or better communication than women currently seeing men physicians, the possibility exists that gender-congruent care might be valued by some women as a matter of privacy or for some other reason having to do with personal comfort levels.

With regard to women's receipt of clinical preventive services, some effects of physician gender were found, but they were not consistent across preventive services or physician specialty groups (Cassard et al. 1997). To test the effect of physician gender, some time frame had to be chosen for each of the screening tests measured in the survey: Pap smears, blood cholesterol tests, clinical breast examinations, and mammography. (Blood pressure readings also were measured, but nearly all women reported receiving them, and there was insufficient variation to analyze physician gender effects.) Because the recommended intervals vary by screening test, a single time frame (e.g., within the last year) would not necessarily reflect appropriate care. Consequently, test-specific intervals were analyzed that generally were recommended at the time of the survey by the U.S. Preventive Services Task Force (1989). Therefore, the hypothesis tested is whether physician gender affects women's receipt of these preventive services within a time frame specified in one set of prevailing guidelines.

Table 4.1 shows the effect of having a regular physician who is a woman on receipt of four key preventive screening services within generally recommended intervals, controlling for physician specialty, seeing an additional obstetrician-gynecologist (and that physician's gender), and the woman's age, education, and race/ethnicity. The odds ratios shown in the table are adjusted for these covariates.[7] Among women whose regular physicians were family or general practitioners, having a woman physician significantly increased the odds of receiving a Pap smear within the last three years and a blood cholesterol test within the last three years. Women ages 40 to 49, furthermore, were more than twice as likely to have received a mammogram in the last two years if their family or general practitioner was a woman, thus confirming the finding of Kreuter and colleagues (1995) that women family practitioners, compared with men in the same specialty, may be more aggressive providers of mammography for younger women. The only other significant physician gender effect was found among women whose regular physicians were internists: having a woman internist increased the odds of receiving a Pap smear within the last three years more than threefold. The gender of obstetrician-gynecologists—as either the regular physician or as an additional physician—had no significant effects on any preventive services. However, seeing an additional obstetrician-gynecologist of either gender significantly increased the odds of receiving Pap smears, breast examinations, and mammograms among the patients of family or general practitioners and internists.

These analyses provide limited evidence of physician gender effects. The most noteworthy findings are the tendency for women who have been treated by a woman physician to prefer a woman physician, and the tendency for women physicians in some specialties to provide more women's preventive services than their male counterparts. With regard to women's receipt of preventive screening, evidence for a gender effect is most consistent among family or general practitioners, who were the regular physicians for most

Table 4.1
Effect of Physician Gender on Women's Receipt of Preventive Services
(Adjusted Relative Odds)[a]

	Specialty of Regular Physician[b]		
	Family or General Practitioner ($N = 1,313$)	Internist ($N = 383$)	Obstetrician-Gynecologist ($N = 318$)
Pap smear, last 3 years	1.75*	3.41*	1.28
Blood cholesterol test, last 3 years	1.60*	1.34	1.51
Clinical breast exam, last year	1.14	1.04	0.78
Mammogram, last 2 years			
Ages 40–49	2.31*	0.48	1.84
Ages 50+	1.09	0.74	—[c]

* $p < .05$

[a] Adjusted relative odds for female physician gender, adjusting for women's age, educational level, race/ethnicity, and the gender of an additional obstetrician-gynecologist seen, if any (for women whose regular physician was a family or general practitioner or an internist). There were no significant gender effects among obstetrician-gynecologists, as either the regular or additional physicians.

[b] Sixteen percent of family or general practitioners, 14 percent of internists, and 31 percent of obstetrician-gynecologists were women.

[c] For women ages 50 and over, those whose regular physician was an obstetrician-gynecologist are omitted because there were too few ($N = 37$) for analysis.

women studied. And because women beyond the reproductive years were less likely than younger women to see an obstetrician-gynecologist in addition to their regular physician, the older patients of male family or general practitioners may be at particular risk for not receiving regular screening.

Even if research cannot support all of the claims or expectations for gender-congruent health care for women, the current state of the evidence, combined with the preferences of many women for women physicians, suggests that the issue continues to be an important one with which the health care delivery system must contend.

HEALTH CARE ORGANIZATIONS FOR WOMEN: A BRIEF HISTORY

Another issue in the health care marketplace is the growth and diversity of separate organizations for delivery of women's health care. These organizations have a long history in the United States. Sometimes these organizations have arisen out of women's health activism, and as we have seen, the creation of new institutions for women's health care is a familiar repertoire of women's health movements. Women's health organizations also have arisen out of entrepreneurial interests in the health care marketplace. Some of the organizational forms currently in evidence had their origins in earlier eras. This brief historical overview provides the context for an examination of current women's health care organizations.

The earliest American organizational entities providing health services exclusively to women were charitable institutions for maternity care. During the colonial period, almshouses established in larger towns provided health care to poor persons who did not have the benefit of family care and were not deemed deserving of "outdoor relief," that is, assistance under the colonial poor laws in private homes (Abramovitz 1988). "Lying in" wards were established in some almshouses for "undeserving" women, including unmarried women and prostitutes. The almshouse was therefore a socially stigmatizing option of last resort as well as an unsafe setting for childbirth, because of the high risk of infection (Lynaugh 1990). The first U.S. hospitals were founded by philanthropists as an alternative to the almshouse for respectable poor persons (Rosenberg 1987). Maternity hospitals trace their origins to Dr. William Shippen Jr.'s lying-in ward and school for midwives founded in Philadelphia in 1765. Scattered maternity hospitals were in evidence in the early 1800s. For example, the Boston Lying-In Hospital, founded in 1832, was the first such facility in New England and restricted admissions to married or widowed women of good moral character (Speert 1980). Hospital births remained rare, however, owing in part to the high risk of infection in institutional settings.

Although originating as services for the deserving poor, women's hospitals evolved during the second half of the nineteenth century, as did hospitals generally, into institutions that also served the training needs of physicians and nurses, and they increasingly accepted paying patients. The growth of specialty hospitals dedicated to obstetrics or gynecology coincided with the development of the modern hospital and with the emergence of gynecology as a surgical field (Moscucci 1990; Speert 1980). The Woman's Hospital of the State of New York, founded in 1855 by Dr. J. Marion Sims with the help of a group of local women philanthropists, was the first hospital in the United States devoted exclusively to the treatment of gynecological disorders. Other women's hospitals of this era, however, were founded by women physicians who faced overt discrimination within the medical profession, based in part on male physicians' fear of competition. Women regular physicians were excluded from many medical societies, hospital positions, and hospital-based training programs. To obtain training, particularly in surgery, and to create employment opportunities, they founded a number of separate institutions, including dispensaries and hospitals specializing in those fields in which women physicians claimed expertise: the care of women and children, especially maternity and gynecological care. The founders sometimes expected these organizations to be showplaces for women's distinctive forms of medical practice.

Examples of institutions established by early women physicians include the New York Infirmary for Women and Children, which was founded by Elizabeth Blackwell and expanded from a dispensary into a full hospital in 1857, and the New England Hospital for Women and Children, founded in Boston by Marie Zakrzewska, a protege of Blackwell's, in 1862. The New England Hospital had three explicit goals: the care of women by women, training women physicians, and training nurses. (Male physicians served on a consulting staff.) Virginia Drachman's (1984) case study of this hospital shows that it provided benefits to women physicians and nurses in the form of training opportunities and colleagueship, but it is not apparent that its "separatism" provided a different therapeutic milieu for patients. Morantz-Sanchez (1985) compared records of maternity cases at the New England Hospital and at Boston Lying-In, a Harvard-affiliated hospital where the physicians were men, for a period in the late 1800s. She found no significant differences between the institutions in the use of forceps, in infant mortality, or in maternal outcome; however, she found that the women physicians at New England Hospital provided significantly more pain medication, particularly postdelivery. One possibility is that the women physicians were more sympathetic than their male counterparts to their patients' pain and need for postdelivery supportive therapy.

By the turn of the century, the appropriateness of separate women-controlled women's hospitals was debated even among women physicians. They weighed the relative benefits and costs of "separatism" versus "assimilation" as strategies for educating and expanding career opportunities for women physicians and for providing optimum women's health care. Most notably, they debated whether specialist women's hospitals, though often born of necessity, could continue to provide adequate training experiences or attract sufficient resources to maintain technical standards (Drachman 1984; Morantz-Sanchez 1985). The women's hospitals that followed were less the creatures of women physicians than of the growth of the hospital maternity market.

The number of women's hospitals has fluctuated over the years. A spurt of growth in maternity facilities occurred in the 1920s and 1930s, when childbirth moved into the hospital in earnest. At the turn of the century, fewer than 5 percent of births took place in hospitals, but by the 1930s, 60 to 75 percent of births in U.S. cities were in hospitals (Wertz and Wertz 1989). New hospitals, maternity wards, and private women's wings built during this period often were marketing devices to attract paying customers to settings providing rest and comfort and also, in some cases, architectural strategies to reduce infections (Leavitt 1986; Wertz and Wertz 1989). The American Hospital Association reported that there were fifty freestanding hospitals in 1987 admitting women exclusively (AHA 1990), but by 1994 the number had declined to 12, reflecting a general decline in the number of specialty hospitals and an increase in hospital mergers.

The diverse medical marketplace in the mid-nineteenth century had produced some other entrepreneurial health care facilities for women. These were services intended for paying customers and often established by women and marketed as gender-congruent services. They included private clinics catering to a variety of "female complaints" that probably included sexually transmitted diseases (STDs). In addition, abortion clinics often were run by "female physicians," as they called themselves, before abortion became illegal. The best known abortion provider was Madame Restell (really Ann Lohman, an English immigrant with no formal medical training), who was based in New York City in the 1830s to 1870s, with branches in Boston and Philadelphia (Brodie 1994; Gordon 1990; Mohr 1978). Water-cure establishments, which thrived between 1840 and 1900, served both women and men, but many had separate residential programs for women that offered respite from routine activities, cures for female complaints, and treatment by women hydropathic physicians (Cayleff 1987).

In the early twentieth century, organizational forms were invented by women reformers to provide services that were not being offered in general medical practice or in mainstream health care organizations. The first of these, prenatal care clinics and birth control clinics, were the inventions of nurses and women social reformers who intended to make these new services available to all women, including underserved, rural, immigrant, or poor women who were not likely to have access to private physicians. The concept of prenatal care to promote infant health had been devised by public health nurses and women reformers, and the first such services were provided as home visits to pregnant women, often organized by maternity hospitals or municipal health departments (Meckel 1990; Thompson, Walsh, and Merkatz 1990). Prenatal care clinics were established in the 1920s, facilitated by the Sheppard-Towner Act of 1921, which provided government funding for nearly 3,000 permanent clinics nationwide. In these clinics, public health nurses and primarily women physicians provided examinations, counseling, and education in hygiene, nutrition, and infant care to local women. As we saw in chapter 2, private physicians began to perceive these services as competing with their practices, and they organized both to incorporate prenatal and preventive care into medical practice and to oppose the renewal of the Sheppard-Towner program. Though the program expired in 1929, some states maintained the services, at least until the Depression reduced their capacity to continue funding, and in 1935, Title V of the Social Security Act again provided grants to states for prenatal and childcare facilities in rural areas. Other programs, such as the Maternity and Infant Care Projects initiated by the federal government in the 1960s, have helped establish and maintain prenatal care clinics for indigent women operated by public health departments, hospitals, community and migrant health centers, family planning centers, and others. The Alan Guttmacher Institute estimated that in 1987–89, there were at most 5,400 clinic sites involved in the delivery of prenatal care to poor women (Singh, Forrest, and Torres 1989).

Birth control clinics in the United States date to 1916. Margaret Sanger's illegal Brownsville clinic in Brooklyn, though in operation for only ten days before its founders were arrested, served as the prototype for a new organizational form. As we have seen (chapter 2), these clinics at first grew slowly, due to the hostile legal climate, but they expanded in number during the 1920s and 1930s after a number of court rulings began to chip away at the legacy of nineteenth-century restrictions on dissemination of birth control information and devices. The early clinics were privately funded, primarily by wealthy women and foundations, but a series of injections of public funding spurred later growth. These included Title V of the Social Security Act, which permitted family planning services in 1942; the Office of Economic Opportunity, created in 1965, a federal program that established community agencies specifically to provide family planning services for low-income women; and Title X of the Public Health Service Act, enacted in 1970, which provided federal support of family planning programs and contributed to the growth of a national network of clinics in the 1970s, including both private and public organizations, in which low-income women and adolescents were priority clients.[8]

By the 1990s, most family planning clinics were sponsored by state and local public health departments. The largest private sponsor of clinics was the Planned Parenthood Federation of America. The Alan Guttmacher Institute estimated that in 1992, there were between 5,460 and 5,960 clinical sites offering family planning services in the United States (Henshaw and Torres 1994).

These clinics generally provided services in addition to family planning and were important sources of cancer and STD screening services for low-income women. Most of these clinics provided limited services to men (e.g., condom distribution, screening or treatment for STDs), and clinics sponsored by public health departments were more likely than other clinics to serve men. The great majority of clients in most family planning clinics were women, however, owing to the predominance of female forms of contraception and the cultural presumption that women are responsible for birth control (Brindis 1994).

The Women's Health Movement of the 1960s and 1970s gave impetus to several new types of organizations invented and controlled by women to provide health information and services to women. These organizations were developed outside established health care institutions as an explicit alternative to mainstream, male-dominated medical care, and they generally were promoted as a political strategy for demystifying medicine and empowering women to take control of their health. Like the earlier prenatal care clinics and birth control clinics, these organizations were perceived as competing with physicians' practices and as challenging the medical profession's authority to establish standards of care. In some cases, these controversies produced accommodations in which the disputed services eventually were incorporated within mainstream institutions, although the separate organizations for women did not disappear altogether.

As we saw in chapter 2, abortion referral services and abortion clinics (some of them illegal) were established in the 1960s, frequently by women, and the number of abortion clinics grew after abortion was legalized in 1973. Carole Joffe (1995) makes the point that the growth of these clinics was facilitated by a combination of hospitals' reluctance to provide elective abortions and the belief that freestanding centers could provide first-trimester abortions at lower cost and greater convenience to women. Self-help and feminist women's health centers also were founded in the 1970s, giving rise to the term "women's health center." These were consumer-controlled freestanding centers that provided some combination of health education, clinical services, referral services, and advocacy in a supportive environment in which women could be active participants in their care and, in some cases, conduct self-examinations (Ruzek 1978; Worcester and Whatley 1988). Most of these centers specialized in contraceptive and gynecological care, although some offered expanded primary care services. Though few of the original cohort of feminist clinics, which originated in Los Angeles in 1971, survive (Morgen and Julier 1991), the Federation of Feminist Women's Health Centers listed approximately 50 affiliated centers nationwide in 1993.

Freestanding birth centers also grew during the 1970s in response to women's increasing dissatisfaction with hospital-managed childbirth and demands for alternative delivery options. The new centers also responded to the needs of certified nurse-midwives for practice opportunities (Rothman 1991; Wertz and Wertz 1989). Although the first of these centers appeared prior to the 1970s in rural communities, where the the need for obstetrical services was greatest, birth centers expanded to urban areas in 1975, when the Maternity Center Association established a childbearing center in New York City. It was promptly opposed by the local chapter of the American College of Obstetricians and Gynecologists, which declared out-of-hospital deliveries to be unsafe for both mother and child (Speert 1980). Demand for such services grew, however, and by 1987 there were about 160 freestanding birth centers nationwide, some of which were operated by physicians (Rooks et al. 1989). The National Association of Childbearing Centers and the Commission for the Accreditation of Freestanding Birth Centers define "freestanding" centers as those meeting a number of criteria for governance, services, and other factors; hospital-sponsored birth centers (including those physically located within the hospital) may be accredited as "freestanding" birth centers if they meet the criteria.

A second wave of women's health centers appeared in the 1980s and 1990s when hospitals began to establish on-site and off-site programs providing a range of educational and clinical services, sometimes including both outpatient and inpatient components and featuring nurses and women physicians in prominent roles (Looker 1993). Unlike the centers previously described, these second-wave women's health centers were developed largely within mainstream institutions and typically did not provide reproductive services exclusively. In response to the increasingly competitive health care environment, many hospitals sought strategic advantage by marketing services to women, since women were perceived as major consumers of health care as well as the health care decision makers and referral sources for their family members (Dearing et al. 1987). In their advertising, some of these hospital-sponsored centers appealed directly to the preferences of some women for a gender-segregated health care environment, for the convenience of "one-stop shopping," or for treatment by experts in women's health, especially women physicians.

Since 1990, the American Hospital Association's (AHA) annual surveys have tracked the number of hospitals that have a women's health center of some type. The AHA (1993) defines a women's health center as "an area set aside for coordinated educational and treatment services specifically for and promoted to women as provided by this special unit. Services may or may not include obstetrics but include a range of services other than OB." In 1990, 19 percent of U.S. hospitals reported having a women's health center, and by 1994, 32 percent of hospitals reported having a center provided by the hospital or a subsidiary; this represents 49 percent growth between 1990 and 1994 in the number of hospitals with centers.[9] A 1990 AHA report described the typical hospital-sponsored women's health center as an ambulatory care center such as that pioneered by Illinois Masonic Medical Center in Chicago in 1982 (AHA 1990). The AHA surveys, however, do not collect information on the types of services provided in these centers.

Another trend in the 1980s and 1990s was the emergence of freestanding and hospital-based breast care centers founded mainly by physician groups or hospitals. These centers were responding both to a growing market for breast cancer screening services and to the need to integrate breast care services across the various medical specialties and other disciplines involved in the care of patients with breast disease. As distinct from mammography screening facilities, of which there were more than 10,000 nationwide in 1995 (U.S. General Accounting Office 1995), breast centers provided various combinations of screening, education, diagnosis, treatment, rehabilitation, and follow-up services for breast disease (Rabinowitz 1994).

The ongoing debate about "separatism" versus "assimilation" has carried over to the women's health organizations created in the 1980s and 1990s. Underlying this debate are different beliefs about the uniqueness of women's health care needs and about the capacity or willingness of mainstream health care institutions to provide gender-sensitive services. Some of these tensions were apparent in feminist criticisms of the early hospital-sponsored women's health centers in the 1980s. For instance, some advocates of women-controlled care were suspicious of the new hospital-sponsored centers and viewed them as marketing strategies that coopted some aspects of the feminist centers of the 1970s without replicating control by women, holistic care, or other features (Morgen and Julier 1991; Worcester and Whatley 1988). Yet the success of a social movement sometimes is judged on the basis of the degree to which its reforms become institutionalized, and the recent growth of hospital-sponsored women's centers could be viewed as one indicator of the influence of the Women's Health Movement on mainstream health care organizations.

ORGANIZATIONAL AND POLICY ISSUES

Organizational theorists have not paid much attention to women's health care organizations, either as examples of specialization in health services delivery or as examples of the impact of consumers on the development of U.S. health care institutions. This neglect of women's health care organizations is particularly surprising given their early appearance, their diversity, their survivability, and their influence on mainstream health care organizations. Studies of women's health care institutions can potentially shed light on how and why new organizational forms are created, how they change over time, and what factors influence their survival in a changing environment. Furthermore, since women are a majority of both the adult population and health care consumers, organizations that are designed for their health care potentially serve a major market and could account for substantial use of health care resources.

Both their creation in different historical eras and their diversity of services and targeted clientele suggest that U.S. women's health care organizations consist of several distinct organizational types.[10] Each of these types may be subject to different environmental dynamics and survival potential. From the perspective of organizational ecology theory (Hannan and Freeman 1989), different types of women's health centers would be understood as having emerged and grown in number in response to new resource opportunities (or "niches") in the health care environment. For example, specific types of women's health organizations might appear in response to increased purchasing power of a particular subgroup of women as health care consumers (e.g., employed women, insured midlife women); changing demographics (e.g., the aging U.S. population in which women are a majority of the elderly and have specific health care needs such as breast cancer and osteoporosis screening and treatment); or availability of public resources to support delivery of specific health services (e.g., federal funding streams for family planning services and for prenatal and childbirth services for low-income women). New markets might also be created by increased demand, among either consumers or providers, because of changing preferences or beliefs about new women's health services or about the advantages of separate health care organizations for women.

The factors promoting the creation of women's health centers within the hospital sector are of particular interest because of the growth and diversity of hospital-owned or -operated centers during the 1980s and 1990s, when environmental conditions were changing rapidly. Strategic marketing approaches suggest that hospitals identify the female population, or segments thereof, as potential clients and develop service lines to attract that clientele. An important motivating factor is the desire to generate new revenue for the hospital by "capturing the women's market," creating "spinoffs" to other programs and services in the hospital, creating an "ongoing relationship" between the hospital and the woman's family, and enhancing the hospital's image within the community (Dearing et al. 1987). The diffusion of women's health centers within the hospital sector also can be understood from the perspective of institutional theory (Scott 1995), that is, as a consequence of the increasing institutional legitimacy of women's health services and of the efforts of hospitals to adapt to a changing normative climate in women's health care in the early 1990s. In this context, hospitals' sponsorship of women's health centers might serve to enhance their images within the community and to attract both clients and practitioners interested in new models for women's health care.

Why and how women's health care organizations change over time is another question with particular policy significance during a period when the survival of various community-based health care organizations is threatened by dramatic changes in U.S. health care. While the absence of a national health care system in the United States probably encourages the growth and diversity of new organizational forms, there is no mechanism for ensuring the survival of unique organizational options or of services essential to a community's health care when environmental conditions change. In the 1990s, a confluence of environmental trends affecting health care organizations included the uncertainties created by the debate over national health care reform, actual or threatened reductions in public funding programs, restructuring of the Medicaid and Medicare programs, increasing responsibilities for health care programs at the state level, continued growth and increasing diversity of managed care organizations and integrated delivery systems, increasing enrollment of Medicaid and Medicare beneficiaries in managed care programs, and growth in the number of uninsured persons. During the debate over national health care reform in the early 1990s, the role and survivability of "essential community providers" (i.e., health care providers such as community health centers, family planning clinics, and public health department programs that traditionally have served as a "safety net" for vulnerable populations such as poor, low-income, or uninsured persons and adolescents) was recognized as an important access issue during transformational phases in the health care environment (Starr 1994). Although national health care reform was not enacted, threats to federal funding and the rapid growth of managed care, including Medicaid managed care plans, has continued to pose a threat to the survival of safety-net providers (Lipson and Naierman 1996; Rovner 1996). Those safety-net women's health centers that can adapt by finding alternative sources of funding, by negotiating managed care contracts, or by joining integrated delivery systems would be expected to have the best chances of survival.

The key policy questions for women's health care organizations therefore have to do both with the uniqueness of their mission and with their survival in a changing health care environment. The old debate about separatism versus assimilation—that is, does it make sense (in terms of patient satisfaction, quality of care, efficiency, or some other factor) to provide separate health care organizations for women—is still relevant. To date, research comparing the quality of care provided in women's health care organizations with that provided in mixed-gender settings is not available to answer questions about the "value added" of gender-segregated care. The basic dilemma posed by women's health organizations is whether their separateness contributes to or ameliorates the fragmentation of women's basic health care. That is, some women's health centers might exacerbate the fragmentation problem by organizationally segregating or "marginalizing" women's reproductive or other health services; others might provide innovative models of how to integrate and coordinate services optimally, consistent with new holistic conceptions of women's health. In the current health care marketplace, an additional question is whether gender-segregated health care organizations can survive financially. Specifically, can those organizations with innovative models in women's health care or that provide essential care for underserved women in the community remain viable given the growth of managed care and of organized delivery networks?

WOMEN'S HEALTH CARE ORGANIZATIONS IN THE 1990S

To describe the types of health care organizations for women currently in operation and to attempt to answer questions about their missions and prospects, a national study was conducted in 1993–96.[11] This project consisted of the National Survey of Women's Health Centers in operation in 1993–94 (Weisman, Curbow, and Khoury 1995) and case studies of eight innovative centers in 1995. For purposes of this study, "women's health centers" were defined as organizational entities, in both the public and private sectors, providing clinical health services designed for and marketed to women in either hospital-based or freestanding facilities.[12] (See Appendix for a description of the survey and case study methodologies.)

Extrapolating from the survey results from 467 responding organizations, it was estimated that there were 3,600 women's health centers in operation in the United States in 1993, serving an estimated 14.5 million women, or about

14 percent of women ages 15 and over in the U.S. population in 1993. Women made over 28 million visits to these centers in 1993, and of those served, an estimated 7.8 million women used these centers as their usual source of health care. The centers therefore were the point of entry to the health care system for many women. Furthermore, since two-thirds of the centers surveyed reported that their client base was growing, it is likely that increasing numbers of women will receive services in one or more types of women's health centers during their lifetimes. Five types of women's health centers were identified in the survey, based on the responding centers' self-classifications. An estimated 71 percent identified themselves as reproductive health centers, 12 percent as primary care centers, 6 percent as breast care centers, 4 percent as birth or childbearing centers, and 6 percent as various other types of centers providing highly specialized or unusual combinations of services. (These five types of centers are described shortly.)

The survey confirmed that hospital sponsorship of women's health centers was a recent and growing phenomenon. With the exception of reproductive health centers, substantial proportions of all types of women's health centers identified in the survey were owned or operated by hospitals. (See Table 4.2 for selected characteristics of the centers and their clients.) In general, the hospital-owned or -operated centers were newer: 76 percent of them had been founded after 1985, compared with 24 percent of nonhospital centers. Nearly all (98 percent) of the hospitals sponsoring a women's health center were accredited by the Joint Commission on Accreditation of Healthcare Organizations (JCAHO), and 55 percent had some type of academic affiliation, since they provided training for physicians, nurses, or other clinical personnel. Sponsoring hospitals were predominantly private and not-for-profit: 72 percent were private and not-for-profit, 18 percent were government owned (primarily Veterans Administration hospitals), and 10 percent were for-profit. Compared with all U.S. hospitals, those sponsoring women's health centers tended to be relatively large (their average bed size was 342).

Overall, the women's health centers that were owned or operated by hospitals were more market oriented than centers that were not hospital sponsored. That is, the hospital-sponsored centers tended to have been created or redesigned to meet needs and maintain financial viability within a local market. For example, 60 percent of hospital-sponsored centers (vs. 30% of others) reported that a market analysis was conducted prior to opening the center; 86 percent of hospital-sponsored centers (vs. 38% of others) used the services of an internal or external marketing department or firm; among those centers planning to add new services within the next two years, 63 percent of hospital-

Table 4.2
Selected Characteristics of Women's Health Centers and Their Clients

	Primary Care (N = 107)	Reproductive Health (N = 106)	Birth/ Childbearing (N = 69)	Breast Care (N = 102)	Other (N = 83)
Year founded*					
Before 1974	18%	49%	9	3	6
1974–1980	10	25	17	4	6
1981–1990	47	18	50	70	57
1991–1993	25	8	24	23	30
Hospital-owned/operated*	52%	13%	46%	82%	88%
Ownership*					
Private not-for-profit	64%	60%	54%	67%	67%
For-profit	12	22	41	22	26
Public	23	18	6	11	6
Managed care contracts*[a]	36%	39%	54%	59%	46%
Revenue sources, FY 1993[b]					
Private insurance	16%	7%	31%	32%	27%
Private managed care	9	5	12	20	20
Public insurance	28	22	34	33	27
Other government	10	16	2	1	5
Out-of-pocket payments	15	42	17	8	18
Other	22	9	4	6	3
Usual source of care[c]	71%	56%	44%	19%	19%
Client ages[d]					
Under 18	7%	15%	10%	0%	6%
18–39	59	73	78	17	43
40–64	27	10	10	60	38
65 and over	8	1	1	23	11
Client race/ethnicity[d]					
White, non-Hispanic	68%	64%	73%	75%	75%
African American	17	20	9	14	14
Hispanic/Latina	10	9	13	7	8
Other	6	6	5	5	4
Client health insurance[d]					
Private indemnity	27%	11%	30%	29%	27%
Private managed care	15	7	13	20	23
Medicaid	19	26	35	9	21
Medicare	7	2	1	28	15
Military/other	17	5	4	6	8
None	15	47	17	9	7

* The cross-tabulation of center type by the given characteristic is statistically significant ($p < .05$) by the chi square test.

[a] Percentage of centers with any formal contracts with HMOs or PPOs.

[b] Mean percentage of revenues from each source. "Other" includes support from the sponsoring institution, if any. Kruskal-Wallis analysis of variance is significant ($p < .05$) for all revenue sources.

[c] Mean percentage of clients who relied on the center as their usual source of care in 1993. Kruskal-Wallis analysis of variance is significant ($p < .001$). In tests for multiple comparisons, the mean for primary care centers was significantly different ($p < .05$) from all other centers, and the means for breast and "other" centers were significantly different ($p < .05$) from all others.

[d] Mean percentages. Kruskal-Wallis analysis of variance is significant ($p < .05$) for all variables except percentage Hispanic/Latina and other race/ethnicity.

sponsored centers (vs. 47% of others) reported that the plans were based on a market analysis; 67 percent of hospital-sponsored centers (vs. 54% of others) reported that "increasing market share" was very important for continued viability; and 58 percent of hospital-sponsored centers (vs. 44% percent of others) reported that "expanding into new markets" was very important for continued viability. Compared with other centers, hospital-sponsored centers were more likely to report targeting employed women (including employees of the hospital), high-income women, privately insured women, midlife women, and senior women; centers that were not hospital sponsored were more likely to target women of reproductive age and subgroups of women who often experience barriers to care, including Medicaid recipients, uninsured women, lesbian women, adolescents, and minority women. Compared with other centers, hospital-sponsored centers received significantly more of their revenue in fiscal year 1993 from public and private health insurance payments or private managed care contracts; other centers received more revenue than hospital-sponsored centers from out-of-pocket patient payments, government grants and contracts, and donations.

An advantage that hospital-sponsored centers had over other centers was their access to the financial, clinical, and administrative resources of the hospital. For example, 85 percent of the hospital-sponsored centers received their start-up funds from the hospital, whereas 85 percent of centers that were not sponsored by hospitals reported that their start-up funding came from private investors, contributions, or government grants or contracts. Hospital-sponsored centers were more likely than nonhospital centers to have on-site pharmacies and radiology departments, as well as the part-time services of hospital physicians and other clinical personnel and an available referral network. Seventy-five percent of hospital-sponsored centers used the marketing department of the hospital, whereas 20 percent of centers that were not hospital-sponsored employed their own marketing director, and 10 percent employed an outside marketing firm. On the other hand, hospital-sponsored centers typically had to demonstrate their financial benefit to the hospital to survive. Seventy-two percent of the hospital-sponsored centers reported that "commitment to attracting women to the hospital" was a core value of the center, and 52 percent of the hospital-sponsored centers (vs. 42% of others) reported that a commitment to "enhanced profitability" was a core value of the center. Among the hospital-sponsored centers, 45 percent had separate accounting for financial purposes (as opposed to be being accounted as part of another department or program within the hospital), and 55 percent had information systems for tracking referrals of patients for outpatient services (e.g., outpatient surgery, radiology) or admissions to the hospital. The latter is important both for patient follow-up and for monitoring revenues generated by center patients in other hospital services.

The women's health centers in operation in 1993 had highly diverse organizational structures, operated in different markets, and confronted somewhat different challenges for the future. The diversity among women's health centers also reflected their historic origins in different periods in the development of the U.S. health care system. The five types of centers (reproductive health, primary care, birth or childbearing, breast care, and others) were characterized by different organizational structures, staffing patterns, service mixes, clientele, financial profiles, mission and philosophies, and approaches to quality improvement, marketing, and planning.

Reproductive Health Centers

Reproductive health centers were the most numerous and oldest type of women's health center (the oldest reproductive health center in the sample was founded in 1925). The sample included both public and private, primarily non-hospital-sponsored centers. The nonhospital centers included Planned Parenthood affiliates, feminist and other independent health centers, public health department clinics, and centers owned by physician groups. The centers all provided contraceptive counseling and family planning services (including a wider range of contraceptive options than primary care centers in the sample), and 90 percent or more provided routine gynecological care, screening and treatment for STDs, and pregnancy tests. While one-third of these centers provided prenatal examinations, only 15 percent provided vaginal deliveries. About one-half of the centers in this sample were abortion providers (vs. 11% of primary care centers), and all centers that provided abortions also provided counseling and clinical services in addition to abortions. Although they served as the usual source of care for, on average, 56 percent of their clients, reproductive health centers were less likely than the primary care centers to provide general physical examinations, certain preventive tests (e.g., blood pressure checks, immunizations, tuberculosis tests), diagnosis and treatment of menstrual problems, and mental health services. Among a set of twelve mental health services measured, the most frequently provided service in reproductive health centers was rape or sexual abuse counseling, but only 27 percent of these centers provided this counseling.

Compared with other types of women's health centers, reproductive health centers served more adolescents and uninsured women. In 1993, nearly half of the women served in these centers had no health insurance or were self-paying, and on average, 42 percent of these centers' revenues in fiscal year 1993 were from direct patient payments. (On average, 26 percent of the patients served in these centers were Medicaid recipients.) Compared with other types of centers, reproductive health centers also provided reduced rates or "no charge" care to a larger percentage of patients. Forty-four percent of these centers received Title X funds, 26 percent received Title V (maternal and child health) funds, and 24 percent received Title XX (Social Services Block Grant) funds. Thus a substantial proportion of these centers could be regarded as "safety net" providers.

The reproductive centers, not surprisingly, reported the bleakest financial picture of all types of women's health centers: 31 percent reported that their fiscal year 1993 financial performance was worse than 1992, and 24 percent projected worse financial performance for fiscal 1994 than for the previous year. Reductions in public funding (e.g., Title X),[13] the growth of managed care, and, among abortion providers, increased expenses to protect the centers from antiabortion violence were all contributing to financial problems in these centers and were jeopardizing their ability to continue to provide uncompensated care. Reproductive centers also appeared to have been slower than other types of women's health centers to adapt to managed care: these centers had proportionately fewer managed care patients than other types of centers and the lowest average percentage of revenues from managed care contracts. This could have been due, in part, to the effects of legislation in the mid-1980s exempting family planning services from the requirements of Medicaid managed care contracts, rather than providing for their integration; though intended to preserve women's freedom to choose their family planning providers, the family planning "carve out" had the unintended consequence of isolating these centers during a critical period in the growth of Medicaid managed care networks (Rosenbaum et al. 1995).

Compared with other types of women's health centers, the reproductive centers planned the most changes within the next two years: 39 percent of the centers planned to acquire new managed care contracts, and 75 percent planned to add new services. Most notably, 26 percent planned to expand primary care services, 22 percent planned to add midlife women's services, 11 percent planned to add new services for men, and 10 percent planned to add pregnancy termination services, including medical abortions. Planned Parenthood centers were significantly more likely than other types of reproductive health centers to report planning to expand primary care services for women, but these centers also were struggling with how to reconcile their traditional mission as providers and advocates of women's reproductive services with the pressures to adapt in an increasingly competitive market.

Of all types of women's health centers, reproductive health centers were the most threatened by changes in the health care system, and their survival has important implications for health care access among the underserved subpopulations of women who rely upon these centers for reproductive health services or for their basic health care. To the extent that these centers make successful transitions to primary care, their clients would, potentially, have access to a wider range of services and to more coordinated health care.

Primary Care Centers

Primary care centers were most likely to integrate the reproductive and nonreproductive components of women's basic health care, but they comprised only 12 percent of women's health centers nationwide at the time of the survey. This percentage could grow substantially, however, if a sizable proportion of reproductive health centers were to make a successful transition to primary care, or if the trend for hospitals to sponsor primary care centers continues. About half of the primary care centers were hospital-owned or -operated, and the hospital-sponsored centers were newer: 39 percent of the hospital-sponsored centers had been founded after 1990, compared with only 5 percent of the nonhospital centers. Hospital-sponsored primary care centers included those in academic medical centers, community hospitals, and Veterans Administration hospitals, where women's health services had begun to be expanded as a result of the Women Veterans Health Program Act of 1992.

Primary care centers provided a wider range of well-woman services than all other types of women's health centers studied, and they came closest to an integrated model of women's comprehensive primary care. These centers served as the usual source of care for, on average, 71 percent of their clients, and they provided general medical examinations, including routine gynecological care and clinical preventive services, as well as a range of other clinical services. Primary care centers were more likely than the other types of centers to provide mental health services: most of these centers provided rape and sexual abuse counseling (59% of centers), screening for anxiety or depressive disorders (58%), and stress management (57%). However, fewer primary care centers provided alcohol abuse counseling or treatment (37%), drug abuse counseling or treatment (31%), or screening and treatment for violent injuries (31%). Primary care centers also were more likely than other types of centers to provide diagnosis and treatment of menstrual problems (91% of centers), menopause counseling (78%), and hormone therapy (68%). With the exception of nutritional counseling, primary care centers were no more likely than other types of women's health centers to provide nontraditional therapies: 81 percent of primary care centers provided nutritional counseling, compared with 41 percent of all others. However, fewer than 10 percent of all types of centers reported providing massage therapy, podiatry, chiropractic services, herbal medicine, naturopathy, or acupuncture.

Comprehensive primary care centers serving women in the general community (as opposed to closed populations of women's college students or women veterans) were of three general types. First, *hospital-sponsored women's primary care centers* typically were owned or operated by academic medical centers or private not-for-profit community hospitals. These centers were located either in dedicated space within the hospital facility or in ambulatory care buildings, and they typically were directed by women internists or obstetrician-gynecologists. Physicians from several specialties were affiliated with these centers, usually on a part-time or contractual basis, and other disciplines such as nursing and psychology also were represented. These centers used other hospital clinical services (e.g., radiology) and administrative services (e.g., marketing, billing), and they coordinated referrals for patients within the hospital. Clients included employees of the hospital as well as women in the community, including women enrolled in managed care plans. Some academically affiliated centers provided medical training in women's health and were involved in women's health research.

The second type of primary care center was the *nonhospital not-for-profit center.* This type included formerly reproductive health centers (e.g., some Planned Parenthood affiliates and feminist women's health centers) that recently had expanded services to include nonreproductive components of women's primary care, as well as other community-based health centers. These centers typically employed primary care physicians and other providers (e.g., nurse practitioners) and had arrangements with local hospitals, physician groups, or community agencies to provide specialized services (such as radiology), backup care, or educational or social services. These centers were more likely than other primary care centers to be safety-net providers, and they often relied on volunteers for some patient and administrative services. The client bases of these centers often included substantial proportions of lower-income, disadvantaged, or adolescent patients. The centers usually had contracts to serve Medicaid managed care patients, sometimes for specialized services, and sometimes served as primary care providers for private managed care enrollees.

The third type of primary care center was the *nonhospital for-profit center.* These centers were founded by physician groups, advanced practice nurses, or other entrepreneurs. Often they distinguished themselves in local markets by featuring women providers or offering unique combinations of services. (For example, the for-profit Spence Centers for Women's Health, which originated in Cambridge, Massachusetts in 1995, combine traditional primary care medicine with nontraditional services [e.g., muscular therapy, acupuncture] [Braus 1997].) Arrangements with local hospitals were common (e.g., contractual arrangements for a hospital to operate the center's radiology service). These centers typically served private and/or Medicaid managed care enrollees as well as patients with private indemnity insurance.

Birth, Breast Care, and Other Centers

Birth or childbearing centers were diverse and included both hospital-sponsored and independent centers. Nearly half of these centers were owned or operated by hospitals, and the hospital-sponsored centers had been established more recently (62% had been founded after 1984 compared with 49% of nonhospital centers). Forty-one percent of birth centers were for-profit enterprises (more than any other type of women's health center), and nonhospital centers were significantly more likely than hospital-sponsored centers to be for-profit. All of these centers provided vaginal deliveries, 45 percent provided cesarean sections, 77 percent provided prenatal care, and 88 percent offered childbirth education classes. Compared with hospital-sponsored centers, nonhospital birth centers were significantly more likely to employ certified nurse-midwives and to provide prenatal, primary, and preventive care, including family planning services. Hospital-sponsored centers, on the other hand, provided more cesarean sections, sterilizations, and other surgical and high-technology care (Khoury, Summers, and Weisman, forthcoming). Birth centers had the most optimistic financial outlook for fiscal 1994 of all types of women's health centers; 68 percent projected better financial performance in fiscal 1994 than in fiscal 1993, possibly because of perceived effects of the Medicaid expansions for pregnant women.

Breast care centers were a relatively new type of women's health center: 78 percent were under ten years old at the time of the survey. Most (82%) were hospital sponsored. These centers were of two types: about 20 percent provided primarily breast screening and imaging services, while 80 percent pro-vided more comprehensive breast care services, including diagnostic and treatment services for benign breast disease and/or breast cancer in inte-grated programs. The philosophy of the comprehensive breast care centers was to provide multidisciplinary services over the continuum of care for breast disease, with attention to the woman's physical, psychological, and so-cial needs. Ninety-five percent of breast centers provided screening and/or di-agnostic mammography (83% had on-site radiology), 93 percent provided breast self-examination instruction, 71 percent provided breast biopsies, 70 percent provided breast ultrasound, 68 percent provided physical breast ex-aminations, 37 percent provided breast cancer treatment, and 19 percent had mobile service units. Breast centers served an older clientele than other types of women's health centers, and an average of 28 percent of their clients were Medicare beneficiaries. Breast centers reported a generally favorable financial picture: 52 percent reported that their financial performance in fiscal year 1993 was an improvement over the previous year, and 56 percent projected im-proved financial performance for fiscal 1994.

The "other" women's health centers were primarily hospital owned or op-erated (88%) and relatively new. They included a mix of models. Nearly half were centers offering specialized combinations of outpatient services (e.g., "breast and bone" imaging). About one in four of the "other" centers provided mainly education and referrals, with minimal clinical services, such as breast examinations or blood pressure checks. These entities often were an "um-brella" coordinating center for the hospital's services for women. Finally, about one in four were hospital inpatient units or pavilions focused primarily on obstetrics and gynecological surgery. Many of the "other" centers had generic names such as "The Center for Women's Health" that did not accu-rately communicate the specialized or limited nature of their services. This was likely to be confusing to consumers, particularly to those seeking more in-tegrated care, and to have contributed to the perception, noted above, that many of the newer hospital-sponsored women's health centers were merely marketing devices to attract women to the hospital.

Summary

Women's health centers are diverse in organizational form, the service mix provided, and the clients served. The number and types of centers, particu-larly in the hospital sector, have grown. Although a variety of highly specialized hospital-sponsored women's health centers have appeared in recent years, a trend toward provision of more comprehensive women's health services was apparent in the growing number of primary care centers and in some reproductive centers' plans for expansion into primary care. Accordingly, women's health centers may include some of the most innovative approaches to primary care available to women in the U.S. health care marketplace.

THE VALUES OF WOMEN-CENTERED CARE

To what extent do women's health centers subscribe to values or orientations that reflect emerging conceptions of what women's health care ought to be? Data to address this question include some quantitative indicators of the dimensions of women-centered care as well as qualitiative information from the case studies of model women's health centers.

Due to the absence of standards or guidelines for women's health centers, the Jacobs Institute of Women's Health convened a 1993 conference "Women's Health Centers: Review, Assessment, and Goals" in part to develop a normative conception of women-centered care. The conference proposed a set of "philosophical core values" for women's health services, regardless of organizational form, level of care, or populations served. The five core values are as follows: (1) mutual respect between women and health professionals (including shared decision making and quality communication), (2) provision of comprehensive care with a prevention and wellness focus, (3) a multidisciplinary team approach that crosses the boundaries of body systems and medical specialties, (4) education as an integral part of women's health (including community programs, education of both consumers and providers in women's health, and women's health research), and (5) quality improvement focusing on clinical outcomes and meeting professional standards (Schaps et al. 1993). (These values might be considered equally relevant to men's health care, but they were specifically responding to the fragmentation and long-standing criticisms of women's health care.) This specification of core values, however, did not explicitly address the inclusion of nonmedical or alternative services that might be relevant to a more holistic approach to women's health care, nor did it address the need to improve women's access to care through outreach to traditionally underserved subgroups of women or by providing expanded hours of operation (e.g., evenings and weekends), transportation, childcare facilities, or culturally sensitive services. These latter topics also could be considered components of women-centered care.

Table 4.3 shows how the five types of women's health centers compare on indicators of core values. There was near uniformity across centers on the value of mutual respect between women and providers. The administrators of nearly all centers, regardless of type, reported having implemented a commitment to shared decision making between women and health professionals, a commitment to a sensitive and caring attitude toward women, and a commitment to empowering women to take control of their health. The case studies provided some insights into how centers operationalized these values. For example, clinical personnel in the case study centers reported that they emphasize the importance of forming "partnerships" with women by encouraging joint decision making about their care; by providing patients with multiple opportunities to talk with their primary providers, both during visits and by telephone or e-mail; by providing adequate time during patient visits for patients to ask questions and receive the information they need; and by providing information to patients—especially about test results and treatment plans—in both oral and written form. Physicians also recognized women's preferences, which the patient focus groups confirmed, to be fully clothed during the "talk" portion of the visit.

Physicians reported increased pressures to shorten visits and to conduct both the "talk" and physician examination portions of visits in the examining room. Providers in a number of centers were concerned about finding ways to preserve time for communication and for patient education and counseling, despite current pressures to conduct visits more efficiently. In all of the case study centers, patients reported in focus groups that their ability to communicate directly with their physicians was among the attributes they appreciated the most about women's health centers, compared with other places where they had previously received health care. Patients valued communication, furthermore, not only for the informational content, but also for the socioemotional benefits (e.g., "the doctor made me feel better," "the doctor told me not to worry about the billing problem").

As to the comprehensiveness of care, differences among centers in the survey reflected their service orientations. Administrators of primary care centers were most likely to report a commitment to primary and/or preventive care, to a holistic approach to care, and to "one-stop shopping." Reproductive health centers were least likely of all centers to report that commitment to primary and/or preventive care was an implemented core value; this could reflect the discrepancy between these centers' plans for change (e.g., expansion of primary care services) and their current status. Breast care centers were the least likely to report a commitment to holistic health care, probably reflecting their highly specialized services, although the more comprehensive breast care centers often espouse a holistic approach to care of the breast cancer patient. Primary care centers reported providing significantly more preventive and other clinical services than all other types of centers, out of a total of 92 services measured, as well as significantly more mental health services.

Commitment to a multidisciplinary team approach to women's health care was reported to be an implemented core value in a majority of all types of centers except reproductive health centers. The staffing patterns of the centers were examined for disciplinary mix by counting the number of physician specialties and the number of other types of providers (e.g., nurse practitioners, certified nurse-midwives, registered nurses, physician assistants, social workers, psychologists, health educators, radiology technologists, nutritionists) employed by the center on either a full-time or part-time basis. With regard to physician specialties, primary care centers were significantly more multidisciplinary than other types of centers, and birth and "other" centers were least multidisciplinary. Reproductive health centers, however, employed a more diverse set of nonphysician providers than all types of centers except primary care centers. In particular, reproductive health centers were significantly more likely than all other types of centers to employ nurse practitioners. Finally, primary care centers were more likely than other types of centers to have any type of mental health provider (psychiatrist, psychologist, or social worker) on staff.

The administrators and providers in all of the case study centers valued a multidisciplinary team approach to care delivery, and several of the centers, including the comprehensive breast care centers, highlighted this aspect of their services in marketing. The informants in the case studies agreed that optimal health care crosses the boundaries of body systems and treats the whole woman, including her physical and psychosocial needs. In addition, there was consensus that both physicians and nonphysicians are required to provide optimum care. In seven of the eight case study centers, patients were served by a team of physicians and nonphysician providers, the latter including primarily registered nurses, nurse practitioners, and physician assistants. (The exception was a center operated by nurse practitioners, in which medical services were provided only through referrals.) In some of the primary care centers, women were given the choice of receiving routine well-woman examinations from either a physician or a nurse practitioner; often a benefit to the patient of opting for a nurse practitioner was a shorter wait for an appointment. In the focus groups, patients reported that they found care by nurse practitioners to be highly acceptable.

Table 4.3
Indicators of Core Values of "Women-Centered" Care in Women's Health Centers[a]

	Primary Care (N = 107)	Reproductive Health (N = 106)	Birth/ Childbearing (N = 69)	Breast (N = 102)	Other (N = 83)
Mutual respect between women and providers					
Commitment to shared decision making[b]	90%	90%	90%	82%	85%
Commitment to sensitive and caring attitude toward women[b]	98%	99%	98%	97%	100%
Commitment to empowering women to take control of health[b]	90%	92%	88%	89%	90%
Comprehensive care: prevention and wellness					
Commitment to primary and/or preventive care	92%	52%	79%	64%	78%
Commitment to a holistic approach to health care	68%	45%	73%	33%	58%
Commitment to "one-stop shopping"	51%	16%	28%	25%	27%
Number clinical services (mean)[c]	37.6	26.8	26.7	7.1	19.7
Provides two or more mental health services	75%	18%	22%	10%	49%
Multidisciplinary team approach					
Commitment to a multidisciplinary team approach	67%	43%	71%	54%	67%
Physician specialties (mean)[d]	1.7	1.3	0.5	1.2	0.8
Other types of providers (mean)[e]	3.7	4.1	3.2	2.2	3.0
Any mental health providers[f]	43%	34%	20%	15%	31%
Education of consumers and providers					
Provides speakers bureau	60%	68%	74%	78%	81%

Provides no-cost community service programs	33%	26%	41%	61%	55%
Provides community agency referral service	92%	94%	78%	77%	88%
Training site for physicians, nurses, or others	58%	67%	82%	45%	42%
Commitment to conducting women's health research[b]	18%	19%	24%	27%	21%
Trains providers in results of women's health research[b]	32%	36%	29%	32%	34%
Quality improvement					
Center is accredited	65%	65%	77%	95%	95%
Physicians who are board certified[g]	83%	71%	70%	92%	74%
Uses quality indicators to assess performance	47%	64%	71%	68%	70%
Monitors patient outcomes	62%	76%	94%	72%	76%

a The five "philosophical core values" of women-centered care are described by Schaps et al. (1993). Cross-tabulations between center type and items are significant ($p < .05$) unless otherwise noted.

b Differences between types of centers are not statistically significant ($p \geq .05$).

c Clinical services provided in centers range from 1 to 74 (out of a possible 92 preventive and treatment services measured). Kruskal-Wallis analysis of variance is significant ($p < .001$). In tests for multiple comparisons, the means for primary care centers and breast centers were significantly different ($p < .05$) from all others.

d Kruskal-Wallis analysis of variance is significant ($p < .001$). In tests for multiple comparisons, the mean number of physician specialties in primary care centers was significantly different ($p < .05$) from all other centers, and the means for birth and "other" centers were significantly different ($p < .05$) from all others..

e Kruskal-Wallis analysis of variance is significant ($p < .001$). In tests for multiple comparisons, the mean number of nonphysician provider groups in breast care centers is significantly different ($p < .05$) from all other centers, and the mean for reproductive centers is significantly different ($p < .05$) from birth, breast, and other centers.

f Mental health providers included psychiatrists, psychologists, or social workers.

g Mean percentage of center-affiliated physicians who are board certified in their principal specialty. The mean percentage for breast centers is significantly different ($p < .05$) from reproductive health and birth centers.

Although the education of consumers and providers could be regarded as a key factor in improving women's health, centers differed in their educational activities. Nearly all of the centers (98%) provided printed health information (e.g., brochures, newsletters) for their patients and, as we have seen, about 90 percent of all centers reported commitment to empowering women to take control of their health. On other educational dimensions, however, there was variation by type of center. Community outreach programs, such as speakers bureaus and no-cost community service programs, were provided most frequently by "other" centers and by breast care centers; this probably reflects both the resources available to these primarily hospital-sponsored centers and their commitment to attracting women in the community to the sponsoring institution. Breast care centers and birth centers were less likely than other centers to provide community agency referral services. Breast care centers and "other" centers were least likely to be training sites for physicians, nurses, or other clinical personnel, and birth centers were most likely to provide clinical training.

There were no significant differences among types of women's health centers on commitment to conducting women's health research (only about one in five centers did so) or in providing in-service training programs on the results of women's health research (only about one in three centers provided training.) Given the recent emphasis on women's health research and educational reforms, these findings reflect surprisingly little commitment within women's health centers to expanding the knowledge base. Most of the case study centers, however, were involved in research and training, and they provided educational opportunities for providers through research conferences, case conferences, or journal clubs. One case study center had a residency training program in women's health. The greater commitment of the case study centers, compared with the surveyed centers, to research and training suggests that the potential contribution of women's health centers in these areas has not been realized.

With regard to quality improvement indicators, accreditation status was strongly associated with hospital sponsorship: 98 percent of hospital-sponsored centers were accredited on the basis of the hospital's accreditation or another type of accreditation, while only 54 percent of nonhospital centers were accredited by some appropriate organization or agency. Probably reflecting their higher rate of affiliation with academic medical centers, breast care centers and primary care centers had the highest average percentage of board-certified physicians. As to quality measurement activities, primary care centers were less likely than other types of centers to use quality indicators to assess the center's performance over time and were less likely to monitor patient outcomes; birth centers were most likely to monitor patient outcomes. The most frequently reported quality improvement activities used by the centers were patient satisfaction surveys and providing continuing education opportunities for clinicians.

In the case study centers, both providers and administrators recognized the need for women's health centers to be able to demonstrate performance—or the "value added" of women-centered care—using methods other than patient retention and satisfaction measures. Until recently, these centers had regarded themselves as successful if they articulated women-centered missions, if patient volume was growing, if patient retention was high, or if they were functioning "at capacity." The growth of managed care and increasing competition in the health care marketplace seemed to be driving the recognition in these centers that to compete, they would need to demonstrate quality in terms of patient care process or outcomes, or their performance in relation to "benchmarks" for women's health care.

Finally, centers differed in their specific efforts to target underserved groups of women and to improve access to care for women in the community. With respect to the specific segments of the female population currently targeted, primary care centers, reproductive health centers, and birth centers were differentiated from breast care and "other" centers primarily by the age groups targeted: the former centers targeted women of reproductive age, and the latter targeted midlife or senior women. In addition, reproductive health centers and birth centers were more likely than other types of centers to target low-income, Medicaid, and uninsured women. Reproductive health centers were more likely than other centers to target minority women and lesbian women. Birth centers were most likely to target rural women. With regard to any new segments of the female population the centers planned to target within the next two years, only reproductive health centers reported substantial plans for change: about one-fourth of reproductive health centers reported planning to target privately insured women, and one-third planned to target midlife or senior women. This was a marketing strategy to enhance revenue by attracting a wider patient population.

Service accessibility also varied by type of center. Primary care centers were least likely to have any evening or weekend hours of operation (49% vs. 71% of other centers) but most likely to provide transportation services for clients (31% vs. 15% of other centers). Reproductive health centers were most likely to provide translator/interpreter services (70% vs. 52% of other centers), even though they did not serve a higher proportion of non-English-speaking clients than other types of centers. Only 10 percent of centers provided any type of childcare facilities, and there was no difference by type of center.

In sum, all types of women's health centers were highly committed to mutual respect between providers and patients, to shared decision making, and to providing health information. On most other indicators of women-centered care, however, there was variation by type of center. Comparing the two types of centers that serve as the usual source of care for most of their clients—primary care and reproductive health centers—the former were more oriented to prevention and wellness and to one-stop shopping; they provided more comprehensive services (including more mental health services); and they were most multidisciplinary, at least with regard to the medical specialties. There was room for improvement in all types of women's health centers on the dimensions of comprehensiveness of care, multidisciplinary teamwork, consumer education and community outreach, involvement in women's health research and training, quality improvement methods, and extending access.

CONTROL BY WOMEN

How women-controlled are women's health centers, and does being controlled by women make a difference in services provided or in the values of women-centered care? In the women's health centers founded during the Women's Health Movement of the 1960s and 1970s, control by women (usually consumers) had been a defining feature and an explicit challenge to male-dominated, mainstream health care. By the 1980s and 1990s, women were gaining influence as health care providers and as managers within mainstream health organizations, and they were thought to serve in key administrative and clinical roles in some second-wave women's health centers.

Table 4.4 presents some indicators of control by women in women's health centers. With regard to leadership, the five types of centers were equally likely to have women administrators, and overall, 87 percent of centers were administered by women. These administrators were most often professional managers or registered nurses. Centers' medical or clinical directors were less likely than the administrators to be female, and primary care centers were most likely to have a woman in this role: 64 percent of primary care centers had a woman medical director, most often an obstetrician-gynecologist or an internist. One-half of the birth centers had a woman medical or clinical director, most often an obstetrician-gynecologist or a certified nurse-

Table 4.4
Indicators of "Women Control" in Women's Health Centers (%)

	Primary Care (N = 107)	Reproductive Health (N = 106)	Birth/ Childbearing (N = 69)	Breast Care (N = 102)	Other (N = 83)
Woman administrator[a]	89	89	81	88	89
Woman medical/clinical director	64	35	50	35	35
Woman board chair[b]	46	70	57	40	36
% Women board members[b]	53	61	48	42	46
% Women physicians[c]	57	33	17	24	18
Commitment to women providers[d]	59	43	60	35	32
Commitment to feminist ideology[e]	33	43	28	12	16

[a] Differences between types of centers are not statistically significant ($p \geq .05$).

[b] Among centers that report to a governing body of some kind (73% of all centers).

[c] Mean percentage of center-affiliated physicians who are women. The mean percentage for primary care centers is significantly different ($p < .05$) from the other groups.

[d] "Commitment to provision of women's health care by women providers" is an implemented core value of the center.

[e] "Commitment to a feminist ideology" is an implemented core value of the center.

midwife. Governance varied by type of center and also depended upon hospital sponsorship. Among the centers that reported to a governing body of some kind (e.g., a board of directors governing the center or its sponsoring institution, or an advisory council, or both), reproductive health centers and birth centers were most likely to have boards chaired by women, and the boards of reproductive health centers had the highest percentage of women voting members. Centers that were hospital-sponsored were less likely than nonhospital centers to have women-controlled boards.

With regard to the providers practicing in the centers, only 16 percent of the centers had all-women medical staffs, and on average, centers reported that 32 percent of their physicians were women. Primary care centers had the highest average percentage of women physicians (57%), followed by reproductive health centers (33%). Centers did not differ with respect to the gender composition of nonphysician clinical staff. On average, 93 percent of these staff members were women. Administrators of primary care centers and birth centers were most likely to report that commitment to gender-congruent care—that is, provision of women's health care by women providers—was an implemented core value of the center. In addition, centers that were not sponsored by hospitals were more likely than hospital-sponsored centers to report commitment to women providers (56% vs. 37%). Contrary to expectations, centers founded after 1985 were more likely than older centers to report a commitment to women providers, perhaps because women physicians were more numerous by the late 1980s than they had been in previous decades; by 1985, women were 15 percent of all physicians, nearly double their proportion in 1970 (AMA 1993). Consequently, newer women's health centers could more realistically expect to recruit women physicians.

Commitment to a "feminist" ideology (which was not defined in the survey question) was associated with center type and with identification with the era of the Women's Health Movement. Most centers (56%) that were founded in the 1960s and 1970s described themselves as committed to a feminist ideology; this was significantly higher than among centers founded before 1960 (36%) or from 1980 on (28%). Centers affiliated with the Federation of Feminist Women's Health Centers or the National Women's Health Network (about 10% of all centers surveyed, primarily reproductive health and primary care centers) were significantly more likely than other centers to report a commitment to a feminist ideology. Overall, the administrators of reproductive health centers were more likely than those in other types of centers to report that commitment to a feminist ideology was an implemented core value. Centers that were not sponsored by hospitals were significantly more likely than hospital-sponsored to report commitment to a feminist ideology (43% vs. 14%).

To determine whether being controlled by women is associated with women-centered values, each center was assigned a score on a four-item index of clinical control by women (having a female medical or clinical director, having an all-woman medical staff, commitment to women providers, and commitment to feminist ideology) and a score on a ten-item index of women-centered values (including selected indicators of comprehensiveness, multidisciplinary team approach, education, and quality improvement from Table 4.3). The score on women-centered values was regressed on a set of predictors including control by women, type of center, year the center was founded, and hospital sponsorship. Greater control by women had a statistically significant, positive effect on women-centered values, independent of the other predictors.

The case studies provided some perspective on how center personnel and patients regard control by women. All eight of the case study centers had either a woman administrator or a woman clinical director, and most of these centers had been founded by women. Clinical and administrative personnel in all of the case studies reported that women providers, particularly physicians, were an asset to a women's health center. This opinion seemed to be based on two beliefs: that some patients were more comfortable with or preferred women physicians and that women physicians gave the centers credibility and were an asset in marketing. Simultaneously, informants recognized that there were insufficient numbers of available women physicians, particularly in the surgical specialties required in breast care centers, to expect to staff women's health centers exclusively with women. Informants in several of the centers expressed the opinion that it was the center's culture, not the gender of providers, that was most important; they believed that if the center did a good job implementing women-centered values, then having some providers who were men would be acceptable to clients. They also believed, however, that having women in leadership roles was essential for creating a women-centered culture.

The patients who participated in the case study focus groups generally expressed a preference for women providers. About 75 percent of these women reported in questionnaires that they preferred to be treated by women. In the 1993 Survey of Women's Health, only 14 percent of women ages 18 and over in the general population reported that they "somewhat" or "strongly" preferred a physician who is a woman. (Seventy-four percent of women in the survey reported that they "didn't have any preferences between male and female physicians.") That women attending women's health centers held a stronger preference than those in the general population for gender-congruent health care suggests that these women had selected themselves into women's health centers in part because of this preference, or that they had formed the preference after experiencing treatment by women physicians within the women's health center.

In sum, many of the women health centers studied had some control by women, and greater control by women was associated with having more of the attributes of women-centered care. A plausible interpretation of these findings is that clinical control by women increases women-centered values, although it is also possible that organizations with these values are more likely to attract women providers. The case studies, however, suggest that control by women, or at least a major female presence on the medical staff, was an explicit strategy both to create a women-centered culture of care and to attract and retain patients.

WOMEN'S HEALTH CENTERS AND MANAGED CARE

A crosscutting issue for women's health centers, regardless of type or region of the country, was the challenge posed by the growth of managed care. The challenges perceived by center administrators and providers were both financial and substantive. The growth of Medicaid managed care, which had caused some women's health centers to lose Medicaid patients to other primary care providers, and the difficulties of obtaining managed care contracts were reported by a number of centers. In addition, the increasing demands for efficiency in managed care were compelling some centers to change some elements of service delivery, such as reducing the amount of time physicians spent per patient visit. Since provider-patient communication is believed to be a critical component of primary care and an aspect of care that is highly valued by women patients, this trend was perceived as potentially threatening some centers' women-centered missions.

Nevertheless, most center administrators reported that they recognized the importance of participation in managed care networks for their center's viability: 55 percent reported that obtaining managed care contracts was "very important" for continued viability, and 26 percent reported that it was "moderately important." Nearly half (46%) of centers had at least one managed care (HMO or PPO) contract at the time of the survey and were serving either public or private managed care patients.[14] Primary care and reproductive health centers were least likely to have managed care contracts, and reproductive health centers, as noted above, had the fewest patients enrolled in managed care plans and the lowest percent of revenues from managed care. Neither region of the country (which reflects different managed care markets), hospital sponsorship, nor accreditation status was associated with whether or not women's health centers had managed care contracts. However, for-profit centers were significantly more likely than not-for-profit and public centers to have contracts. In addition, centers that had acquired managed care contracts were significantly more likely than other centers to have undergone, or to be planning, other organizational changes. Strategic changes included forming alliances with community organizations (80% of centers with managed care contracts, compared with 71% of other centers); joint ventures with hospitals (49% of centers with contracts, compared with 40% of others); joint ventures with physician groups (48% of centers with contracts, compared with 36% of others); joining multi-institutional systems (30% of centers with contracts, compared with 19% of others); or merging with another organization (26% of centers with contracts, compared with 16% of others). Women's health centers with managed care contracts therefore appear to have been more proactive generally, and the organizational changes undertaken may have enhanced the centers' attractiveness to managed care plans or may have been required by the plans.

From both the survey and case study results, four strategies were identified that were being used by centers to acquire managed care contracts, and some women's health centers were transforming themselves to participate in managed care networks (Weisman, Curbow, Khoury 1996). The first strategy, which was observed in reproductive health centers, was expanding primary care or midlife women's services to obtain contracts as a primary care provider for privately insured women or Medicaid enrollees. This strategy required hiring primary care physicians, expanding services to include the nonreproductive components of women's primary care, and arranging for backup and referral services. Although there were some cases of successful transitions of reproductive health centers into primary care centers, it is not yet known how widespread these transformations will be or how these transformations might affect women's access to the services traditionally provided by reproductive health centers.

Second, some primary care centers sought to qualify as family primary care providers by extending primary care services to men and/or children. In some cases, centers pursuing this strategy changed the center's name by removing the word "women," which had the added advantage of reducing community perceptions that the center was an abortion provider. In centers that had recently broadened their patient populations, however, the large majority of patients continued to be women, and new patients tended to be the male partners or children of these women. It was not yet known how the patient mix might change and whether these centers would maintain their women-centered missions in the long run.

Third, some reproductive health and primary care centers contracted with managed care plans to provide specialty reproductive services in which the center was expert and had established a niche as an essential community provider for uninsured women or women on medical assistance. Examples of such services were surgical abortions and routine gynecological examinations for physically or developmentally disabled women, which require special equipment and counseling services. Although this strategy provides a mechanism for delivering services that might not otherwise be available to women in the community, it also could exacerbate the problem of fragmentation in women's basic health care in two ways. First, women enrolled in managed care plans who are required to obtain specialty reproductive services from another site incur additional costs and inconvenience. Second, if services are obtained separately from the primary care provider, coordination of the woman's overall care is complicated. Some women's health centers that had contracted with managed care plans to provide specialty services experienced difficulties obtaining necessary referrals or attempting to coordinate care with primary care providers located elsewhere.

Fourth, a strategy identified among hospital-sponsored primary care and breast care centers was incorporating the center as a featured service in the hospital's managed care marketing plan and, in some cases, negotiating special rates or package pricing for services provided. The primary care women's health centers, in particular, were perceived as enhancing the sponsoring hospitals' ability to market their primary care capacities and integrated services. In this strategy, successful women's health centers were viewed by both center and hospital administrators as helping the hospital attract managed care contracts.

Despite the challenges of managed care exemplified in many of these centers, women's health centers and managed care are by no means incompatible concepts. On the contrary, women's health centers that have developed innovative models of comprehensive primary care or of integrated care for a specific condition could be highly compatible with managed care. The capacity to realize efficiencies through organizational coordination of gender-appropriate services, to provide well-woman care in fewer visits per patient, and to motivate women to take an active role in maintaining their health may be optimized in certain types of women's health centers. These attributes could be particularly attractive to capitated managed care plans. Women's health centers, therefore, could serve both as contracted primary care providers for patients enrolled in managed care plans and as models for women's health care within managed care plans.

CONCLUSION

Within U.S. health care, the appropriateness of gender-congruent health care for women has been debated for about two centuries, and there also has been a long tradition of separate health care organizations for women. In the current health care system, these issues are expressed in debates about the possible benefits to women of being treated by women physicians—who are increasingly available in primary care practice—and about the role of a variety of types of women's health centers. These debates also highlight the issue of women's ability as health care consumers to act on their preferences for women providers or for women-centered service settings. The policy implications of these issues are far reaching; they affect health professionals' education and training as well as the design of health care organizations and delivery systems.

Women's health centers are particularly interesting and relevant. Some, such as family planning centers, originated in women's historical efforts to legitimize new services and were sustained through government programs designed to extend services to underserved groups. Some reproductive health centers currently serve as the usual source of care for many women, and some are expanding services to provide more comprehensive well-woman care. At the same time, the continued specialization of some of these centers tends to perpetuate fragmented care. The newer comprehensive primary care centers are providing innovative models of well-woman care in women-centered settings that ostensibly reduce access barriers associated with fragmented care. Some of these centers serve as primary care providers for women enrolled in managed care plans. Such centers may serve as models for women-centered care within managed care or other health care delivery organizations. Still unknown, however, is how the process and outcomes of care, client satisfaction, and costs of care compare between primary care women's health centers and other models of primary care delivery for women. Research has not investigated whether these centers provide the quality of care women want, at the same or lower price, compared with other models of care delivery.

In short, many unanswered questions remain about the benefits and costs for women of gender-congruent care and of care in separate health care organizations. The persistence of interest in these phenomena, however, and the continuing growth of women's health centers, suggests that an expanding market exists for models of care that are gender sensitive, treat women holistically, and integrate services for women.

5

Transforming Women's Health Care Policymaking

IF HEALTH CARE policy is defined to include all decisions made by society, through both governmental and nongovernmental means, to define and allocate health care resources and to shape health care institutions, then it is clear that American women have always been involved in health care policymaking. The waves of the women's health megamovement are the most conspicuous examples of women's influence on health care policy, but since the 1970s, women's health advocacy and interest groups have become prominent members of the health policy community. Yet there is no consensus on how to incorporate gender in health care policymaking, what the role of women's health groups ought to be, or which women's health issues might form the basis of a policy agenda within the changing health care environment.

The prospects and opportunities for continued collective action in women's health care appear to be great, however. Because women are a majority of health care consumers and tend to be responsible for the health care of their families, they are likely to be among the first consumers to experience problems as the health care delivery system evolves. In addition, the post–World War II baby-boom generation of women, which provided the grassroots organizers of the Women's Health Movement of the 1960s and

1970s and many of the leaders of the women's health agenda of the early 1990s, began to enter midlife in the 1990s. These women are likely to be assertive and well-informed consumers as they confront menopause and other conditions of aging. What is more, as the middle-class members of this cohort contend with changes in their health insurance status, interact with increasingly diverse types of managed care organizations, and become caregivers of aging parents, they may expand their concerns to include the system-level issues of organization and financing of health and long-term care. Similarly, the growing influence of a historically unprecedented number of women in medicine, biomedical and health services research, and all branches of government is likely to continue to be felt in both the public and private sectors as these women seek to reshape health care institutions and correct perceived gender inequities. The continued proliferation of women's health care delivery organizations and of women's health advocacy and interest groups provides an organizational base for women to be informed and mobilized around a variety of health issues. To the extent that these groups can broaden their constituencies, furthermore, the more diverse their issues could become. Regardless of the issues they define, however, women in their various stakeholder positions now expect health care institutions and government to respond to their needs, and they expect to be involved in health care policymaking.

Yet American society is conflicted about how gender should enter public policy. While gender is one of several underlying social factors that affect individuals' status and opportunities, decision makers do not always acknowledge this when they formulate policies or programs. The dominant (though not universal) ideology of gender equality sometimes creates blind spots about gender inequities in society at large and produces skepticism about responding to women as an "interest group." Those who attempt to expose gender inequities, furthermore, often are conflicted about the appropriate policy instruments for remedying them. Ignoring gender or failing to remedy gender inequities can, in fact, be policy decisions. (As Linda Gordon [1990b:10-11] points out, "policy is as much constructed by denials of needs as by meeting them.") On the other hand, gender may be explicitly incorporated into public policy in ways that harm women. When policy attempts to reinforce what are perceived to be traditional gender-based roles in ways that encourage women's dependency, choices and opportunities may be curtailed for many women.

In the case of health care policy, because both access to health care and health care delivery have gendered structures, policy inevitably is involved with gender issues, whether it explicitly addresses gender or not. Explicit consideration of gender, furthermore, inevitably raises the topic of human reproduction and related moral concerns about sexual behavior, fertility-control practices, and family roles. Reproductive issues have been linked, historically, with women's health concerns and continue to be the focus of some of the most contentious policy debates. In health care policymaking, therefore, the stakes are particularly high for women's capacity to pursue their personal objectives and for gender equity in society generally.

FRAMEWORKS FOR INCLUDING GENDER IN POLICY

There is no consensus in American society about how gender issues should be addressed in public policy. Gender differences, of course, are not inherently problematic; differences first have to be constructed as social problems requiring public attention to arise on the policy agenda. Once on the agenda, gender-based problems may be addressed in different ways. Two contradictory frameworks have been used for incorporating gender in policy: the "gender-neutral" approach, in which policy is intended to be gender-blind and nondiscriminatory, and the "gender-specific" approach, in which targeted policies are formulated to provide special benefits or protections to one gender. Demands for gender equity in recent decades have resulted in policymaking based on both of these approaches. The different assumptions, ethical and moral concerns, and relative advantages and disadvantages of these approaches have been actively debated, exposing variations within feminist thought.[1] The issues, furthermore, are quite relevant to health care policymaking.

Gender Neutrality

The gender-neutral approach to policy is based on the assumptions that women and men are, or should be, socially equal and that public policy should be gender blind so as not to advantage or disadvantage one gender with respect to the other. This approach became prominent during the 1960s and 1970s and has been used to ensure equal access for women and men to opportunities or social resources. In this framework, the "equal treatment" of women and men—nondiscrimination—is the goal.

Kirp, Yudof, and Franks (1986), for example, are proponents of gender-neutral public policy who argue that women have generally been harmed by gender-specific policies designed to protect them. They argue that paternalistic policies, such as protective labor legislation, deny women the opportunity to make autonomous decisions and relegate women to specific social roles, dependency, and marginal statuses relative to men. They also argue that result-oriented affirmative action, such as court-ordered gender-based employment quotas, harms women by treating them as members of a class, rather than as individuals, and by undermining individual choice. Asserting that equal liberty is the basis of sound gender policy, they state that the basic principles of such policy are "the *opportunity* [for all individuals] to choose, the *capacity* to make choices, *information* on which to base preferences, and a climate of *tolerance* in which to explore alternatives" (Kirp, Yudof, and Franks 1986:131). Government support, they argue, should be nonobtrusive, enabling autonomous individuals to make their own choices rather than dictating what those choices should be.

This approach to policymaking can be criticized on several grounds. The most obvious is that it equates ends and means. In formulating intendedly gender-neutral policy, decision makers may overlook gender-based differences (e.g., in biology, socioeconomic circumstances, or caregiving responsibilities) that have important consequences for individuals' capacities to make choices or to act on those choices. In doing so, more often than not, they take the male experience as the normative standard and thereby perpetuate female disadvantage. Gender-neutral policymaking has particular difficulty dealing with gender-linked conditions, of which the clearest example is pregnancy. Although pregnancy occurs only to women, some public policies related to pregnancy have been framed in gender-neutral terms, with negative consequences for women. For instance, court decisions involving pregnancy discrimination in the 1970s sometimes, ironically, ignored gender and referred to "pregnant women and non-pregnant persons" in upholding employers' exclusion of pregnancy from insurance coverage (Rhode 1989:118). Similarly, the Pregnancy Discrimination Act of 1978, which required that pregnancy be treated as any other temporary disability in employment, failed to acknowledge that pregnancy is gender specific and that pregnant women might confront problems, in the workplace or elsewhere, that temporarily disabled men do not face (Eisenstein 1988; Gonen 1993).

Gender neutrality also has been criticized for failing to acknowledge the gendered cultural context within which intendedly gender-neutral policies are formulated and implemented. It does not, for example, provide a basis for addressing the possibility that men are dominant in most policymaking bodies and therefore might fashion agendas and policies that privilege their position. Or again, it does not recognize that women and men have differential access to economic resources and that the institutions in which they negotiate options or purchase services (such as the health care marketplace) might have historically conditioned gendered structures. Some feminist scholars also have argued that gender-neutral policy that views humans as autonomous decision makers is based on a male model, since it ignores the social circumstances in which women have less decision latitude or are more strongly tied than men to communal caregiving responsibilities (Sherwin 1996). Gender-neutral policy, in short, tends to assume a level playing field and to be unconcerned about the potential for differential impact by gender.

In health care, a common assumption seems to be that if a proposal or policy is stated in gender-neutral terms, it will be gender neutral in impact. One example is the generally gender-neutral discourse on primary care. Despite pervasive gender differences in primary care needs and delivery, as described in chapter 3, a 1996 report by the Institute of Medicine's Committee on the Future of Primary Care did not directly address women's primary care needs or acknowledge gender-specific issues in delivery of adult primary care (Donaldson et al. 1996). Another example is the gender-neutral language used in many assessments of the impact of the Human Genome Project, despite the facts that women predominate among those undergoing prenatal genetic screening and that because only women's bodies house fetuses, only women undergo fetal therapies and pregnancy terminations (Mahowald 1996).

An illustration of the potential for differential impact by gender of supposedly gender-neutral health policy may be found in recent proposals for restructuring Medicaid and Medicare. Debate around such proposals often fails to acknowledge the predominance of women among the beneficiaries of these programs and that women's health care needs, access to other socioeconomic resources, and family caregiving responsibilities differ systematically from those of male beneficiaries. Consequently, increases in premiums, reductions of benefits, changes in eligibility requirements, or relaxation of federal requirements regarding state management of benefits would differentially affect women and men, as both patients and informal caregivers. Another example may be found in proposals for age-based health care rationing that would favor younger persons in the allocation of resources, particularly with respect to life-extending technologies.[2] Feminist bioethicists have pointed out that because women live longer than men and predominate in the oldest age groups, age-based rationing would unjustly burden women (Nelson and Nelson 1996).

A related phenomenon is the assumption among some analysts of women's health care issues that universalistic health care policies—that is, policies that apply to all, rather than to targeted underserved subgroups—necessarily benefit women. Universalism, however, does not guarantee equitable treatment of women and men for all of the reasons noted above. Even enactment of universal single-payer health insurance coverage for all Americans—including a comprehensive basic benefits package—would not be experienced similarly by women and men unless health care delivery organizations also were redesigned to integrate women's health services and to address gender-based needs. This is not an argument to avoid universalism, but rather to consider the impact of universalistic policies on social groups for whom special considerations might be needed.

Gender Specificity

A contrasting framework is the gender-specific approach, an example of what Iris Young (1990:173) calls "group-conscious" policy. This approach is based on the social construction of some gender differences as social problems that require specific public responses. (Deborah Rhode [1989] argues for reframing discussions of "gender differences," which tend to use men's experiences as the standard, to "gender disadvantage," which focuses on how to eliminate gender inequalities that disadvantage either women or men.) Given the current dominant ideology of gender equality, gender-specific policies resulting in differential allocations of public resources by gender are likely to be perceived as just if they reduce differences in opportunities or outcomes between women and men. They are likely to be perceived as unjust if they exacerbate gender inequalities in opportunities or outcomes (for example, by giving what is perceived to be unfair advantage to one gender) or if they increase overall societal costs.

Historically, gender-specific policymaking has been used both to reinforce socially valued gender differences (as in the case of early twentieth-century maternalist social policies intended to protect the role of motherhood) and to redress gender inequities (as in the case of policies to protect women's jobs during pregnancy or maternity leaves). Separate women's institutions, such as women's colleges and women's hospitals, sometimes have been created because of beliefs about women's unique needs, vulnerabilities, or capacities and sometimes to compensate for women's exclusion from mainstream institutions. Today, invoking gender-based needs as a basis for policy is politically charged, because assertions about these needs may be confused with conservative efforts to preserve what are perceived to be traditional gender roles.

Typically, the gender-specific approach to policymaking refers to the formulation of policies that constitute women as a vulnerable group and provide special benefits or protections to women. Justifications for such policies might be based on perceptions of women's specific biological or social vulnerabilities or, as in the case of affirmative action policies, on a desire to remedy past inequities that unfairly disadvantaged women. Examples of so-called benign discrimination include protective labor legislation targeted to women, workplace fetal protection policies targeted to women, and policies pertaining to maternity leaves that do not also provide for paternity leaves. Also included are policies targeting women for which there are no policy analogues for men—such as legislation requiring counseling or waiting periods prior to obtaining abortions, mandated health insurance coverage of maternity care or of minimum hospital stays following delivery, and legislation designating obstetrician-gynecologists as primary care providers for women.

A proponent of group-conscious social policy, Young (1990) argues that policy according special treatment to oppressed social groups (such as women) promotes social justice. Recently, some women's health advocates have supported gender-specific policies to redress past injustices. Debra De-Bruin (1994), for example, argues for the preferential treatment of women subjects in biomedical research to compensate for the neglect of women's health problems in prior research and for the exclusion of women from clinical studies. As we have seen, such arguments often were successful in the 1990s in attaining increased federal spending on women's health research and establishing new offices and programs for women's health within government agencies.

There are a number of potential problems with gender-specific policymaking. For one, it is often based on assumptions about the essential (i.e., biologically determined) nature of gender differences and may serve to reinforce traditional gender roles and stereotypes or to limit women's autonomy or capacity to improve their socioeconomic circumstances. Another potential problem is that gender-specific policies, even if enacted to redress injustice, tend to homogenize women and to ignore the diversity of women's experiences and preferences. By lumping all women together as a class, they may deny differences in the social situations and needs among subgroups of women defined by socioeconomic status, race/ethnicity, age group, sexual orientation, or other circumstances; vulnerable subgroups of women could therefore be neglected. (On the other hand, lumping women may be a more politically expeditious approach, since policies emphasizing potential benefits for all women—including white, middle-class women—are likely to sustain more political support than those targeting disadvantaged subgroups of women.)

Another criticism of gender-based policymaking is that it does not necessarily provide mechanisms for ensuring that institutions change over time so as to minimize the gender inequities that the policies may have been designed to correct in the first place. Some policy initiatives rely on financial incentives to bring about institutional change—as, for example, when federal funding for women's health research is increased in an effort to attract more academic researchers to the study of women's health problems. In this example, however, additional mechanisms would be needed to ensure that academic researchers do not revert to form when the funding is expended or that research results are readily translated into health care practices that benefit women. Similarly, establishing separate women's institutions may, in some cases, create effective competition with mainstream institutions that spurs them to adopt innovations that benefit women or, in other cases, may merely perpetuate gender inequities.

EXAMPLES OF GENDER-SPECIFIC HEALTH CARE POLICY

Some examples of gender-specific health care policy will illustrate these points. A distinctive feature of many of the enacted gender-specific public policies related to women's health is a focus on maternity, that is, on the health of women as mothers or potential mothers. This reflects a pattern in which women's health traditionally has been attended to in public policy on the basis of reproductive issues that distinguish women from men. This pattern, as we have seen in chapter 2, was not a simple function of male policymakers' biases about women or their attempts to control women; it also resulted from women's agency in different eras and from women's changing conceptions of their maternal role. Policies focusing on maternal health have taken two forms: the development of categorical public programs in which economically disadvantaged women become eligible for health benefits on the basis of their maternal status (that is, by being pregnant or by being the mother of dependent children); and policies designed to protect the health of women to ensure healthy children. These policies, furthermore, have had mixed consequences for women.

The earliest example of health care policy for pregnant women may be found in the colonial poor laws, which made provision in local communities for midwifery services for morally deserving poor women (Abramovitz 1988). However, the modern policy linkage of women's health with maternity can be traced to late nineteenth-century protective labor legislation targeted to women and to the Progressive Era, when "maternalist" social reformers supported a number of social policies intended to protect idealized conceptions of motherhood and the family at a time when motherhood, as Gordon puts it, was "the quintessential female labor" (Gordon 1994:38).[3] Examples of Progressive Era maternalist policies include mothers' pensions—which were intended to enable poor, widowed women to support their children, avoid institutionalization, and preserve the family unit—and programs to improve the health of mothers and children through maternal education and direct services, including prenatal care, as exemplified by the activities of the Children's Bureau and the programs initiated under the Sheppard-Towner Act. Although the maternal and child health programs were universal, in that they were not intended only for socioeconomically disadvantaged women, they were institutionalized in subsequent social welfare programs that targeted needy women. These included Title V, the maternal and child health provisions of the 1935 Social Security Act; the Emergency Maternity and Infant Care program during World War II; the Medicaid program; and the Women, Infants, and Children program, established in 1972 and administered by the Department of Agriculture to provide nutritional supplements to low-income, nutritionally disadvantaged pregnant and lactating women and to young children.

In all of these public programs, women became eligible for the health benefits—for example, prenatal care, obstetrical care, nutritional services, and general preventive services or medical care—by being poor or having low incomes *and* by being pregnant or having young children. Hence, needy non-pregnant women and non-needy pregnant women were not eligible for benefits. Both the exclusion of non-needy pregnant women from an entitlement to health insurance coverage and the policy linkage of health benefits for needy women with their maternal status can be criticized for reflecting a muddled conception of family health. For one thing, the linkage of poor women's health care with maternity implies that their health is socially valued only when they are reproducing, and it perpetuates the presumption that only mothers (not fathers) are responsible for child health and caregiving. Family well-being, it could be argued, depends upon parental caregiving and the health of both parents throughout the child's development to adulthood. Among maternal and child health experts, furthermore, there is growing recognition that women's health status prior to conception, as well as during pregnancy and the postnatal period, is relevant to outcomes for both mother and child (Hughes and Simpson 1995; Wise 1995). This broader understanding of "maternal health" provides a rationale for ensuring continuous basic health care and other social resources for all females, beginning at birth.

Well-meaning proposals for health care reform that put "pregnant women and children first"—or that focus on child health by providing services to mothers (usually prenatally)—tend, often unintentionally, to perpetuate the linkage of maternal status with women's health, normative assumptions about parental roles, and fragmented women's health care. Proponents of such policies often appeal to justice for vulnerable groups, point out that the technology is currently available to treat many maternal and infant health problems at relatively low cost, or argue that maternal-child health issues are a good first step toward more broadly based health care reform. History, however, provides little evidence to support the contention that maternal-child health programs open the door to broader health benefits.

The linkage of mother and child health also is apparent in policies designed to protect women and their potential children from perceived health hazards, such as the risks of the workplace or participation in clinical trials of new drugs or medical devices. The historical concern has been to protect the health of women, pregnant or not, to ensure healthy newborns. The implicit view of women in such protectionist policies is that they are perennially potentially pregnant. Once again, the policy origins of this approach may be found in Progressive Era protective labor legislation designed to regulate women's employment to protect reproductive health. When the U.S. Supreme Court upheld the constitutionality of maximum hours for female workers in *Muller v. Oregon* (1908), the decision included the statement that "as healthy mothers are essential to vigorous offspring, the physical well-being of woman becomes an object of public interest and care."[4] Later public policies to protect the health of women and their potential children included provisions governing research on human subjects and inclusion of women in testing of new pharmaceuticals and medical devices. These were exemplified in 1977 Food and Drug Administration (FDA) guidelines recommending that all women of childbearing potential, not just pregnant women, be excluded from early phases of drug trials, except in cases of life-threatening diseases. These policies, as we have seen in chapter 2, arose as a result of some highly publicized cases of harm to women or fetuses—the thalidomide, DES, and Dalkon Shield IUD episodes—and of efforts during the Women's Health Movement of the 1960s and 1970s to bring public attention to inappropriate experimentation on women (Johnson and Fee 1994). In addition, post–*Roe v. Wade* abortion politics included a growing concern for fetal rights among an increasingly organized antiabortion countermovement during the 1980s.

Cynthia Daniels (1993:4) argues that more recently "the rhetoric of protectionism has fundamentally shifted from maternal to fetal health." During the 1980s, a combination of antiabortion ideology and new medical technologies, including fetal surgery, led to a new conception of fetal rights separate from those of the pregnant woman and to policy intended to protect the fetus by intervening on the mother or potential mother.[5] To illustrate the point, Daniels uses three benchmark court cases dealing with fetal rights in which attempts were made either to portray the interests of pregnant women and their fetuses as oppositional or to define women's citizenship rights contingent upon fetal rights. The first was the case of Angela Carder, a pregnant, terminally ill cancer patient who underwent a court-ordered cesarean section delivery, against her own and her family's wishes, at George Washington University Hospital in 1987. Both the baby and the mother died following the procedure, and the family brought legal action against the hospital.[6] The second was the 1991 case of Johnson Controls, a Vermont battery manufacturer that excluded all fertile women (defined, interestingly, as all women under the age of seventy) from jobs exposing them to lead. Ostensibly to protect potential children, this employer's policy applied to women, but not to men. The third was the case of Jennifer Johnson, a Florida woman convicted in 1989 of delivering cocaine to her unborn children through the umbilical cord. She was sentenced to one year of treatment in a residential drug rehabilitation program, fifteen years' probation, and temporary loss of custody of her children. Each of these cases eventually was decided in favor of women's rights, but they reflect ongoing debate about the nature of the linkage between maternal and fetal health, about the value of women's health for its own sake, and about women's autonomy as decision makers on behalf of their potential children as well as their own health and health care.

The legacies of public policies focused on maternity therefore are mixed. On the one hand, they reflect society's—and women's health advocates'—efforts to improve maternal and child health by assisting women in need of governmental protection, special services, or health insurance. On the other hand, they have sometimes reinforced women's dependency or marginal status by taking an essentialist view of gender roles, and they have sometimes limited women's autonomy to make decisions about their health or social functioning. It is often observed that gender-specific policymaking cuts two ways: it may offer special benefits to women, but it may also perpetuate gender-based disadvantages. The latter outcome often awaits a subsequent policy cycle in which interest groups of women, whose consciousness of their circumstances has changed, become advocates for change.

TRANSFORMING HEALTH CARE POLICYMAKING

The challenge is to attend to women's health care needs without creating social distinctions or programs that contribute to women's dependency or
care-seeking burdens. In other words, health care policy should be constructed so as to reduce, rather than to perpetuate, gender-based disadvantages in the health care delivery system and in society at large. Developing
policy that is responsive to women's health problems, as well as to how they
experience health care, requires the direct involvement of women who can
articulate their viewpoints and help implement change. Women's health activists, as we have seen, have a tradition of organizing to influence health care
institutions. Nevertheless, ensuring that information about women's diverse
experiences and needs are given voice in health care policymaking requires
transforming the institutional context within which health care policy is
formulated and implemented. There are at least two approaches for accom-
plishing this. One is to increase the representation of women in policymaking bodies, both public and private, that are responsible for decisions related
to health and health care. Another is to structure ways in which women's
health advocacy and interest groups can participate as partners in public policymaking.

Increasing Representation

The representation of women in policymaking bodies may be improved
both by increasing the number of women who are legislators and members of
legislative staffs and by ensuring women's participation in government and
private-sector groups responsible for health care decision making.[7] The proportionate representation of women, in relation to their numbers in either the
general population or in the population affected by policies under consideration, is one possible approach to ensuring that women's viewpoints are included in policymaking. This has been proposed by the philosopher Mary
Mahowald (1993, 1996), who argues that proportionate representation is a re-
medial strategy that not only ensures the democratic participation of women
and other nondominant social groups in policymaking, but also avoids to-
kenism (that is, the tendency to assume that one person or a small number of
persons represents a social group). The mathematics of proportionate representation quickly become cumbersome, however, when considering that individuals always are members of multiple social groups simultaneously, that

not all women will recognize a collective identity based on gender, and that there is no single "women's viewpoint." For example, both women's health care needs and their patterns of health care utilization vary by age, socioeconomic status, race/ethnicity, and other factors, and these variations are likely to produce different perspectives among women on problem identification and the selection of strategies for change in the health care system.

In addition, the viewpoints and interests of women consumers may differ from those of women health care professionals and biomedical researchers. With the growing numbers and increasing seniority of women physicians and other professionals, women's health consumer advocates will increasingly encounter women in leadership roles in elite health care institutions and policymaking bodies and will have to contend with differences in viewpoints deriving from their different social statuses and stakeholder positions. Women physicians, nurses, and biomedical researchers may be allies of consumers and highly credible spokespersons for some policy objectives that fall within their areas of expertise, such as expanding the biomedical research agenda in women's health and developing more effective screening tests, treatments, or service delivery models for women. However, their interests in promoting biomedical research and clinical services may not necessarily coincide with consumers' interests in, for example, expanding attention to the psychosocial aspects of health care, promoting nonclinical approaches to maintaining their health, protecting women from overutilization, or expanding access to health services for disadvantaged social groups. A case in point is that women physicians and women consumers did not always agree on the issues during the health care reform episode of the early 1990s. For example, separate Times Mirror surveys conducted in June 1994 found that women physicians were significantly less likely than women in the general population to support the Clinton health care reform plan: 22 percent of women physicians favored the plan, compared with 33 percent of all women (Pew Research Center for the People and the Press 1994).

Nevertheless, the principle of including more women in health policymaking is a sound one that could be implemented by ensuring the participation of women of diverse social statuses and in different stakeholder relationships with the health care delivery system. These diverse subgroups of women could be included as members of, for example, internal review boards overseeing biomedical research studies and informed consent procedures; boards of directors of health insurance companies, managed care organizations, hospitals and other health care delivery organizations, community health agencies, and pharmaceutical and medical device manufacturing companies; governing boards of trade associations, accrediting commissions of health care organizations, and associations of health professionals; legislatures and legislators' staffs at all levels of government; the leadership of government agencies (including their offices on women's health) responsible for health care policy, research, and regulation; and government commissions and advisory panels. In addition, the creation of women's health offices in a number of government agencies, as discussed in chapter 2, has increased both the number of women responsible for women's health programs and their visibility within these agencies.

Involving Advocacy and Interest Groups

The participation of women's health advocacy and interest groups in health care policymaking is not new, but including them as partners in public policymaking is another approach to transforming the context within which health care policy is formulated and implemented. This approach can help ensure the participation of diverse groups of women and can help facilitate communication between policymaking bodies and the constituents of women's health groups representing a broad range of interests. The strategy has the added benefit of facilitating communication among women's health groups who may be adept in pursuing their constituents' interests but less experienced in balancing the interests of diverse groups in pursuit of broader objectives for the social good.

Current women's health advocacy and interest organizations are quite varied, both in structure and in the issues they advocate, and some have sustained a presence in the health policy community for more than two decades. They range from local advocacy groups of patients or survivors of specific diseases to national multi-issue public interest groups whose members often include both consumers and health professionals. (Men may be members, too, but the leadership and overwhelming majority of members typically are women.) These organizations may provide members with social support, health information, or opportunities for political action at the local, state, or national level on behalf of a particular disease, issue, or set of issues. Some groups are involved in multiple activities. Many of these groups may not be broadly representative of the female public because they tend to be organized and financed by middle- and upper-income women.[8] However, because they represent members who have a special interest in health-related matters, are better informed on their issue than is the general public, have often donated time or money to the organization, and are likely to be politically active, the groups are likely to represent opinion leaders on their issues.

The politically active women's health advocacy and interest organizations are increasingly sophisticated in the use of the media and lobbying for getting their message out. Although most of these groups do not have large budgets and some rely on volunteers for much of their work, they are increasingly professionalized, in the sense that they are administered by paid staff, have boards of directors, and sometimes hire public relations, lobbying, or consulting firms to influence legislators, coordinate media or fund-raising campaigns, or organize rallies or conferences. Some have also been quite successful in obtaining financial support from corporations—both within the health industry (e.g., pharmaceutical firms) and outside it (e.g., cosmetics manufacturers)—that see a public relations benefit in supporting women's health causes. Member organizations often have newsletters and large mailing lists for communicating with and activating members. On-line services are becoming more common as well. In addition, the national offices of these organizations typically are located in Washington, D.C., in proximity to legislators and federal health program offices. These organizations are important resources for policymakers in that they can provide information, report feedback from their constituents, and often mobilize members in local communities through linked organizations.

A taxonomy of recent women's health advocacy and interest groups reveals both community-based and regional or national organizations. At the community level are self-help and advocacy groups organized around specific conditions (e.g., breast cancer advocacy groups) as well as chapters of national interest groups such as NARAL.[9] Networks of like-minded groups may form at the local, state, or regional level around specific issues, such as the Coalition for Reproductive Freedom in Boston (Boston Women's Health Book Collective 1992). At the national level are federations of local or state chapters of single-issue groups (e.g., NARAL), organized networks of like-minded groups (e.g., the National Breast Cancer Coalition [NBCC]), organizations providing primarily educational and informational services (e.g., the Boston Women's Health Book Collective), multi-issue political action organizations (e.g., the National Women's Health Network), and associations of professionals concerned with women's health research, delivery system issues, or policy (e.g., the Society for the Advancement of Women's Health Research, the Jacobs Institute of Women's Health, the Institute for Research on Women's Health). Members of these organizations typically receive regular informational mailings in the form of newsletters, legislative updates, or calls to action. When political opportunities arise, these organizations can readily mobilize their members (e.g., to provide funding, contact legislators, or participate in other activities), and they may form temporary coalitions to pursue their interests. For example, in 1994 during the national health care reform episode, the National Women's Health Network, with over 20,000 individual and organizational members, issued a "call to action" in its newsletter urging members to contact their representatives in Congress to urge reform. Also during this episode, the Campaign for Women's Health (discussed in more detail below) was organized as a coalition of multiple groups to promote women's interests in national health care reform.

Although some of these groups—most notably, the breast cancer organizations—have become important participants in recent efforts to influence the health policy agenda, there is no consensus about which groups "fit" in the public policymaking process or what their role should be. Among legislators and their staffs, groups pushing programs for specific diseases or health problems, who often are referred to as "the disease-of-the-month club," are viewed with ambivalence. Sometimes these groups are seen as a nuisance, and sometimes as politically helpful. For example, groups advocating for increased federal funding for breast cancer research in the early 1990s provided some politicians with a way to curry favor with female voters while avoiding more controversial issues such as abortion. The tendency to view consumer or public interest groups as threats to the authority of professional experts also is common within the health policy and biomedical communities, including among women physicians and other professionals. Advocacy groups often are seen as promoting "policy by anecdote," in that they may highlight statistically unrepresentative, egregious cases to make a point about the need for protective policies. Professional groups also often accuse consumer groups of advocating unproven treatments, yet many of the medical practices and technologies now in common use were not subjected to scientific research prior to their adoption into practice and sometimes continue to be used on the basis of tradition rather than accumulated evidence of effectiveness. Consequently, the values of medical science and practice are not inherently privileged in policymaking, and recent attempts to integrate advocacy groups into formal policymaking processes promise the development of avenues through which advocacy and biomedicine can inform each other.

Women's health advocacy and interest groups can fill various functions as partners in policymaking. They can draw the public's and policymakers' attention to gender-specific health problems or gender inequities in health care that need to be "on the agenda"; they can help identify and choose among policy alternatives; they can help assess the potential for differential impact by gender of proposed policies or programs; they can help policymakers avoid unintended consequences that would be detrimental to women; and they can help mobilize support for (or opposition to) policy options. They also can help clarify the positions or various stakeholders attracted to women's health issues. Because women's health has become a good political issue for groups with varied interests, women's health groups face, simultaneously, increased opportunities to coalesce broad-based support for their issues and increased risks of losing control of the public agenda in women's health. Other interest groups, such as physicians' associations or trade associations of health care organizations, may promote their own causes as "women's issues" for political expediency. Politicians may support legislative or programmatic efforts framed as "women's health issues" if they believe that by doing so, they stand to improve their credibility with women constituents. Including women's health advocacy and interest groups in policymaking is one way to clarify and balance the diversity of interests in health care policymaking.

CASE STUDIES IN ADVOCACY AND POLICYMAKING

Two cases of the ways in which women's health advocacy and interest groups have been involved in recent health care policymaking provide illustrative examples. The case of breast cancer organizations illustrates how a national network of single-issue groups responded to the political opportunities created by the women's health agenda in the early 1990s and had major influences on breast cancer policy. The case of the Campaign for Women's Health from 1990 to 1994, illustrates how a temporary, broad-based coalition of women's interest groups attempted to influence national health care reform. Although national health care reform failed, the coalition advanced a women's health agenda within health reform and created a new repertoire of action in women's health activism.

Breast Cancer Advocacy

Breast cancer activism provides a case study of how health advocacy organizations have worked with government both to achieve specific policy objectives and to attempt to transform the policymaking process. Breast cancer activism had an extended history of grassroots organizing before national networks were formed and were able to take advantage of the political opportunities opened by the women's health agenda episode of the early 1990s. This history of organizing and the linkage of local and national groups contributed to the successes of the breast cancer advocacy community in the early 1990s.

The first example of women's organized activity related to breast cancer was the American Cancer Society's Reach to Recovery Program, founded in 1952 by Terese Laser, a New York woman who had undergone a mastectomy, which was then standard treatment. In this program, breast cancer survivors were trained as volunteers to visit postmastectomy patients in the hospital and to provide support services, including prostheses so that a woman could "leave the hospital looking as close as possible to the way she looked before she went in" (Altman 1996:294). Organized in local affiliates, this program was essentially an adjunct to medical practice and had to be "ordered" by the patient's physician. The program did not attempt to reform services or to affect public policy.

The climate changed during the 1970s because of the combined effects of the Women's Health Movement, which was focusing attention on women's health issues generally, and media attention to several prominent women who were diagnosed with breast cancer—notably, Shirley Temple Black, Happy Rockefeller, and Betty Ford. In addition, several studies and exposés questioned the appropriateness of radical mastectomy as standard treatment and pointed to the need for informed consent procedures prior to breast surgery (Altman 1996; Love 1995; Ruzek 1978). Grassroots breast cancer groups began to appear in many communities in the late 1970s and early 1980s, often organized by breast cancer patients or their survivors. These groups generally were organized around what John McCarthy (1994) calls "identity opportunities" for victims, that is, the creation of a collective identity facilitated by such factors as media attention to famous victims and local community concerns about breast cancer clusters. Examples of these varied advocacy groups include the Susan G. Komen Breast Cancer Foundation, founded in Texas in 1982 by the sister of a woman who had died of breast cancer, to raise funds for research and services through such programs as Race for the Cure sponsored by foundation chapters throughout the country; Arm-in-Arm, organized in Baltimore in 1987 to provide information and support services to breast cancer patients and their families and to draw attention to the need for services and research on breast cancer; and Kendall Lakes Women against Cancer, which formed in a Florida community in 1985 to investigate a breast cancer cluster thought to be associated with environmental contamination (Altman

1996; Love 1995; McCoy et al. 1992). The organizers of these groups, typically, were middle-class women, some with professional careers or political connections, who were savvy about public relations, fund-raising, and lobbying. National networks were soon being created. In 1986, the National Alliance of Breast Cancer Organizations (NABCO) was formed to provide "information, assistance and referral to anyone with questions about breast cancer" and to act "as a voice for the interests and concerns of breast cancer survivors and women at risk" (NABCO 1994). In 1994, NABCO was a network of more than 350 organizations providing breast cancer services. The National Breast Cancer Coalition (NBCC) was formed in 1991 to influence public policy on breast cancer. Several cancer and breast cancer organizations, including advocacy groups, formed the NBCC, with NABCO administering the planning committee. The coalition soon had members in all fifty states, and by 1994, nearly 300 organizations were affiliated with the NBCC (Love 1995).

As we saw in chapter 2, during the early 1990s episode of women's health activism, the breast cancer organizations "caught the wave" and were well positioned to work effectively with the Congressional Caucus for Women's Issues to obtain increased federal funding for breast cancer research (in the National Institutes of Health (NIH) and the Department of Defense), to influence the topics of research, to extend access to screening mammography, and to enact quality standards for mammography screening. Several members of Congress, as well as other public officials, had personal or family experiences with breast cancer, which increased their receptivity to the breast cancer groups. In addition, gender politics played a role in the breast cancer groups' ability to garner support in Congress. In the early 1990s, some members of Congress saw breast cancer as a politically "safe" issue that could help them with women constituents, and breast cancer was a good women's issue for both antiabortion and abortion rights legislators. For example, Senator Arlen Specter, an abortion rights supporter who, as a member of the Senate Judiciary Committee had aggressively interrogated Anita Hill during the Clarence Thomas confirmation hearings and found himself in trouble with women voters, became a key advocate of breast cancer initiatives.

The breast cancer groups were effective not only because of their organizational base and ability to work with government, but also because their issue resonated with many women. The key to this was their successful reframing of their issue from a focus on victimization to a focus on gender equity. Consistent with the overall theme of the contemporary episode in women's health activism, the breast cancer groups argued that women's health was disadvantaged, relative to men's, because of inadequate allocation of public resources to the breast cancer problem. Furthermore, they argued, this was not only a problem for victims: all women were "at risk" for breast cancer and required information and screening. This framing emphasizing generalized risk was facilitated by demographics: the post–World War II baby boomers were now older and more receptive to information about cancer risk. As one observer put it, "baby boomers who were nursed in 60's activism are increasingly at risk for breast cancer [in the 1990s]" (Ferraro 1993:58). The broad appeal of the issue to women is reflected in the breast cancer groups' success in attracting funding from corporations, particularly in the cosmetics and fashion industries, for breast cancer advocacy, research, and services.

Interestingly, despite the long history of organized women's health activism in the United States and the women's health movement episode in which they were participating, many breast cancer advocates credited grassroots AIDS activists with providing the model for their framing of the problem and for their political action (Altman 1996; Dickersin and Schnaper 1996; Eagan 1994; Ferraro 1993; Love 1995; Soffa 1994). They admired AIDS activists' success both in directing public attention to a heretofore taboo disease and in successfully making the claim that the level of government funding for AIDS research was inadequate. Like the AIDS activists, the breast cancer activists' zealousness was sometimes criticized (e.g., for exaggerating the risk of the disease, particularly among younger women, or for deflecting funding from other research priorities), but their impact on members of Congress was generally acknowledged.

In addition to their successes in achieving research funding, new programs, and mammography quality standards, the breast cancer groups also transformed the policymaking process. They demanded direct involvement of consumers in the research agenda–setting process, including decisions on research funding. For example, the NBCC called for representation of women with breast cancer in such bodies as the National Cancer Institute's National Cancer Advisory Board. The NBCC also called for a national strategic plan to fight breast cancer. In October 1993, breast cancer activists presented President Clinton with petitions signed by 2.6 million persons asking for a national plan to end breast cancer. In response, the Secretary's Conference to Establish a National Action Plan on Breast Cancer was convened by Donna Shalala in December 1993 to establish priorities in health care, research, and policy, and it was attended by government officials, health care providers and researchers, and breast cancer activists. One of the actions recommended in the conference was to "involve advocacy groups and women with breast cancer in setting research priorities, in evaluation, and in patient education" (NIH

1994:21). When it received $10 million in federal funding for small grants for breast cancer research in 1995, the National Action Plan—which had been designed as a public-private partnership coordinated by Susan Blumenthal, Deputy Assistant Secretary for Women's Health, and Fran Visco, president of the NBCC—included members of advocacy groups on grant application review committees. The Department of Defense breast cancer program also included consumers on review panels. These partnerships of advocates and scientists in program coordination and the peer review process provided an opportunity for breast cancer survivors to influence which research topics were selected for funding and to sensitize researchers to some issues in research design, such as the possible reactions of women to treatment options.[10] With regard to research topics, advocacy groups tend to be particularly interested in areas they perceive to have been neglected, such as breast cancer etiology (including environmental and lifestyle factors), primary prevention (as opposed to screening), and health care delivery issues (including overuse of mammography and ethical-legal issues involved in genetic testing).

The participation of advocates in grant reviews, however, also raised the prospect of increasing tension between scientists and lay persons over research priorities and grant funding decisions (Erikson 1995). Professionals typically claim that consumers do not appreciate the value of basic research that is not focused on a specific disease application and that consumers are untrained in research design and methods. Consumers, in turn, may feel insecure about expressing their opinions in groups composed of both lay and professional members. To address these issues, the NBCC instituted a program in 1995 to train breast cancer activists for their new roles as participants on review panels and advisory boards. Project LEAD (Leadership, Education, Advocacy, and Development) trained 125 women in intense four-day workshops held around the country during the project's first year of operation (Dickersin and Schnaper 1996). Conducted by biomedical researchers and NBCC Board members, the workshops addressed such topics as the epidemiology of breast cancer, basic science relating to the cell, and research design and methods. This program provides a model for preparing consumer advocates for expanded roles in health care policymaking.

In sum, the well-organized breast cancer groups, with both local and national organizations, were able to take advantage of the opportunities for action on their issue that were opened by the episode of women's health activism in the early 1990s. By reframing the issue from a focus on victims to a focus on equity for women, they were able to argue for a greater allocation of public resources to breast cancer research and treatment and for a larger role for breast cancer patients in research agenda setting. They also established formal mechanisms for working with government, including the Office on Women's Health. In doing so, they created institutional changes in the policymaking process.

National Health Care Reform and Women's Health Advocacy

The national health care reform debate of 1992–94 provides another case of the participation of women's health advocacy and interest groups in the health care policymaking process. This case illustrates how these groups participated in a policymaking episode that was not focused exclusively on women's health concerns but provided a political opportunity to advance a women's health agenda. In addition, although there had been previous health reform episodes throughout the twentieth century, this was the first time that women's organizations emerged as prominent advocates of systemwide change in health care and of universal health insurance.

By the time the Clinton administration elevated health care reform on the national agenda, women's health advocates inside and outside of government were actively pursuing a well-publicized legislative agenda in Congress, as well as a number of private initiatives, on health issues of concern to women. As described in chapter 2, these efforts focused mainly on expanding biomedical research on women's health problems and redressing gender inequities in medical treatment. The organizational readiness around women's health issues, the activist subculture and its action repertoires, and the heightened public awareness of women's health concerns should have provided the basis for a natural transition into health care reform efforts among women's groups. Did this happen?

The Center for Public Integrity (1994:1) calls health care reform "the most heavily lobbied, legislative initiative in recent U.S. history," and it identified over 650 groups that spent over $100 million in 1993 and 1994 to influence the outcome of the health care reform debate. Women's health advocacy and interest groups were but a small part of this unprecedented surge of organizational influence. The women's health groups were active, however, and attempted to articulate a women's health agenda within the context of national health care reform. They supported reform—though not necessarily a specific health reform bill—as a way of improving women's access to care and attending to women's specific health care needs.

While the Clinton Health Security Plan was being formulated and a variety of alternative health care reform proposals was introduced in Congress, the various women's health groups framed women's interests in health care reform around two key issues: universal access to health care and the comprehensiveness of basic health insurance benefits. The groups crafted positions in support of universal access to health insurance coverage and the specific health care concerns of women. Financing universal health insurance, however, was a politically charged issue, and it was therefore difficult for bipartisan groups in general (not just women's groups) to endorse a particular plan for universal coverage. Groups were also politically astute enough to recognize that throwing early support to a specific reform plan could limit their influence in later stages when compromises were likely. Therefore, although many of the women's groups were advocates of a Canadian-style single-payer system, they tended to focus their public efforts on advocating universal access to care and defining the scope of benefits that should be guaranteed to women within the basic benefits package under any reformed health insurance system. They took an expansive approach to this task, including a wide array of both medical and nonmedical services of specific concern to their various constituencies. They did not attempt to prioritize these services, to consider the evidence for their effectiveness, or to confront the thorny issue of the financial costs of the benefits they were proposing.

The key coalition that emerged to forge a women's health agenda within health care reform was the Campaign for Women's Health. The campaign was formally established in 1990 and was given space in the offices of the Older Women's League in Washington, D.C., under the direction of Anne S. Kasper, a sociologist, women's health activist, and cochair of the first board of directors of the National Women's Health Network. The campaign had evolved, however, out of a core group of organizations with a longstanding interest in national health insurance and the foresight to recognize that a new window of opportunity was likely to open for this recurring issue. These organizations formed a planning group in the 1980s including representatives from the American Association of University Women, the American Nurses' Association, the American Federation of State County and Municipal Employees, the Services Employees International Union, the National Black Women's Health Project, the National Women's Health Network, the National Women's Law Center, and the Older Women's League. As health care reform emerged as a national issue during the presidential campaign of 1992, the membership of the Campaign for Women's Health quickly exploded. Eventually, it became a broad-based coalition of over 100 national, state, and grassroots organizations representing over eight million individuals.

The organizations that constituted the coalition included women's rights and advocacy groups, professional associations (including groups of nurses and women physicians), labor unions, religious groups, and health care and policy organizations. The women's health groups affiliated with the campaign included both first- and second-generation single- and multi-issue organizations, such as the Boston Women's Health Book Collective, the Jacobs Institute of Women's Health, NARAL, the National Asian Women's Health Organization, the National Black Women's Health Project, the NBCC, the National Women's Health Network, and the Society for the Advancement of Women's Health Research. The second-generation women's health organizations—including the Jacobs Institute of Women's Health, the NBCC, and the Society for the Advancement of Women's Health Research—were being founded at about the same time the campaign was forming, and they had less experience and fewer resources than some of the other members of the coalition. Yet they were able to contribute their expertise on the core issues confronting the coalition.

The campaign's first task was the formulation of a set of principles to articulate the coalition's position. Defining health care reform as "a unique opportunity to redress many of the inequities women have faced securing health care for themselves and their families," the campaign endorsed universal access to quality health care; comprehensive health benefits; availability of women's health care from a variety of physician and nonphysician providers (e.g., advanced practice nurses, lay midwives) in a variety of health care settings (e.g., community health centers, family planning clinics, the home); system accountability to women; full health care information for women; an expanded research agenda on women's health; and increased opportunities for women in research careers (Campaign for Women's Health 1993:7). The campaign made an explicit decision not to include children's health in its agenda, so that women's health would not be subsumed by other issues.

The campaign also formulated a comprehensive "model benefits package" for women that received coverage in the national media and may be the best available collaborative statement of what women want in their health care. The package, described in an eight-page document, included primary, preventive, reproductive, and long-term care services in addition to services for the treatment of illness or disease. Asserting that "all services which are necessary or appropriate for the maintenance and promotion of women's health should be included in a benefits package," the campaign explicitly challenged some prevailing notions of "medical necessity" that limit coverage of services to treatment of disease or injury and do not include health promotion and disease prevention (Campaign for Women's Health 1993:1).[11] The package called for a comprehensive set of primary and preventive services in both reproductive and nonreproductive health, including, for example, a periodic history and examination; clinical preventive services; mental health screen; dental, vision, speech, and hearing checks; prescription drugs and devices; evaluation for lifestyle risks; a full range of family planning services; abortion; infertility treatment; maternity care; and menopause counseling and services. It also included long-term care services in the home, community, and institutional settings. Finally, the package called for women's health care to be available in a variety of settings (including in community-based centers accessible to women where they live, work, or attend school) and from a range of providers (including women providers, physicians, advanced practice nurses, lay midwives, and home care workers).

Despite the expansive list of covered services, its authors believed that much of basic health care consists of low-technology, hands-on services and that "the majority of health care for women is basic care which can be provided in low-cost settings by a range of efficient providers" (Campaign for Women's Health 1993:7). The campaign's package therefore implied that provision of appropriate primary and preventive services for women could help reduce health care costs overall. Although health care reform efforts were being driven largely by the need to control national health care costs, this is as close as the campaign came to confronting the financial implications of its benefits program.

Activities of the campaign included analyses of the various health care reform proposals, congressional briefings and testimony, public education, coordinating national and state-based meetings and briefings on women's health, background research on women's health problems, and, beginning in late 1993, grassroots organizing to educate women nationwide to advocate for their needs in health care reform. While it did not officially endorse a particular health care reform bill, the campaign consulted informally with the President's Task Force on Health Care Reform, including meeting with Hillary Rodham Clinton and her staff, and it worked with the task force's working group on benefits coverage to define the services women want and need and to ensure that women would have a voice on the various boards that would make decisions about covered services. In addition, the campaign briefed the Congressional Caucus for Women's Issues, which, as we saw in chapter 2, adopted a set of principles for health care reform based on the campaign's principles. The campaign also worked with the caucus on a "town meeting" on women's health problems and health care reform held in Washington,

D.C., in the summer of 1994, which was well attended by women from around the country but received little media attention.

The campaign confronted some obstacles in its attempt to get its message out and to exert influence. Because the campaign operated on a small budget and relied on donations (it did not require financial contributions from its member organizations), it did not have the resources to devote to a national media campaign or to widespread grassroots organizing. And because the campaign was newly formed to work on health care reform, it did not have the lead time to organize a fund-raising effort. (Campaign organizers were concerned, furthermore, about the propriety of accepting funding from pharmaceutical or insurance companies, whose primary interests might be to market their products to women.) In addition to financial constraints, the diversity of the groups composing the campaign presented both opportunities and obstacles. On the one hand, the groups tended to view health care reform issues within their own agendas and to seek to be responsive to their particular constituencies. These varied interests tended to broaden the health issues addressed, including the range of services to be included in the basic benefits package. On the other hand, some groups saw the campaign as a way of furthering their reproductive rights agenda, particularly abortion rights. While the campaign did endorse abortion coverage within the basic benefits package and held firm to its position that this would not be compromised as negotiation over the benefits package proceeded, there was a constant tension between the reproductive rights agenda and the broader vision of women's health being advocated by some members of the coalition. The diverse groups in the coalition did not necessarily disagree on the objectives, but rather on where to commit political effort.

Other women's health advocacy and interest groups, some of them members of the campaign, also issued reports or position statements articulating women's issues within health care reform. For example, the National Women's Health Network worked with the campaign on the model benefits package and endorsed universal coverage for all U.S. residents, including undocumented immigrants (Parsons 1994). Groups such as the National Women's Health Network, the Boston Women's Health Book Collective, and the National Black Women's Health Project endorsed single-payer financing of universal health insurance coverage (Norsigian 1993). The Commonwealth Fund Commission on Women's Health (1994) presented seven goals for health care reform, including affordable health care coverage for all Americans. The Jacobs Institute of Women's Health drew attention to the need for comprehensive covered benefits for women and the need to preserve publicly funded providers of last resort in a newly reformed health system (Brown 1994). Several women's interest groups provided analyses of the impacts of the various health care reform proposals on women. For example, the National Women's Law Center (1994) assessed the impact of the Clinton plan on women, and the Women's Research and Education Institute (1994b) compared the various health reform proposals with regard to coverage for women's reproductive and preventive services.

Kasper believes that the key accomplishments of the Campaign for Women's Health were its success in linking the goal of advancing women's health with health care reform and using the model benefits package as an educational tool to illustrate what women want and are entitled to in their health care. The major weakness of the campaign, according to Kasper, was its inability to build a grassroots movement quickly, in support of health care reform. This, however, was a problem shared by many proreform groups, who were hampered not only by limited resources but also by an inability to explain and interpret the highly complex health financing proposals, particularly the Clinton Health Security Plan, for their constituents (Skocpol 1996).

The extent to which the women's health organizations influenced the opinions of women in the general population on the issue of health care reform is difficult to assess. Although the largely middle-class members of the various women's organizations that participated in the campaign are likely to have been aware of the official positions adopted by their groups, these positions did not receive wide coverage in the national media. The impact of these positions, furthermore, might have been diluted within the deluge of persuasive communications designed by many other organizations to influence public opinion during the health care reform debate. Most notably, the series of "Harry and Louise" television ads, sponsored by the Health Insurance Association of America at a cost of about $15 million, featured a middle-aged, middle-class married couple lamenting the bureaucracy and high costs of the Clinton plan, and they were extremely effective at turning public opinion against the plan. The ads, moreover, fostered the impression that women and men shared the same interests and concerns in health care reform.

Yet the health care reform debate addressed issues, such as extending health care to the growing number of uninsured persons and families, that generally are believed to be of concern to women and to draw women into social reform activities (West and Blumberg 1990). Conventional wisdom of gender-gap politics has it that women are generally more supportive than men of social reforms to protect children, the poor, the elderly, or other disadvantaged groups. Some attribute this to women's altruism, care-based ethics, or socially prescribed caregiving roles; others attribute it to women's self-interest, since women tend to live in more precarious economic circumstances than men and are more likely than men to depend on publicly funded safety-net programs (Schlesinger and Lee 1994). In the case of the national health care reform episode, because women were more dependent on public health insurance programs than were men, were less likely than men to have health insurance through their own employment, and were more likely than men to be family caregivers, they would have been expected to be more supportive of reforms that extended insurance coverage to all, dissociated health insurance from employment, and protected families from loss of insurance. Was this true?

Public opinion polls conducted during the health care reform episode did not reveal substantial or consistent differences between women and men on support for specific health care reform proposals or for specific components of reform, such as universal health insurance coverage. Many reports of polling results did not present breakdowns by gender because no significant gender differences were found.[12] Examples of single items from various polls can be identified in which women were significantly more likely than men to favor reform, or some aspect of reform, but these examples are scattered, and the gender differences typically are small. One of the larger gender differences occurred in a Gallup poll of 1,519 adults conducted in January-February 1994 for the American Medical Association, in which 82 percent of women and 68 percent of men reported that ensuring "every American has health insurance" was a "very important" issue in health system reform (AMA 1994a:5). The significant effect of female gender held after controlling for other sociodemographic variables (including age and income), access to health care, and perceptions of the health care system (Shapiro, Jacobs, and Harvey 1995). In the same survey, no significant gender differences were found on the importance of other issues in health reform, such as choice of doctors, access to medical technology, personal health care costs, or waiting time to receive treatment.

In addition, the opinions of women and men tracked similarly over time. In Gallup polls conducted from late September 1993 through the summer of 1994, the percentage of both women and men reporting that they favored the Clinton plan to reform health care rose and fell in tandem. For both women and men, support for the Clinton plan peaked in late 1993 (at about 60 percent in favor) and declined to less than half the population by early 1994. In nine Gallup polls conducted during 1993-94, women consistently were more likely than men to favor the Clinton plan, but the average gender difference was only 4.4 percentage points.[13]

Also, there is no evidence that women in the general population were more involved politically in health care reform than were men. One study found that women were less politically active than men on the health care reform issue; that is, women were less likely to give money, contact public officials or the media, join an organization, or attend a forum on health care reform (Brodie 1996). One possibility, of course, is that pro-reform women were already engaged in women's health advocacy or interest groups by the time of the health care reform episode. If health was already an important issue for many women, then the debate about health care financing options might not have motivated women to join additional groups or to take other actions. Indeed, the Brodie study also found that in general, those who were most active on health care reform tended to be persons most likely to *oppose* reform, including self-identified conservatives.

Taken together, the evidence from the activities of organized groups and from public opinion polling shows that women's health organizations were active in health care reform efforts, along with a multitude of other groups, and that women and men generally responded similarly to polls on health reform issues. Thus, although the women's health advocacy and interest groups supported health care reform, this did not translate into a gender gap in the polls. There are several possible explanations for this. For one, while many of the women's health advocacy and interest groups, including the Campaign for Women's Health, endorsed some form of universal health insurance coverage, they apparently did not succeed in framing universal access as a "women's issue" for the public or in publicizing gender-based inequities in access to health care. Instead, they took universal access as a "given," and preferring to focus on care rather than on costs, they concentrated their efforts on defining basic services for women. The campaign's model benefits package did receive national media coverage (e.g., in the medical journalist Leslie Laurence's syndicated column, "Her Health"), but the elaboration of expansive benefits may have unintentionally heightened public concerns about the ultimate costs of any health care reform plan.

Perhaps the most public attention on women's issues within health care reform was focused on abortion coverage (Leigh 1995). Including abortion as a basic benefit, as we saw in chapter 2, was controversial and ultimately might have threatened the political viability of specific reform proposals in Congress. On this issue, furthermore, the dominant coalition of women's groups might have been out of step with the female public: a June 1994 Times Mirror poll found that women were less likely than men to think that abortions should be included in a basic health benefits package: 22 percent of women, compared with 31 percent of men.[14] While most of the public—both women and men—support legal abortion under at least some circumstances (Bowman 1996), they do not necessarily conflate abortion rights and abortion financing as matters of public policy.

Finally, the various health care financing proposals, which tapped into ideological differences about the role of government and fears of higher costs to consumers, probably divided women as much as men along partisan and socioeconomic lines. Ultimately, the politically charged financing proposals and the massive mobilization of anti–health reform forces limited the ability of the women's health coalition to activate support among the female public. It is also possible that women were less interested in financing issues than in improving health care services and that they perceived the financial focus of the health reform debate as deflecting attention from issues of care. This may have dampened women's enthusiasm for reform.

In sum, the women's health advocacy community drew on its organizational base to participate in a dominant coalition, the Campaign for Women's Health, that was actively involved in the policymaking process during the health care reform episode. The coalition brought together a diverse set of organizations and by doing so widened the base of organized interest groups on women's health. By the time national health care reform failed in 1994 and the campaign went "on hiatus," it had achieved a historically unprecedented consensus on a number of points, including universal access to care and the contents of a comprehensive benefits package for women, and it had influenced the public debate and the content of health care reform proposals. Although it did not forge a consensus on how to finance universal health insurance or its proposed benefits package, it familiarized women's groups with a new vocabulary (including "universal coverage" and "comprehensive benefits") that implied the need for fundamental delivery system changes. In addition, the broad-based coalition that formed as the Campaign for Women's Health was a new repertoire of action for women's health activists that could serve as a model for future efforts to secure national health insurance.

CHALLENGES FOR WOMEN'S HEALTH CARE POLICYMAKING

Vigilance on women's issues is particularly important during periods of fundamental changes in health care financing and delivery systems when other agendas—such as slowing the rate of growth of health care expenditures—can easily deflect attention from social equity issues related to access or quality of care. The United States remains alone among major industrial nations in failing to provide financial access to basic health care for all of its citizens. Recent trends in U.S. health care organization and financing include a growing number of uninsured and underinsured persons; a decline in the percentage of nonelderly Americans covered by private employment-based health insurance; the growth of managed care organizations of various kinds; the growth of for-profit health care organizations; the consolidation of health care delivery systems serving larger and more diverse populations; and the restructuring of public financing of health care with the prospect of fewer safety-net providers and greater variation across states in the administration' of public programs. These trends are reshaping the ways in which both women and men experience health care, and they are likely to arouse consumers' concerns about their health care generally. They also have gender-specific implications.

There are numerous issues with which women's health care policymaking might contend in the changing health care environment. They extend well beyond expanding the biomedical research agenda or developing new medical treatments for specific women's health problems. They also include basic questions of whether and how women will be able to access health information and services that enable them to maintain or improve their health. Recent women's health movement waves have been characterized by the dual demands for access to more gender-appropriate health services and for protection from unnecessary, ineffective, or unsafe services. Although these two themes sometimes appear contradictory, they can be understood as complementary approaches to improving women's health care by ensuring women's access to care, designing women-centered health services, and empowering women to maintain or improve their health and well-being.

Ensuring Women's Access to Care

A major challenge confronting women's health advocates and other participants in the policymaking process is to ensure that all women—regardless of age, reproductive status, race/ethnicity, employment status, or other socioeconomic circumstances—have access to comprehensive basic health care in their communities. This includes reducing both financial and nonfinancial barriers to care among all segments of the female population. It also includes ensuring that women do not face additional access burdens by virtue of their reproductive status. Nonpregnant women and women who are not the mothers of young children are as entitled to access to health care as are pregnant women and women who have young children; conversely, pregnant women should not lose their entitlement to health care or be assumed to have diminished capacity to make health care decisions because they are pregnant.

Financial access to basic health care is a critical policy issue confronting Americans in the absence of some form of national health insurance. Although universal health insurance coverage that is not means tested, that uncouples health insurance and employment, and that includes a basic gender-appropriate benefits package for all Americans remains the most straightforward approach to ensuring financial equity of access, the health care reform debate of the early 1990s demonstrated that there is no national consensus on this approach. Instead, a series of incremental health insurance reforms, regulation of managed care, and restructuring of the Medicaid and Medicare programs has ensued, with various implications for women.

Women's ability to obtain health care depends, in part, upon their access to affordable health insurance coverage without restrictions for preexisting conditions (including pregnancy) and with a benefits package covering both reproductive and nonreproductive services. Women, as we have seen, are less likely than men to obtain health insurance through their own employment and are more likely than men to rely on a family member's employment-based insurance or on public programs, especially Medicaid. Women therefore have much at stake in incremental private health insurance reforms that affect, for example, portability, coverage of employees' dependents, coverage of preexisting conditions, and mandated benefits. They also have much at stake in the decisions made by private employers regarding health insurance coverage of employees and their dependents and the nature of benefits provided. Finally, they are directly affected by continuing debates about restructuring Medicaid and Medicare and by state-level decisions regarding the administration of Medicaid.

Nonfinancial barriers to access also are critically important to women. The availability of a full range of women's basic health services, including both reproductive and nonreproductive services, remains a key problem in some communities and in some organized delivery systems. The survival and system integration of safety-net providers—especially family planning clinics that serve as the usual source of health care (albeit for a limited range of services) for many uninsured and adolescent women—have important implications for access to at least a minimal level of care. Inconvenient hours of operation and lack of transportation and childcare also are barriers to care for many women, particularly if they must seek services outside their communities or in multiple service settings. Legal restrictions on access—such as requirements for parental consent for reproductive health services or limitations on pregnant women's rights to make health care decisions—are additional barriers that impede women's access to services.

The women's health advocacy community in the 1990s was more successful in drawing attention to specific diseases and health problems of women than to the systemic problems many women have obtaining a basic standard of care. One barrier to framing access as a women's issue may be the middle-class hegemony of women's health advocacy. Obtaining better information about the number and characteristics of uninsured, underinsured, and intermittently insured women—including their experiences in accessing care and their unmet needs for care—would help define the situation. Broadening the constituency of advocacy and interest groups to reflect a range of access problems confronting women of all socioeconomic levels and racial and ethnic groups also could help define an "access agenda." Similarly, including more older women who confront the special access burdens of women enrolled in Medicare is critically important as the population ages. More fundamentally, however, advocacy groups will have to contend with conceptualizing what a basic standard of care is for women and how to ensure that it is available to women within their communities.

Designing Women-Centered Health Care

Ensuring access to health care is not sufficient in itself to enable women to maintain or improve their health. In the case of women's health care policy-making, issues of health care access cannot be separated from consideration of the question, "access to what?" The fragmented nature of women's health services, the wide variation in primary care patterns for women, and concerns about the effectiveness of treatments for women raise important questions about the appropriate content of women's health care and its organization and delivery. Another challenge for policy therefore is to ensure the availability of women-centered services that correct the deficiencies in women's health care resulting from a legacy of inadequate research and of clinical and system fragmentation. The creation of delivery models that provide comprehensive, coordinated, and effective health care for women should be a key policy objective.

Recent normative definitions of women-centered health care, as discussed in chapter 4, have suggested what the characteristics of these delivery models might be. Ideally, they would integrate reproductive services with the non-reproductive components of women's care, including prevention and treatment, to lower the risks of gaps or redundancies in services, to ease the burdens of care-seeking for women, and to reduce the costs of additional visits. Women's health care would be provided in accessible community settings and coordinated across providers and over time by primary care practitioners with excellent communication skills who are knowledgeable about, and sensitive to, women's health care needs at different stages of the life span. Women providers would be available in these settings in response to some women's preferences for gender-congruent care. "Carve outs" in health insurance plans that require women to seek selected services in settings apart from the regular source of care would be avoided as much as possible because they tend to fragment care, disrupt patient-provider relationships, inconvenience women, and, in some cases, present confidentiality problems for women seeking sensitive services.[15] Finally, women-centered care would combine clinical services of demonstrated effectiveness for *women* with health information and self-help strategies that enable women to maintain or improve their health through their own actions.

The concept of integrated health care for women inevitably raises the question of fertility-control services and their role within primary care. Fertility control, as we have seen, is a fundamental women's health concern that has been in evidence in all waves of the women's health megamovement, and women's demands for fertility-control sometimes have provided the impetus for new services and health care delivery organizations. Women-centered care would treat women's ability to control their reproductive lives as fundamental to their health and social well-being, and fertility-control information and services would be incorporated into basic care according to the woman's needs and preferences. In addition, women's ability to protect themselves from unwanted sexual intercourse and its consequences would be viewed as fundamental to health maintenance. Consequently, screening for sexual abuse, emergency contraception, follow-up mental health services, and referrals for appropriate social services also would be integral components of primary care.

Several strategies, which are not mutually exclusive, are available for designing women-centered health care. One strategy is to create a practitioner, who could be a physician or an advanced practice nurse, with specific training and competencies in women's health who would serve as a primary care provider for women. This provider would assume responsibility for performance—or for coordinating a multidisciplinary team's performance—of basic well-woman services, including screening and preventive services, routine gynecological and prenatal care, routine acute care, and health education. This provider also would coordinate referrals to specialists or community services and would monitor the woman's health care, including her schedule of periodic screening services, over time.

Within the medical profession, proposals for a new interdisciplinary medical specialty in women's health exemplify this approach. The new specialist has been envisioned as combining the expertise of, for example, the general internist or family physician, the obstetrician-gynecologist, and the psychiatrist in a life-span approach to women's health care (Hoffman and Johnson 1995; Johnson 1992). The main concern that has been raised about a new specialty is that it might further marginalize women's health care rather than encouraging other specialists to incorporate it into their practices (Harrison 1992). Nevertheless, some proponents view the new specialty as a strategy for transforming medical practice generally, by compelling the profession to acknowledge and integrate women's viewpoints and information on women's health, much as the creation of women's studies programs influenced scholarship in traditional academic disciplines during the 1980s (Rosser 1994).

An additional option within medicine is to provide expanded training in women's health in undergraduate or graduate medical education or in postgraduate, continuing education for physicians in practice. The Council on Graduate Medical Education (1995), calling for "a new paradigm in women's health," has specified themes and competencies to guide curriculum reform. While little curriculum reform has occurred at the undergraduate level, residency training programs and fellowships in women's health have been established in some graduate medical education programs in internal medicine, family practice, and obstetrics-gynecology. Some of these programs have been offered in conjunction with primary care women's health centers. Continuing education in women's health has expanded substantially in recent years. The American Medical Women's Association (Wallis 1993), for example, developed a core continuing-education curriculum on women's health that specifies content areas for women's primary care in different life phases. One policy objective might be to ensure that all physicians, regardless of specialty, who are credentialed to serve as primary care providers for women within managed care organizations or other delivery systems be required to demonstrate appropriate training and competencies in women's health care.

Another strategic approach to women-centered care focuses on the delivery organization rather than the primary care provider. In this approach, the providers and other resources needed to offer comprehensive primary care to women are brought together in teams or in organizational entities sponsored by hospitals, managed care plans, or provider groups. The organizational approach is embodied in the concept of the multidisciplinary comprehensive primary care women's health centers (as described in chapter 4), but it also could be realized in other team-based integrated practices or in managed care organizations with the capacity to physically link providers and services. The primary care women's health centers combine medical services, nonmedical clinical services, and health information and education in a team-based "one-stop shopping" approach to health care delivery. Currently available in only a limited number of communities, these centers promise efficiencies in care delivery, particularly under capitation, because they can provide basic well-woman services (including clinical preventive services) in fewer visits per patient and coordinate a woman's total care. Some of these centers are hospital sponsored, thus providing an organizational basis for on-site referrals for specialized services (e.g., diagnostic mammography), and some provide community outreach services including health education and delivery of services to underserved groups.

The provision of clinical preventive services illustrates how primary care women's health centers might be positioned to improve women's health care. By concentrating providers and services in one place, by coordinating a woman's care, and by emphasizing patient education and well-woman care, these centers may enhance comprehensive preventive screening for women. As discussed in chapter 3, different preventive services typically are offered by different types of physicians and in different settings, requiring many women to make multiple visits for a full array of age-appropriate preventive services. Furthermore, the recommended screening intervals for various preventive services (e.g., Pap smears, mammography, cholesterol tests, stool guaiac tests, immunizations) do not coincide, so that women and their providers might have difficulty keeping track of their screening schedules and coordinating services. Although reminder systems (e.g., written or telephone contacts) have been shown to improve screening rates among women in some practices (Commonwealth Fund Commission on Women's Health 1996b), these strategies typically have focused on individual tests rather than on comprehensive preventive visits appropriate for a woman's age and risk status. Primary care women's health centers may be better positioned organizationally to coordinate a woman's screening schedule and to provide comprehensive preventive services in one visit.

The main concerns raised about primary care women's health centers are that they may be costly to establish or maintain and that they might contribute to increased duplication or fragmentation within the health care system as a whole. To date, no research has compared the efficiency or effectiveness of these centers with that of other models of care delivery for women. As more of these centers serve women enrolled in managed care plans, one way to study the "value added" of centers, while controlling for the effects of selection, would be to compare the care received by women served in women's health centers with care received by women in other practice models within the same managed care plans.

Despite the absence of comparative research on delivery models, there are at least three arguments in support of public policy to encourage the development or maintenance of comprehensive primary care women's health centers in all communities. The first is that some of the existing centers are safety-net providers that serve as the usual source of care for traditionally underserved segments of the female population, particularly poor and low-income, uninsured, minority, and adolescent women. Consequently, policies that support the survival of these centers are likely to preserve some women's access to basic health care during a critical period of change in the health care delivery system. The second argument is that primary care women's health centers provide a preferred health care option for women of all socioeconomic levels who seek comprehensive services in one location from providers who are expert in and committed to women's health care and information needs. Consequently, policies that support the creation or maintenance of these centers help preserve the option of women-centered care and increase choice for consumers. Third, primary care women's health centers provide innovative models of care. There is little evidence that managed care organizations are adopting the characteristics of women-centered care pioneered by these centers or that employers consider the possible benefits of these centers or of team-based approaches to care when they negotiate contracts with health insurers. Consequently, policies that support the integration of primary care women's health centers into managed care networks could help provide useful models for managed care organizations.

These issues raise the important question of how to define and measure quality in women's health care. In research to assess which organizational approaches to women-centered primary care provide the highest quality of care, all approaches to quality measurement would be relevant, including process of care, patient satisfaction and retention, clinical outcomes, functional status, and quality-of-life outcomes. Available measures of quality, however, are limited in their ability to capture distinctive features of the process and outcomes of care for women and to include women's perspectives. The leading indicators of the care process in women's health focus on provision of readily measured clinical preventive services (e.g., the percentage of women receiving Pap smears and mammograms and the percentage of pregnant women receiving early prenatal care). Measures are needed for the comprehensiveness of preventive services provided (appropriate to the patient's age and risk status) and for other process features of women's primary care, such as the coordination of the reproductive and nonreproductive components of care and the amount and quality of communication between providers and patients.

Outcome measures, furthermore, tend to focus on disease management; however, because of historical fragmentation of services and the wide variation in delivery of women's primary care, there is also a need to assess the outcomes of well-woman and preventive care. Such outcomes might include, for example, the degree to which women are protected from unwanted pregnancy, are supported in lifestyle changes to promote health, are confident in their ability to engage in self-care, receive appropriate counseling and follow-up for positive screening tests, or are free from undetected domestic-violence injuries or undiagnosed episodes of depression. Another issue is that measures intended for use in both genders, such as multidimensional patient satisfaction or health status measures, might not include items of particular importance for women and therefore might not be sensitive to differences across organizational settings in the quality of women's health care. For example, patient satisfaction measures may not include items tapping providers' sensitivity to women's psychosocial needs (e.g., the need for respite from caregiving), the quality of provider-patient communication along dimensions important to women (e.g., not being "talked down to"), or the ease of scheduling one visit for comprehensive well-woman care. Health status measures might not include such items as confidence in one's protection from unwanted pregnancy, level of functional incapacities associated with the menstrual cycle, sense of control over one's bodily integrity, or confidence in one's capacity for self-care.

In addition, assessing the effectiveness of specific clinical services is particularly important in women's health care. Women's health advocates since the 1960s have been effective in drawing attention to the medicalization of women's health and bodily functions and to the health risks and other costs to women of untested, invasive, or overused medical procedures. Recently, advocates have argued for expanded research on women's health so that interventions can be based on evidence from studies of women subjects. The need for effectiveness data applies not only to new technologies, but also to many services that have become the standard of practice in women's care. For example, what is the effectiveness—in terms of early detection of treatable disease—of routine annual pelvic examinations and Pap smears, which generate numerous visits by well women? What is the effectiveness—in terms of reduction of unintended pregnancies—of family planning programs? What is the effectiveness—in terms of avoidance of poor birth outcomes—of routine prenatal care visits for low-risk mothers? Are there less costly alternative therapies or lifestyle changes that are as effective as hormone therapy for the treatment of menopausal symptoms or for postmenopausal prevention of heart disease or bone loss?

The women's health advocacy community could promote women-centered delivery models by supporting a diversity of health care delivery models in their communities, by organizing to influence the purchasers of health benefits for women, by lobbying for funding of research on women's health services, and by demanding accountability (from health plans, employers, and government) for the outcomes of women's health care. Increasing the investment in effectiveness research in women's health is an important policy objective. This includes research on the effectiveness of specific treatments and preventive services, as well as research on the quality of care provided within different delivery models. Evaluating new delivery models, such as primary care women's health centers or teams and various types of managed care organizations, will be important for designing women-centered health care and for supporting evidence-based policymaking in women's health.

Empowering Women

Another challenge for policymaking is to improve women's capacity to maintain or improve their health and to make informed decisions on their use of health care services. One objective is to ensure that women receive accurate and complete health information, including information about the effectiveness of services and treatments, the latest research results, the availability of health and social services in their communities, their health plan options, and the political processes shaping their health and health care. Another objective is to safeguard women's autonomy to make informed decisions about their health care, including their right *not* to use health services. A third objective is to decrease the ratio of medically controlled to consumer-controlled services.

One of the enduring themes in the women's health megamovement, and in women's health advocacy generally, has been women's demands for information and education about their health and bodies. Women's health advocacy and interest groups all seek, in one way or another, to empower women with respect to their health and health care, and many of them regard information dissemination—through newsletters, topical pamphlets, telephone hotlines or on-line information or referral services—as part of their missions. (The National Women's Health Network, for example, reports that its information clearinghouse responded to over 8,000 information requests in 1995.) Although these groups traditionally have focused on information about lifestyle factors, clinical services, medical products, and pharmaceuticals, recently they have begun to respond to women's needs for information about health insurance plans and health care delivery options within the changing health care marketplace. In addition to women's health advocacy organizations, women obtain health information from a number of sources, including their health care providers, friends and family members, the mainstream media, commercial women's health newsletters, the professional literature, and, increasingly, direct marketing to women by pharmaceutical companies and other commercial interests. What sources women use, how they distinguish among these sources with respect to the accuracy or usefulness of the information, and how they discern the vested interests of the communicators can all affect their health care decisions.

Public policy can support dissemination of health information by ensuring that the results of health research are communicated directly to the public—through such channels as mainstream media, on-line services, information clearinghouses, or government publications—in a timely and accurate manner. Policy could also provide for integrated health information to consumers. That is, because much biomedical research is disease-focused, there is a great need among consumers for information that integrates findings across diseases and provides women with state-of-the-art information about lifestyle strategies that enhance overall health, about the combination and schedule of clinical preventive services that is most effective for their age group, and about the relative benefits and risks of new interventions. The groups of women for whom information needs might be greatest include, for example, those in the contested age or risk groups for specific screening tests who are confused about how recommendations apply to them; perimenopausal women who are confused or skeptical about the benefits of hormone therapy in relation to the risks; and elderly women for whom the perceived benefits of clinical preventive services, in terms of increased life expectancy or quality-adjusted life years, may not exceed the costs (both financial and nonfinancial) of obtaining them. Public policy also can regulate communications by commerical enterprises that increasingly advertise their products or services directly to consumers. Regulation would help ensure that a balanced picture of benefits and risks of interventions is provided.

Enhancing women's capacity to make informed health decisions is not only a matter of information dissemination, however. Women's responsibilities for making health care decisions on their own behalf need to be defended and protected as a matter of policy. Historical and current policies can be identified that are antithetical to the principle of empowering women as decision makers in matters of their health and health care. These include regulations that limit the acquisition of new information about women's health, such as restrictions on pregnant women's participation as subjects in clinical studies; regulations that restrict communication of health information, such as policies limiting adolescents' access to school-based health education programs or clinics, or the notorious abortion "gag rule" of the Reagan-Bush era that sought to eliminate abortion counseling in family planning clinics receiving federal funding;[16] policies that interfere with the privacy of health communications between provider and patient, such as some states' parental notification requirements for adolescents seeking abortion or family planning services; and policies that presume pregnant women or terminally ill women to be incapable of informed decision making, such as legal restrictions on their rights to refuse medical treatment. Policies that restrict the content of provider-patient communication or that limit the patient's rights to make health care decisions are, by definition, disempowering.

Women also could be empowered by vesting greater control over health and body matters in women themselves, rather than in health professionals. Because women's health has often been regarded as overmedicalized and because women continue to consume health services in greater quantities than men, it is reasonable to ask in what ways it might be "demedicalized" by removing certain conditions or services from medical control.[17] Women's health provides several historical examples of demedicalization in which consumers have taken control of some conditions or services. These cases tend to occur under certain conditions: when the power imbalance between providers and consumers is unacceptably onerous; when the level of distrust of providers is too high; or when the financial or nonfinancial burdens of access through the formal system become too great. A classic example of demedicalization, although it did not produce widespread change, was the attempt by some consumers during the 1970s to redefine childbirth as a natural process that could take place in the home, under the control of the family and attended by a lay midwife.[18] Another example is the case of lay-provided menstrual extractions for abortion in the pre–*Roe v. Wade* era when obtaining a legal abortion required a formal, stigmatizing approval process. A third example is women's performance of artificial insemination on themselves using turkey basters and a donor's semen (Wikler and Wikler 1991).

Approaches to demedicalization that vest more control in consumers and reduce burdens of access might include transferring some services normally provided by physicians—such as routine physical examinations, prenatal care, or childbirth—to other health professionals, such as nurse practitioners or certified nurse-midwives. As noted earlier, routine well-woman, gynecological, and prenatal examinations are frequently the target of such substitution of personnel in managed care plans and in some women's health centers, reflecting, among other things, a recognition that the women so served are not diseased. This approach could be said to empower women by increasing the range of providers available to deliver needed services, by increasing their access to female providers, and by reducing their dependence on physicians. In some states, this strategy would require reduced legal restrictions on the scope of practice of advanced practice nurses.

Demedicalization could also include providing consumers with direct access to pharmaceuticals or medical devices previously available only from physicians or by prescription, so that they no longer are medically mediated or require a health care visit. Home diagnostic tests, such as pregnancy tests and HIV tests, are prominent examples. In women's health, an interesting case is the debate about whether oral contraceptives ought to be available over the counter (OTC) in the United States, as they are in some other countries (Grimes 1993; Laurence and Weinhouse 1994; Samuels and Smith 1994; Trussell et al. 1993). More than 50 million outpatient prescriptions for oral contraceptives were dispensed in the United States in 1992 (Schondelmeyer and Johnson 1994), and most of these prescriptions probably generated a health care visit. The OTC debate has focused on the safety of hormonal contraception (a traditional concern of women's health advocacy groups, including the National Women's Health Network), on implications for women's receipt of other services frequently provided in the same visit when oral contraceptives are prescribed (e.g., blood pressure screening, Pap smear, STD screening), and on the possible effects on access to oral contraceptives. On the one hand, OTC status could increase access (and women's control of their fertility) by making oral contraceptives more convenient to obtain, since women would not be required to make repeated visits to a prescribing provider. Furthermore, one study suggests that the price of oral contraceptives might decline somewhat if they became available without prescription (Schondelmeyer and Johnson 1994). On the other hand, OTC availability could decrease access (and disempower women) because health care insurers are not likely to cover nonprescription medications, and many women may not be able to afford oral contraceptives if they are required to pay the full cost out of pocket. Currently, however, most private health plans do not fully cover the cost of oral contraceptives. Absent from this debate has been information about women's preferences.

Demedicalization, of course, does not necessarily empower consumers; in some cases it might subject them to greater health risks, in some cases it might result in denial of health insurance coverage or other benefits for previously covered conditions or services, and in some cases it might impose a particular caregiving burden on women. However, as long as nonmedical alternatives to current patterns of care are not perceived as eliminating an entitlement, do not substantially increase risks, and do not increase caregiving burdens, they may be not only socially acceptable, but socially preferable and empowering to women.

CONCLUSION

Women's health care is structured differently from men's. It also is highly susceptible to shifting governmental priorities and funding streams, and it is increasingly delivered in managed care arrangements designed by purchasers and providers who may not be particularly attuned to women's health concerns. In addition, large numbers of women remain outside the health care system, at least during episodes when they are uninsured, and they neither receive adequate care nor have an organized voice in policymaking. Some women seek information or care options that are not available in their communities. The challenge is to attend to women's health care needs without perpetuating women's dependency or burdens in seeking care. Policy objectives in three areas are important within the context of the changing health care environment: ensuring women's access to care, designing women-centered models of care delivery, and empowering women to maintain or improve their health.

Since the 1970s, the number and diversity of women's health advocacy and interest groups have grown, and as we have seen, they were especially influential in the health policy community during the 1990s wave of women's health activism. Although there is no societal consensus on how gender should be incorporated in public policy, the formal participation of these groups in health care policymaking processes is one way to ensure the inclusion of women's viewpoints and to promote policies that do not disadvantage women. As we enter the twenty-first century, women's health advocacy and interest groups are positioned to participate as partners in policymaking on a historically un-precedented scale. It remains to be seen whether health care policymaking will be transformed by the participation of these groups and by the growth in the number and influence of women physicians, researchers, legislators, and government officials. What seems certain, however, is that there will be many issues with which women's organizations will contend in the changing health care environment. Health care is likely to remain a social arena in which gender issues are prominent and in which women's social equity concerns continue to be played out.

Appendix

Data Sources

The 1993 Commonwealth Fund Survey of Women's Health

Methods

The Survey of Women's Health was conducted by Louis Harris and Associates for the Commonwealth Fund in February and March, 1993 (Louis Harris and Associates 1993; Falik and Collins 1996). The telephone survey consisted of a national cross-section of U.S. households, excluding Alaska and Hawaii, using a multistage sample stratified by geographic region and metropolitan versus nonmetropolitan residence. Oversamples of African American and Hispanic women were included to ensure representation of these subgroups. Excluded were military personnel, prisoners, hospital and nursing home residents, residents of religious and educational institutions, homeless and phoneless persons, and those who did not speak English or Spanish. The data were weighted by age, race, education, insurance status, and census region, using March, 1992 U.S. Census Bureau data, so that results are representative of the 94.6 million women and 86.7 men ages 18 and over. (Analyses reported in this book use unweighted data.)

In all, 2,525 women and 1,000 men ages 18 and over were interviewed. The completion rate (defined as the number of completed interviews divided by the number of completed interviews plus refusals plus terminated interviews) was 56 percent. No data are available on the reasons for nonresponse or comparing the sociodemographic characteristics of nonrespondents and respondents. However, telephone surveys in general are likely to underrepresent persons who do not reside in households with access to a telephone (estimated to be less than 8 percent of households [Corey and Freeman 1990]).

The weighted age and race/ethnicity profile of the female sample is as follows: 55 percent were ages 18 to 44, 26 percent were ages 45 to 64, and 18 percent were ages 65 and over; 84 percent were white, 13 percent were African American or black; and 3 percent were another race or ethnicity; 8 percent were of Hispanic descent.

Interviews were conducted by female interviewers, and 5 percent of the interviews were conducted in Spanish. The 25-minute women's interview included questions about the relationship between the respondent and physicians, health insurance, access to and use of health services, health habits and counseling, knowledge about health risks and protection measures, work and role stress, social support, self-esteem and depressive symptoms, crime/battering/rape/abuse, health habits, and sociodemographics. (The men received an abbreviated form of the interview.)

Sampling error is approximately ±2 percentage points.

Data Quality

Only 1 percent of interviews were terminated before completion. Missing data are minimal. The highest refusal rate occurred for a question on household income (9 percent of respondents either refused to answer or responded "not sure.") On the questions about physician specialty, 3 percent of women could not identify their physicians' specialties. On questions pertaining to health insurance coverage, fewer than 1 percent were "not sure" on questions about employer-based health insurance and Medicare; 2 percent or fewer were "not sure" about Medicaid, HMO, or other private coverage. Telephone surveys are thought to underrepresent the uninsured (Corey and Freeman 1990); however, the percentage of uninsured women in this survey is comparable to estimates from other sources. For example, this survey found that 17 percent of women ages 18 to 44 were uninsured, compared with 19 percent of women ages 15 to 44 in estimates for 1993 based on the 1987 National Medical Expenditures Survey (Women's Research and Education Institute 1994a).

For some of the utilization variables, comparisons with other recent national survey results can be used to assess consistency. For example, in the 1993 Survey of Women's Health, 80 percent of women and 72 percent of men reported having a regular source of care; this compares with 83 percent of women and 73 percent of men ages 18 and over in the 1987 National Medical Expenditures Survey (Collins et al. 1994:141). In the Survey of Women's Health, women reported an average of 5.2 physician visits in the last year, and men reported 4.1 visits. This compares with a mean of 5.9 visits reported by women and 4.8 visits reported by men in 1989 (Aday 1993a) and with 6.8 nontelephone physician contacts by women and 4.6 by men in the 1993 National Health Interview Survey (computed from data in Benson and Marano 1994).

On reports of clinical preventive services received in the last year, respondents in the 1993 survey generally reported higher levels of services received than were reported by women in the 1992 National Health Interview Survey (Makuc, Fried, and Parsons 1994). The largest difference was for mammography among women ages 65 and over: 39 percent of women in the 1992 NHIS and 54 percent of women in the 1993 survey reported having a mammogram in the last year. These differences could reflect differences in the sample or interview procedures of the two surveys or changes in screening rates between 1992 and 1993. Screening rates for cervical and breast cancer improved in the general population between 1991 and 1994, according to the National Center for Health Statistics (1996b).

The Study of Women's Health Centers

This study consisted of two phases: the National Survey of Women's Health Centers and a set of case studies of innovative women's health centers. The project was conducted at the Johns Hopkins University School of Hygiene and Public Health, Department of Health Policy and Management, with support from the Commonwealth Fund (grant no. 94-54). The investigators were the author, Barbara Curbow, and Amal J. Khoury. Consultants on the project included Barbara Bartman, Herbert R. Hansen Jr., Patricia Looker, and Sheryl Burt Ruzek.

Survey Methods

The National Survey of Women's Health Centers was conducted in 1994 (Weisman, Curbow, and Khoury 1995). The target population for the survey was all organizational entities, in both the public and private sectors, providing any clinical services designed for and marketed to women in either hospital-based or freestanding facilities in 1993-94. Clinical services were defined broadly to include screening or preventive services, acute or chronic care services, and inpatient or rehabilitative services. Excluded were centers that offer only nonclinical services (e.g., resource centers providing education or physician referral services), single-provider practices, women's hospitals (of which there were only 12 at the time of the survey in 1994), and patient advocacy groups.

Because no national listing of women's health centers was available, the sampling frame for the survey was constructed by collecting and merging multiple national listings of women's health centers obtained from fourteen organizations during January to March, 1994. The limitations of this approach are that the sample does not include centers that were unknown to those compiling the source lists nor types of centers for which no lists were available. It is not possible to assess the impact of these limitations.

National listings were obtained from the American Hospital Association, Family Life Information Exchange, Federation of Feminist Women's Health Centers, National Abortion Federation, National Alliance for Breast Cancer Organizations, National Association of Childbearing Centers, National Association of Women's Health Professionals, National Consortium of Breast Centers, National Osteoporosis Foundation, National Women's Health Network, National Women's Health Resource Center, National Women's Mailing List, Planned Parenthood Federation of America, and Women's College Coalition. Additional organizations that assisted in identifying source lists were the Boston Women's Health Book Collective, Family Planning Councils of America, Jacobs Institute of Women's Health, National Family Planning and Reproductive Health Association, Office of Research on Women's Health (NIH), and State Family Planning Administrators.

The national lists were prescreened to eliminate obviously ineligible organizations (e.g., marketing firms, professional associations, advocacy groups) and duplications. In all, these lists identified over 6,500 organizations potentially eligible for this study. The organizations were grouped into mutually exclusive strata for sampling purposes: birth centers, breast diagnostic or treatment centers, reproductive health centers (including family planning and abortion centers), hospital-based centers not otherwise classified, and nonhospital centers not otherwise classified. (It was not possible to classify some of the organizations by type of service on the basis of the information on the source lists.) Centers were then sampled disproportionately (larger strata had smaller sampling fractions), screened for eligibility by telephone (to verify that it was a women's health center of some kind and that it was in operation), and surveyed by mail. Surveys were mailed to the center's administrator, who was identified in the telephone screening. Telephone follow-ups were made to all centers that had not responded within four weeks of the original mailing.

Some centers in each sampling stratum were found to be ineligible. Ineligibility rates and reasons for ineligibility varied by stratum. The ineligibility rate was lowest among birth centers (24 percent) and reproductive health centers (25 percent) and highest among nonhospital centers not otherwise classified (66 percent). About two-thirds of ineligible birth centers had either closed or could not be located; about half of ineligible breast centers were either general radiology departments not focusing on women's services or education/support groups providing no clinical services. Over half of the ineligible reproductive health centers were either single-provider practices or not administratively distinct organizational entities. Among hospital-based centers not otherwise classified, over 60 percent of ineligibles were hospitals in which no women's health center of any kind could be located after telephone inquiries to several offices within the hospital.

(It is possible that hospital-sponsored women's health centers have a high mortality rate, accounting for our inability to locate centers in some of these hospitals; in attempts to locate a center, a protocol was used that involved telephoning the main hospital number, the CEO's office, the public relations office, and the Department of Obstetrics and Gynecology, if any.) Among nonhospital centers not otherwise classified, 37 percent of ineligibles provided no clinical services, and 23 percent did not regard themselves as women's health centers because they also served children or men.

A 26-page self-administered survey questionnaire was developed and pretested on seven subjects who had administrative experience in women's health centers of various kinds. The questionnaire covered seven topic areas: organizational characteristics and staffing, services provided, clients/patients, finances, mission and philosophy, quality, marketing and planning. Because the survey was conducted during a period of heightened expectations for national health care reform, questions were included about how centers were positioning themselves for various changes in the health care system, including managed care. Most questions were closed-ended, and some required reporting numbers or percentages. The instructions included with the questionnaire indicated that although the survey had been mailed to the center's director for completion, it was appropriate for others in the center who had specialized knowledge of a specific area (e.g., finances) to complete those sections.

The overall survey response rate was 56 percent ($N = 467$ centers). Response rates varied by stratum: birth centers had the highest rate (79 percent), and hospital-based centers not otherwise classified had the lowest (48 percent). There was no response bias by region of the country or, among hospital-sponsored centers, by type of hospital ownership.

For population estimates (e.g., number of centers, number of women served), weights were assigned to each center on the basis of the stratum-specific sampling proportions, eligibility rates, and response rates. Unweighted data are used to compare types of centers.

Case Study Methods

The second phase of the project consisted of case studies of eight innovative women's health centers conducted during the spring and summer of 1995. A standard protocol was used in site visits to the centers to obtain in-depth information from the multiple perspectives of administrators, providers, and patients/clients. The case studies provided an opportunity to test some ideas, based on the survey findings and organizational theory, about center characteristics likely to be associated with successful performance. Discussions with center personnel during the site visits provided some insight into the history and evolution of the centers, as well as their expectations for the future. The general hypotheses guiding the case studies were that model women's health centers would exemplify the core attributes of women-centered care identified in the 1993 Conference on Women's Health Centers organized by the Jacobs Institute of Women's Health (Schaps et al. 1993) and would be actively engaged in efforts to adapt to and influence the changing health care environment.

A multiple embedded case study design was used, in which the cases should be viewed as replications of "experiments" to test ideas about women's health centers, rather than as a set of representative observations (Yin 1994). Using data from the survey as well as information obtained from knowledgeable informants, eight women's health centers were selected for case studies. Three types of centers were targeted for the case studies: primary care centers, reproductive health centers that had transformed themselves into primary care centers, and comprehensive breast care centers. These types of centers were chosen because they represented innovative models of care that attempt to integrate and coordinate services, either comprehensive primary care services or breast care services, in a women-centered setting. The selected centers were four primary care centers (one in an academic medical center, one in a VA medical center, one private-not-for-profit independent center, and one for-profit center owned by a nurse practitioner); two reproductive health centers that had expanded to primary care (one feminist women's health center and one Planned Parenthood affiliate); and two comprehensive breast care centers (both in academic medical centers). The centers that gave us permission to identify them are Women's Health Associates at Massachusetts General Hospital in Boston (primary care); T.H.E. Clinic, Inc., in Los Angeles (primary care); Planned Parenthood of Sacramento Valley in California (primary care, formerly reproductive health); University of Michigan Breast Care Center in Ann Arbor; and Revlon/UCLA Breast Center in Los Angeles.

The centers selected generally were well established and had demonstrated their capacity to maintain operations over time: all but two of the centers (the VA center and the Revlon/UCLA Breast Center) had been in operation ten years or more at the time of the site visit, and the youngest center had been in operation about three years. The case study centers were located in the northeastern, middle-Atlantic, north central, and western regions of the country and therefore reflected different health care marketplaces.

The director of each center was contacted by telephone and gave consent to the case study. A site visit was conducted at each center by a two- or three-person team over a period of one or two days. The following information-gathering activities were conducted:

1. Review of center documents (e.g., annual reports, personnel manuals, brochures, media coverage, professional publication)

2. A tour of the center and completion of a checklist describing center facilities and physical location

3. Semi-structured interviews with center administrators (including the center director and, if applicable, the chief financial officer and marketing director)

4. Semi-structured interviews with center clinicians (including the medical or clinical director, if any, and a mix of disciplines, if applicable)

5. Focus groups with established patients/clients (sometimes stratified by age group)

6. Self-administered questionnaires completed by patients participating in the focus groups

The semi-structured interviews lasted between thirty minutes and one hour, and focus groups lasted two hours, during which refreshments were served. The interviews and focus groups were audiotaped.

A case study report was prepared for each center, following a uniform format. Each report was sent to the center director for review for accuracy, and minor revisions were made. An integrated case study report was prepared that addressed the case study hypotheses (Weisman, Curbow, and Khoury 1997).

Notes

Chapter 1: The Social and Historical Context of Women's Health Care

1. For discussions of the various meanings of "gender," see Andersen (1993), Connell (1987, 1995), and Hess and Ferree (1987).

2. The interaction of gender and race/ethnicity in determining health status for women of color in the United States is discussed by Bayne-Smith (1996). For a discussion of racial issues in the study of women's health, see Gamble and Blustein (1994) and Ruzek, Olesen, and Clarke (1997).

3. In 1994, 59 percent of U.S. women ages 16 and over were in the labor force, compared with 75 percent of men. Among women, those ages 35 to 44 were most likely to be in the labor force (77%), and those ages 55 to 64 were least likely (49%). Among all workers, women were more likely than men to work part-time (28% vs. 11%, respectively) (Herz and Wootton 1996). Women's labor force participation rate has increased steadily since 1960, when 38 percent of all women were in the labor force, and it is projected to reach 63 percent in 2005 (Costello and Stone 1994).

In 1994, women full-time workers ages 16 and over earned 76 percent of what men earned; the 1994 median weekly earnings of full-time women workers was $399, compared with $522 for men (Herz and Wootton 1996). In 1993, the median annual family income for female-headed families with no spouse present was $17,413, lower than that for married-couple families and families headed by a man with no spouse present. Nearly half (46%) of female-headed families with no spouse present and children under age 18 fell below the poverty level in 1993. Women are more likely than men to be poor at all ages. In 1993, 15 percent of women ages 18 and over lived in poverty, compared with 10 percent of men; among persons ages 65 and over, women were nearly twice as likely as men to be poor (15% vs. 8%, respectively) (Costello and Krimgold 1996). Goldin (1990) argues that the "feminization of poverty" is the result of a combination of factors, including women's lower earnings than men, divorce, and paternal default.

4. For discussions of how these concepts relate to studies of men's health and illness, see Sabo and Gordon (1995). A key concern among men's health activists is men's less frequent care-seeking behavior, particularly for clinical preventive services.

5. For a discussion of whether "new" social movements are really new and of women's rights movements as examples, see Calhoun (1995).

6. Recent scholarship has begun to document the social welfare activism, including that on health issues, of minority women, particularly African Americans, from the 1890s on (Gordon 1990b, 1994).

7. Although nineteenth-century women physicians sometimes challenged medical orthodoxy with regard to women's health, particularly with respect to beliefs about the negative health effects of education for women, they joined their male colleagues in opposing contraception and abortion (Morantz-Sanchez 1985). Contemporary women's rights activists perceived contraception and abortion as encouraging promiscuity and the exploitation of women; instead, they supported married women's rights to control their fertility by abstaining from sexual intercourse, which they were presumed not to engage in for any purpose other than procreation (Gordon 1990a). These topics are discussed further in chapter 2.

Chapter 2: The Women's Health Megamovement

1. No comprehensive social history of women's health care in the United States is available. Consequently, the historical material in this chapter draws on several different areas of scholarship that intersect in their relevance for women's health. These include studies of gender role ideology and of women's changing social roles; studies of changing conceptions of women's health and illness; histories of the American medical profession, of other health care providers (e.g., midwives), and of health care organizations; histories of specific women's health services (e.g., childbirth practices); and analyses of social welfare policy related to health care. Social and medical historians and sociologists have made important contributions in each of these areas, particularly since the 1970s. Two important collections of historical analyses are edited by Rima Apple (1990) and Judith Leavitt (1984).

Key works on gender role ideology and women's social roles from colonial times to the present include Cott (1977), Kerber (1986, 1995), Rothman (1978), Smith-Rosenberg (1985), and Welter (1983). Key histories of the American medical profession include Duffy (1993), Kett (1968), Rothstein (1992), Shryock (1966), Stevens (1971), and Starr (1982). Histories of obstetrics and gynecology include Dally (1991), Moscucci (1990), and Speert (1980). Women in the medical profession have been studied by Morantz-Sanchez (1985) and Walsh (1977). Histories of specific women's health issues and services include studies of childbirth practices (Leavitt 1986; Rothman 1991; Wertz and Wertz 1989), studies of family planning and abortion practices and policy (Brodie 1994; Gordon 1990a; Luker 1984; McCann 1994; Mohr 1978; Petchesky 1990; Reed 1978; Staggenborg 1991), and studies of mental illness (Brumberg 1989; Showalter 1985). Others have provided histories and critical analyses of the medical profession's discourses on women's nature and women's health (Ehrenreich and English 1973a; Fee 1978; Haller and Haller 1974; Smith-Rosenberg and Rosenberg 1984; Vertinsky 1994). Several case studies are available of women's health institutions or enterprises, including a case study of the New England Hospital for Women and Children (Drachman 1984), a case study of an illegal abortion referral service and practice (Kaplan 1995), and a case study of the Lydia E. Pinkham Medicine Company (Stage 1979). Studies of the history of social welfare policy in the United States from the perspective of women's issues, sometimes including health care, include Abramovitz (1988), Gordon (1994), Ladd-Taylor (1990), Muncy (1991), Rothman (1978), and Skocpol (1992).

2. Regina Morantz-Sanchez has contributed the most comprehensive analysis of women's role in the Popular Health Movement (Morantz 1977; Morantz 1984; Morantz-Sanchez 1985). Martha Verbrugge has contributed a case study of the Ladies' Physiological Institute of Boston and Vicinity during the 1850s (Verbrugge 1979). Susan Cayleff (1987) analyzed the water-cure movement from the perspective of women's health. Discussions of sectarians and the medical paradigms they promoted may be found in Duffy (1993), Kett (1968), Numbers (1977), Rothstein (1992), Shryock (1966), and Starr (1982).

3. Several scholars have described the medical theories of women's health promulgated during the second half of the nineteenth century, including Drachman (1976), Ehrenreich and English (1973a), Fee (1978), Haller and Haller (1974), Morantz-Sanchez (1985), Smith-Rosenberg and Rosenberg (1984), Rothman (1978), and Wood (1984). Consideration of the role of women physicians with respect to prevailing theories and treatments may be found in Dally (1991), Drachman (1976), Morantz (1985), Morantz-Sanchez (1985), Shryock (1966), Vertinsky (1994), and Walsh (1977). Discussions of antiabortion and anticontraception activities during this period may be found in Brodie (1994), Gordon (1990a), Luker (1984), Mohr (1978), and Petchesky (1990).

4. At the time, however, tuberculosis could not be effectively treated. Although the tuberculosis bacillus was discovered in 1882, treatments would not be developed until the twentieth century. Sheila Rothman (1994) describes how the social category of "invalid" attached to persons with tuberculosis in the nineteenth century and how the standard medically prescribed regimens differed by patient gender. Men, for example, were more often advised to travel to salutary climates, whereas women were advised to remain within the domestic circle.

5. It is not clear what effect, if any, regular physicians' campaign against contraception and abortion had on their ultimately successful effort to consolidate

the medical profession. Rivalry among the various medical practitioners continued until the various sects and specialists became dependent upon each other for
referrals and for access to hospital facilities. Mutual dependence also led to general support for medical licensing laws (Cassedy 1991; Rothstein 1992; Starr 1982).
By 1901, all states had licensing laws requiring at least a medical diploma for the
practice of medicine. Thereafter, homeopaths and eclectics declined in number
and eventually were absorbed into mainstream medicine.

6. Protective labor legislation to restrict the hours or conditions of women's
and children's employment began in earnest in the 1890s but peaked during the
Progressive Era. (Women were 25% of industrial workers in 1900 [Kessler-Harris
1995].) Forty-one states had passed women's hours laws by 1921 (Skocpol 1992).
Women's health was not the only rationale for this legislation. Some supporters
saw it as an opening wedge for improving the working conditions of all workers,
regardless of gender (Skocpol 1995). Florence Kelley, for example, saw focusing on
women as a strategy of "appealing to the sympathy of the masses for the welfare
of helpless working women and children," whereas men were thought to evoke little public sympathy because they could vote (Sklar 1995:258). However, some
scholars and contemporaries, including Kelley, observed that protective labor
legislation was sometimes intended to preserve men's jobs and wages by restrict-
ing women's participation in male-dominated occupations (Goldin 1990; Kessler-
Harris 1995; Sapiro 1990). Indeed, women's jobs such as paid domestic labor and
nursing were not regulated.

7. These two reform movements are rarely considered together. Studies of the
maternal and child health reformers during the Progressive Era and after World
War I have been provided by Meckel (1990), Muncy (1991), Rothman (1978), and
Skocpol (1992). Discussions of the birth control movement may be found in
Chesler (1992), Gordon (1990a), McCann (1994), Reed (1978, 1984), and Rothman
(1978). McCann (1994) provides the most direct comparison of the two groups of
reformers and their relations with other feminist causes of the period; she also lo-
cates both groups within Progressive Era ideology and tactics. Rothman (1978)
compares the medical profession's reactions to the Sheppard-Towner programs
and to the birth control movement. Different interpretations of Margaret Sanger's
feminism in the context of the birth control movement are provided by Gordon
(1990a), McCann (1994), and Petchesky (1990).

8. Several scholars have pointed out that legalization of abortion had no political support at the time and, in fact, that the medical profession continued to use
the abortion issue to assert its professional authority during its Progressive Era
campaign against lay midwifery (Borst 1995; McCann 1994). After 1880, an influx
of immigrants from eastern and southern Europe led to a resurgence of the practice of midwifery in urban areas and caused heightened concern among physicians,
public health officials, and infant welfare activists (Meckel 1990). Leslie Reagan
(1995) shows how obstetricians in Chicago, including women obstetricians, at-

tempted to obtain state regulation of midwives by charging that immigrant midwives were abortionists who contributed to the problem of maternal mortality.

9. Amendments in 1942 to Title V, which focused on maternal and child health services, permitted, but did not require, the use of program funds for family planning services because of the perceived connection between child spacing and infant health (Burt 1993). This provided the first policy linkage of the services advocated by the maternal-child health advocates and by the birth control advocates.

10. Sheryl Burt Ruzek (1978) provides the most comprehensive history of the Women's Health Movement of the 1960s and 1970s and a discussion of its properties as a social movement. Other accounts include Eagan (1994), Fee (1975), Marieskind (1975, 1980), Rothman (1978), and Zimmerman (1987). Rodwin (1994) compares this movement with other movements to hold physicians accountable to patients. Discussions of the component of the Women's Health Movement focusing on reproductive rights, particularly abortion, may be found in Gordon (1990a), Luker (1984), Petchesky (1990), and Staggenborg (1991). Lesley Doyal (1983) describes the contemporary women's health movement in Britain.

11. For more detailed accounts of the Finkbine case, see Garrow (1994) and Luker (1984).

12. The emergence of the antiabortion countermovement in the late 1970s and protests aimed at abortion providers are discussed by Joffe (1995), Luker (1984), Meyer and Staggenborg (1996), Petchesky (1990), and Staggenborg (1991).

13. This discussion of the early 1990s episode relies on a few published accounts of some of the events as well as interviews with fifteen key participants in its early stages. Published accounts include Auerbach and Figert (1995), Howes and Allina (1994), Laurence and Weinhouse (1994), and Schroeder and Snowe (1994). Discussions of some of the key issues addressed during the 1990s episode may be found in Dan (1994) and Rosser (1994). The following individuals were particularly helpful in providing information: Lesley Primmer, executive director of the Congressional Caucus for Women's Issues from 1989 to 1995; Susan F. Wood, science advisor and later deputy director of the Caucus (to 1995); Ruth Katz, who served for twelve years (until 1995) as counsel to the Subcommittee on Health and the Environment in the House of Representatives; and Tracy L. Johnson, who served as program director for the Society for the Advancement of Women's Health Research from 1990 to 1994. The interpretations presented, however, are entirely my responsibility.

14. An inventory of NIH expenditures was often cited to make this point. The inventory found that 13.5 percent of the total NIH budget in 1987 went to women's health problems; what was not generally reported was that only 6.5 percent went to diseases unique to men (Kirchstein 1991; Mann 1995). Most funds were expended on diseases that affect both sexes or on basic research for which the applications were not yet known.

15. For example, a 1992 GAO report found that women had been underrepresented in trials of new cardiovascular drugs approved from 1988 to 1991 and that only 12 percent of new drug studies analyzed hormonal interactions in women (USGAO 1992). In 1993, the FDA lifted its 1977 restrictions and issued new guidelines for inclusion of women in the clinical evaluation of drugs (Sherman, Temple, Merkatz 1995).

16. The 1986 NIH policy on inclusion of women in research dated to the 1985 Report of the Public Health Service Task Force on Women's Health Issues. The task force had been appointed "to identify those women's health issues that are important in our society today and to lay out a blueprint for meshing those issues with the priorities of the Public Health Service" (USPHS 1985:74). The report made fifteen specific recommendations, five of which had to do with conducting research and evaluation on a wider range of women's health problems across all age groups and in the context of women's multiple social roles. The report led to the establishment of advisory committees on women's health for each PHS agency and to a new policy, published in the NIH *Guide for Grants and Contracts*, urging applicants to "consider" the inclusion of women in study populations and the analysis of gender differences. The policy was to go into effect in 1987. In 1987, the NIH Women's Health Advisory Committee called on NIH to both implement its policy on inclusion of women and increase its investment in women's health research.

17. Most observers think that health care reform failed because of a combination of politics and public antipathy. Political opponents were able to portray the highly complex Clinton Health Security Plan as a case of "big government," and the public became convinced that their health care choices would be unacceptably constrained under the plan and that the costs of the program would be too high. Alternative or compromise plans became politically infeasible. For analyses of the fate of the Clinton health care reform plan, see Blendon, Brodie, and Benson (1995), Drew (1994), Johnson and Broder (1996), Skocpol (1996), and a set of papers in the spring 1995 issue of *Health Affairs* (vol. 14, no. 1).

Chapter 3: Patterns of Health Care Use

I would like to thank Sandra D. Cassard for her assistance with this chapter.

1. For a discussion of the gradual decline in maternal mortality in the United States that began in the late 1800s, including the factors contributing to the decline, see Leavitt (1986), Loudon (1992), and Shorter (1991). Racial differences persist, however. The age-adjusted maternal mortality rate in the United States in 1993 was 6.7 deaths per 100,000 live births, but rates were substantially higher for black women (20.0 deaths per 100,000 live births) than for white women (4.2 deaths per 100,000 live births) (NCHS 1996a). A study of pregnancy-related mortality in the United States between 1987 and 1990 found a fourfold excess risk

among black women (Berg et al. 1996). In the early 1990s, the U.S. maternal death rate was higher than that of fifteen developed countries, including Canada (Adamson 1996).

2. A number of general purpose national surveys are available for comparing women and men on some basic indicators of health services use (Horton 1995). These data sources have a number of limitations, however. For one thing, the measures typically are not rich enough to characterize problems in accessing care, to identify use of multiple sources of care, to differentiate visits for primary or preventive care from visits for treatment for illness, to link specific services received with specific types of providers, to analyze the theoretically relevant determinants of utilization, or to track trends in access or sources of care. Use of alternative health services and nonmainstream sources of care, furthermore, is rarely measured. In addition, the standard data reports do not use consistent age categories and sometimes group all persons of one sex together, including children and adults. (When all ages are grouped, the terms "females" and "males" are used instead of "women" and "men.") In addition, data reports generally do not provide analyses controlling for both gender and socioeconomic status. Finally, the potential of gender bias is present in many surveys, since women and men may perceive and report on health care use differently.

The typical indicators of health care use that are measured in surveys include having a regular source of health care, the number of physician contacts (in person or otherwise) or physician outpatient visits per year, the number of inpatient hospital episodes per year, and receipt of prescription medications. In some surveys the data are self-reported in household interviews, as in the National Health Interview Survey, a continuing survey that is representative of the civilian noninstitutionalized population of the United States (Benson and Marano 1994). In other surveys the data are reported by health care providers, as in the National Ambulatory Medical Care Survey of a probability sample of nonfederally employed physicians' office-based practices, excluding the specialties of anesthesiology, radiology, and pathology (Woodwell and Schappert 1995).

3. Many national health data sources report statistics by age group, with the ages between 15 and 44 (or 18 and 44, if only adults are surveyed) representing the "reproductive" or "childbearing" years. The National Survey of Family Growth, which provides data on "fertility, contraception, infertility, and other aspects of maternal and infant health that are closely related to childbearing," focuses exclusively on women ages 15 to 44 (Chandra 1995). This age group, however, reflects neither the entire period of women's lives when they are capable of becoming pregnant nor the stage of life when they are most likely to become pregnant. In the United States in 1988, the median age at menarche was 12.5, and the median age at menopause was 48.4. Only four years typically elapse between the birth of a woman's first and last children, and 75 percent of women have completed their desired family size by age 35 (Forrest 1993). The peak reproductive years, for purposes

of identifying women's use of health services related to pregnancy and child-bearing, might be between 18 and 35, but national surveys do not report consist-ently for this age group.

4. For discussions of the definition and classification of nontraditional or al-ternative therapies, see Fugh-Berman (1996), Kronenberg, Mallory, and Downey (1994) and Wardwell (1994). This is also a dynamic area in which some previously conceived "alternative" therapies, such as acupuncture, are being adopted by some mainstream providers and covered by some health insurance plans. Often, yesterday's "alternative" therapies are today's "complementary" ones.

5. There is variation among women, however, in the prevalence of insurance coverage. Among nonelderly women, members of racial and ethnic minorities are more likely than white women to be uninsured: in 1993, 13 percent of Anglo women ages 18 to 64 were uninsured, compared with 20 percent of African Amer-ican women, 32 percent of Latina women, and 21 percent of Asian women (Wyn and Brown 1996).

6. The Personal Responsibility and Work Opportunity Reconciliation Act of 1996 could have important implications for Medicaid coverage for both pregnant and nonpregnant women. This welfare reform legislation repealed the AFDC program, under which women had automatically qualified for Medicaid, and re-placed it with a block grant that could be administered differently by the states. The act also denied Medicaid benefits to certain noncitizens for five years fol-lowing entry to the United States. See Rosenbaum and Darnell (1977) for an analy-sis of the act's health-related provisions.

7. In a 1995 survey of 1,037 private and public employers with 200 or more workers, pre-existing condition limitations were reported by 56 percent of em-ployers in conventional (indemnity) insurance plans, in 56 percent of point-of-service plans, and in 76 percent of preferred provider organizations; health main-tenance organizations typically did not limit or exclude coverage for pre-existing conditions of new enrollees (KPMG 1995). The Health Insurance Portability and Accountability Act of 1996, known as the Kennedy-Kassebaum bill after its lead sponsors, included provisions for coverage of pregnancy-related care, as of en-rollment, for women obtaining group health insurance coverage through an em-ployer or union (Women's Legal Defense Fund 1996).

8. According to the 1988 National Survey of Family Growth, 57 percent of all pregnancies in 1987 were unintended (i.e., unwanted at the time of conception or mistimed), and about half of all unintended pregnancies ended in abortion; among married women, 40 percent of pregnancies were unintended, and 26 per-cent ended in abortion (Forrest 1994). Women most likely to have unintended pregnancies were unmarried, low-income, or at the earliest or latest stages of the reproductive years. The health consequences of unintended pregnancies for women have received less attention than those for infants. Research shows that women with unintended pregnancies receive later and less adequate prenatal care,

are more likely to smoke cigarettes and consume alcohol during pregnancy, and may be at higher risk for depression during and after pregnancy and for domestic violence during pregnancy (Brown and Eisenberg 1995).

9. Specifically, residency programs in obstetrics-gynecology were required to provide residents with "education and experience managing the complications of abortion" (ACGME statement, July 31, 1995). Programs with religious or moral objection to abortion were not required to perform abortions within the institution or to provide training in induced abortions, but such programs were required to ensure that residents received training in managing abortion complications, either inside or outside the institution. Attempts were made in the 104th Congress to prevent the ACGME from requiring abortion training (Chavkin 1996).

10. For discussions of health care as a social good and of ethical principles related to its allocation, see Beauchamp and Childress (1994), Daniels (1985), Daniels, Light, and Caplan (1996), and Nelson and Nelson (1996).

11. The term "fragmentation" has been used to characterize U.S. health care generally, as well as specific components of the health care system, such as the mental health services sector or child health services. The high degree of medical specialization, the tendency to separate preventive and curative care, the complex relations between private and public sectors, and the general lack of coordination among providers, financing programs, and organizations have all been identified as elements of system fragmentation (Aday 1993b; Edmunds 1995; Grason and Guyer 1995; Shortell et al. 1996; Starr 1982; Stevens 1971). Because of the bifurcation of reproductive and nonreproductive care, however, women's basic health care is fragmented in ways that men's is not. The intention here is to focus on specific indicators and consequences of fragmentation in women's health care.

12. California, Maryland, and New York were the first states to pass legislation, in 1994, on the role of obstetrician-gynecologists as primary care providers. The New York law applied to HMOs only, whereas the California and Maryland laws applied to all insurers. All three laws required that women have direct access to an obstetrician-gynecologist without prior authorization from a gatekeeper. Women's groups were involved in these efforts in California and New York. Resolutions were introduced in the 104th Congress stating that obstetrician-gynecologists should be designated as primary care physicians in federal legislation relating to health care provision (Women's Policy, Inc. 1996b).

13. In response to the question "Is there one place in particular you usually go to when you are sick or want advice about your health, or isn't there," 80 percent of women answered "yes." Among those with a usual source of care, 75 percent reported that they go to a physician's office or HMO, 17 percent to a clinic, 5 percent to a hospital emergency room, and 2 percent to some other place. Fewer than 0.5 percent reported using a nurse practitioner or nurse-midwife as the usual source of care. In follow-up questions, the survey focused on the types of physi-

cians used for regular care and did not include specific questions about non-physician providers seen (e.g., nurse practitioners, certified nurse-midwives, physician assistants). More comprehensive questions about women's patterns of health care use might focus on use of multiple service sites as well as different types of providers.

14. Some comparisons with men in the 1993 Survey of Women's Health are noteworthy. While 90 percent of women and 85 percent of men reported that they had a "regular doctor," men were more likely than women to report seeing a family or general practitioner as the regular physician (65% of men, compared with 56% of women). Also, men visited fewer physicians than women. The average number of different physicians visited in the last year was 1.9 for men, compared with 2.1 for women (a statistically significant difference of means, $p < .01$). The median number of physicians visited was one for men and two for women. For men, the average number of physicians seen increased with age, whereas for women, the average number of physicians held steady, at just over two physicians, across age groups.

15. The overall percentage of women in the survey reporting that their regular physician was an internist was 16 percent, while 56 percent reported that their regular physician was a general or family practitioner. The women who reported seeing internists were more likely than women seeing family or general practitioners to also see an obstetrician-gynecologist (56% vs. 43%).

16. These findings may be related to physician supply. In 1993, 87 to 90 percent of physicians in medical and surgical specialties were located in metropolitan areas, compared with 72 percent of family or general practitioners, and 89 percent of nonfederal obstetrician-gynecologists were in metropolitan areas. Also, the highest physician-to-population ratios in 1992 were found in the New England and Middle Atlantic states: 334 and 317 physicians per 100,000 civilian population, respectively (AMA 1993, 1994b).

17. Clinical preventive services have been defined to include individual risk assessments; counseling about lifestyle, self-care, and services; screening tests to detect disease, disability, or genetic predisposition; immunizations; and provision of chemoprophylactic regimens (U.S. Preventive Services Task Force 1996). Primary preventive services (e.g., immunizations, preventive postmenopausal hormone therapy) are provided to prevent the onset of a condition; secondary preventive services (e.g., Pap smears, screening mammograms, genetic screening) are provided to detect a condition before it has developed or early in its development when it is most easily treated. Many screening tests are periodic, in that they are recommended at regular intervals over time, depending on an individual's age, gender, and risk status.

18. For example, among women in the 1993 Commonwealth Fund Survey of Women's Health who had not received at least one preventive service in the last year, lack of a physician recommendation was reported as the reason by 23 per-

cent of women. (The most frequently reported reason for not receiving screening was cost, by 29% of women.) Part of the influence that physicians have might stem from the fact that guidelines for women's screening sometimes are contradictory and confusing, and women are likely to rely on their physicians for interpretations and recommendations in their own cases.

19. The American College of Obstetricians and Gynecologists and the American Academy of Pediatrics recommended a postpartum hospital stay of 48 hours for an uncomplicated delivery and 96 hours for cesarean delivery, to ensure adequate time for care of both mother and newborn and for maternal instruction in breastfeeding and infant care (ACOG 1995).

Chapter 4: Women and Health Care Delivery: Providers and Organizations

1. Of course, as opportunities for women to receive gender-congruent primary care were increasing, opportunities for men to receive gender-congruent care were, potentially, decreasing. Less attention has been paid, however, to the implications of more men receiving health care from women physicians. With regard to specialty care associated with the reproductive system, there is no precise parallel for obstetrics-gynecology in the case of men's health care. Few women are specialists in urological surgery, a specialty that treats both men and women. In 1995, only 0.2 percent of women physicians were in the specialty, and only 2 percent of urologists were women. By contrast, 70 percent of obstetrician-gynecologists were men (AMA 1997).

2. Overall, women are at least 75 percent of the total health care work force, 96 percent of registered nurses (the largest health occupation), and a majority of several allied health occupations that provide direct patient services (Butter et al. 1987; Moses 1994). In 1990, for example, women were 74 percent of physical therapists, 75 percent of radiological technicians, 94 percent of occupational therapists, and 99 percent of dental assistants (Muller 1994). Women also predominate among informal caregivers. In addition to their care of children, women provide most of the unpaid health care to frail elderly family members, including spouses (Brody 1994). According to the 1982 National Long-Term Care Survey, over 70 percent of those giving informal care to the disabled elderly were women (Stone, Cafferata, and Sangl 1987). This pattern reflects both the traditional caregiving role of women and their longer life expectancies. Another illustration of women's caregiving role is their predominance among legal surrogates designated to make health care treatment decisions for incapacitated relatives or loved ones. In a recent study of end-of-life decision making by patients with a variety of terminal conditions and their surrogates, most surrogates were found to be women, even among homosexual male AIDS patients (Sulmasy et al. 1996).

3. Historically, women physicians had worked fewer hours than men and

fewer years during their professional careers. Although there was evidence that work patterns for women and men in medicine were tending to converge, particularly among younger cohorts of physicians (Freiman and Marder 1984), concerns were raised during the 1970s and 1980s that forecasts of a physician oversupply (except in primary care specialties) needed to be adjusted downward to account for the increasing proportion of women entering medical practice. For recent discussions of trends in gender differences in physicians' practice patterns, see reports by the AMA (1991) and the Council on Graduate Medical Education (1995).

4. Professional groups issuing guidelines for screening sometimes disagree on indications or periodicity for the same services. With regard to Pap smears, for example, the U.S. Preventive Services Task Force (1996) recommends routine screening at least every three years for all women who have been sexually active and who have a cervix. However, a consensus recommendation for annual Pap smears for all women who are or have been sexually active, or who have reached the age of 18, has been adopted by the American Academy of Family Physicians, American Cancer Society, American College of Obstetricians and Gynecologists, American Medical Association, National Cancer Institute, and others (American Cancer Society 1993). With regard to mammography, the major recent controversy has surrounded the appropriateness of screening for women between the ages of 40 and 49. The U.S. Preventive Services Task Force (1996) recommends routine screening mammography every one to two years for women ages 50 to 69, but not for women in their forties or over the age of 70. The National Cancer Institute concluded in 1993 that research did not support routine mammography for women in their forties, but reversed itself in 1997 and recommended mammograms every one to two years for women in this age group. Other groups that recommend mammography screening for women beginning at the age of 40 include, for example, the American Cancer Society, American College of Obstetricians and Gynecologists, American College of Radiology, and the American Medical Association.

Although studies of women's use of screening sometimes assume that more screening (or more frequent screening) is better than less screening, the inconsistencies in guidelines reveal disagreement among experts. Indeed, too frequent screening may carry risks to individuals. Louise Russell (1994) provides an important discussion of the benefits and costs of routine preventive screening for cervical cancer, prostrate cancer, and high blood cholesterol. She identifies a key "human cost" of screening to be false-positive test results, which subject patients to stress, repeated tests, and follow-up procedures that may carry risks. In the case of Pap smears, she estimates that a woman's lifetime chance of one or more false positives is greater than her chance of developing cervical cancer.

5. The 1993 survey did find, however, that women report more lifetime dissatisfaction than men with their physicians. Forty-one percent of women, compared with 27 percent of men, reported that they had ever changed doctors

because of dissatisfaction with the doctor (gender unspecified). When asked the reasons for their dissatisfaction, women were more likely than men to report problems with communication, such as the doctor "didn't listen to me." Overall, 2 percent of women, but no men, reported that they had changed physicians because of a preference for a physician of the other gender.

6. The youngest women surveyed, those ages 18 to 34, were significantly more likely than the oldest women, those ages 65 and over, both to have a regular physician who is a woman and to prefer a woman physician. Younger women may be more likely than older women to seek out a woman physician; however, they would also be more likely to receive care from a woman even without seeking it, because younger women are establishing their health care patterns at a time when more women are practicing medicine. In all age groups, however, having a woman physician was significantly associated with reporting a preference for one. These findings may indicate that there will be a growing preference for women physicians among women patients as more women receive care from women physicians.

7. A limitation of this data set for testing the effects of physician gender on preventive services is the absence of information about physicians' ages. The demography of medical practice means that younger women physicians typically are compared with older men physicians, and younger physicians are thought to be more prevention-oriented. At the time of the survey in 1993, 70 percent of women physicians in office-based practices were under the age of 45, compared with 43 percent of men (AMA 1994b). Two recent studies of physicians' screening practices, however, suggest that physician age might not have the expected effects. Turner et al. (1992) conducted a 1985-86 survey of 298 general internists, obstetrician-gynecologists, and cardiologists and found no differences in physicians' reported breast cancer screening practices by year of medical school graduation. Lurie et al. (1993) did not find a consistent pattern of screening practices by physician age; among men, younger physicians (ages 45 and younger) provided less screening by Pap smear and mammography than older physicians; among women, physicians around age 50 provided less screening than both younger and older physicians.

8. Federal programs, in addition to Title V and Title X, that provide funding for family planning services include Medicaid and Title XX of the Social Security Act, the Social Services Block Grant. The history of the major federal programs supporting family planning services is described by Martha Burt (1993). Because some privately owned family planning providers, including Planned Parenthood centers, may be heavily dependent on government funding such as Title X and Medicaid, they may be regarded as quasi-public organizations that are highly susceptible to shifts in public policy.

9. The 1994 data were provided by the AHA Health Statistics Group.

10. Some types of women's health organizations originated outside the United

States (e.g., Dutch birth control clinics provided the model for Margaret Sanger's clinics), and some other developed countries currently have successful women's health centers of a specific kind (e.g., Swedish prenatal care clinics [Miller 1988] and Australian women's health centers promoting a social model of health [Doyal 1995]). However, women's health organizations in the United States appear to be more diverse in form and more entrepreneurial than those in other countries. Three sociohistorical factors might account for this. First, as we have seen in chapter 2, the activism of voluntary associations of U.S. women and of women health care providers has produced a variety of new organizational forms for women's health education and health care. No other country has experienced the recurring waves of women's health movements, with their associated organizational innovations for health care, to the degree experienced in the United States since the 1830s. Second, the absence of a U.S. national health system with centralized control over health care resources has created both needs and opportunities for organizational experimentation in health services delivery. New organizations in women's health care, furthermore, have been supported by both private and public funds, thus increasing possibilities for local variations. Even though women's health movements have appeared in Great Britain, for example, Doyal (1995) points out that few services have been created outside of mainstream organizations, in part because the National Health Service results in a limited market for private health care. Third, a surplus of health care resources in the United States, especially with respect to clinical personnel, has sometimes helped make new women's health services possible. For example, the availability of women physicians who faced educational and employment discrimination in the late-nineteenth and early twentieth centuries was an important factor in the staffing of early prenatal care and birth control clinics. Similarly, the growing number of certified nurse-midwives in the 1970s helped facilitate the growth of freestanding birth centers. In recent years, excess supply in the hospital sector has contributed to the development of hospital-sponsored ambulatory care services of various kinds, including women's health centers.

11. The Study of Women's Health Centers was conducted at the Johns Hopkins University School of Hygiene and Public Health, Department of Health Policy and Management, with the support of grant no. 94–54 from the Commonwealth Fund (see Appendix). The views presented here are those of the author and not those of the Commonwealth Fund, its directors, officers, or staff. I am grateful to my co-investigators, Barbara Curbow and Amal J. Khoury, who contributed to the analyses reported here.

12. The term *women's health center* originated during the Women's Health Movement of the 1960s and 1970s and referred to freestanding, consumer-controlled reproductive health or primary care centers. In current usage, however, the term refers to a much more diverse set of organizational entities, including both hospital-sponsored and independent facilities providing a range of health care

services for women, for which there are no formal criteria (Chez 1993; Looker 1993). One of the purposes of the survey was to identify and describe the various types of women's health centers.

13. Title X of the Public Health Service Act, created in 1970, enjoyed bipartisan support and increased funding through the 1970s, in part because it was viewed as a means of preventing abortions and reducing adolescent pregnancies. Even though Title X funds may not be used for abortion services, the program has been a victim of abortion politics in Congress. Beginning in the 1980s with the Reagan administration's conservative agenda of "pro-family" values and cuts in federal domestic spending, Title X came under attack and was repeatedly threatened with repeal, folding into block grants to the states, various restrictions on use of funds, and reductions in funding (Burt 1993). By 1991, Title X had declined as a source of revenue for family planning programs (Ku 1993).

14. The survey did not identify any women's health centers operated by HMOs or other managed care entities. At the time of the survey in 1994, the Group Health Association of America had no information on HMO-sponsored women's health centers.

Chapter 5: Transforming Women's Health Care Policymaking

1. Legal scholars and social scientists have discussed these frameworks in relation to legislation and court decisions pertaining to gender. See, for example: Bem (1993), Eisenstein (1988), Kirp, Yudof, and Franks (1986), MacKinnon (1989), Minow (1990), Rhode (1989), and Samuels (1995). Bioethicists also have considered the different implications of these frameworks for health care practices and policies. See, for example, DeBruin (1994), Sherwin (1992), and Tong (1996).

2. Discussions of age-based rationing may be found in Beauchamp and Childress (1994), Brock (1989), Callahan (1988), and Daniels (1985).

3. The term *maternalist* has been used in different ways by scholars interested in the history and traditions of social policy. Two usages are relevant here: the concept of a maternalist ideology of women's roles shared by Progressive Era social reformers (and by women across all segments of society), and the concept of maternalist social policies. As an ideology, maternalism referred to a concept of womanhood that emphasized maternal capacities and responsibilities, within both the domestic and public spheres. The maternal role was construed broadly to include the nurturing of families and the care and moral guardianship of communities, particularly the poor and immigrant components of those communities, through social and political action. The maternal role, furthermore, was assumed for all women; those who did not bear children, including some of the most prominent settlement workers and women social reformers, were regarded as "public mothers" (Smith-Rosenberg 1985:263). Gordon (1994:55) notes that maternalists believed that women were uniquely qualified to lead social reform ef-

forts because of "their work, experience, and/or socialization as mothers." Skocpol (1992:36) describes maternalist reformers as groups of women "devoted to extending domestic ideals into public life." The social policies advocated by maternalist reformers were intended to protect the idealized conception of motherhood, to preserve the normative family, and to promote child welfare. These policies were targeted to women and children as a special class. Women without children generally were regarded as potential mothers and were therefore included in the class of protected persons.

4. This quote is from Justice Brewer's opinion, writing for the majority, in *Muller v. Oregon* 208 U.S. 412 (1908). See Freeman (1990) and Rhode (1989) for discussions of the fate and legacies of protective labor legislation targeted to women.

5. The implications of new medical technologies for women's health and women's rights also are discussed by Mahowald (1993), Petchesky (1990), Raymond (1993), Rodin and Collins (1991), Rothman (1986), and Rowland (1992).

6. Another contemporary example of disregard for pregnant women's capacity to make decisions on behalf of their health is described by Karen Rothenberg (1996). The State of Maryland's 1985 "living will" statute stipulated that a woman's living will would not be honored during pregnancy, thus limiting pregnant women's rights to terminate life support. The Maryland Health Care Decisions Act of 1993 provided for advanced directives that included an option for women to provide special instructions for the case of pregnancy. George Annas (1994) observes that women in general, pregnant or not, tend to be treated differently than men in cases involving the right to refuse medical treatment.

7. Recent scholars have provided evidence that as more women are elected to legislative office, they tend to draw attention to distinctive women's issues and to work successfully on those issues (Gelb and Palley 1996; Mandel and Dodson 1992; Thomas 1994).

8. Age-based selection also can be a factor. Cindy Pearson, executive director of the National Women's Health Network, reports that most members in 1996 were between the ages of 35 and 50. This reflects the demographics of the post–World War II baby-boom generation.

9. Theda Skocpol (1992) describes the historical role of the "translocal federation" model of women's groups in promoting women's policy interests. The Women's Christian Temperance Union in the 1870s and the General Federation of Women's Clubs from the 1890s to about 1910 provide examples of highly effective women's groups organized at the local (sometimes church-based), state, and national levels. The advantages of this organizational model include broad-based support that can be mobilized to influence elections and policy at all levels of government and an expansive network of organizations to provide continuity of communication and activity over time. Although today's women's health interest groups tend not to be organized so hierarchically, they sometimes consist of both national and state or local affiliates.

10. Dickersin and Schnaper (1996) provide a discussion of the ways in which consumers can contribute to the research process, for example, by suggesting new research questions and hypotheses and by helping improve informed consent and other study procedures.

11. See Bergthold (1995) for a discussion of the term *medical necessity* and how it was interpreted in the context of health care reform plans.

12. I am grateful to Mollyann Brodie, Mark Cottrell, Larry Jacobs, and Mark Schlesinger for providing their analyses and observations about gender differences, or the lack thereof, in public opinions on health care reform.

13. These Gallup poll data were provided by the Roper Center at the University of Connecticut.

14. These data were provided by the Pew Research Center for the People and the Press.

15. "Carve outs" have been studied primarily in terms of their economic rationales and financial impact, rather than in terms of their impact on quality of care. The problems for women patients associated with "carve outs" for specific reproductive health services, including abortion, were noted in chapter 4. Stephen Shortell and colleagues (1996) provide a discussion of why carved-out benefits and programs generally (e.g., for mental health services and substance abuse services or for cancer care) are inconsistent with the principles of clinical integration of care. These authors also point out that because of changing demographics, increasing numbers of older patients with multiple chronic conditions are likely to exacerbate the clinical and administrative problems associated with carve outs.

16. NARAL (1996) reports that in 1995, four states had "gag rules" preventing state-employed providers or entities receiving state funds from counseling or referring women for abortion services.

17. "Demedicalization" can be construed in a number of ways. According to Peter Conrad (1992), it refers to a social redefinition of a previously medicalized problem as a nonmedical one that no longer requires medical treatment. Further, he argues, it usually is achieved only after some type of organized social action challenging medical authority. He does not consider cases where services normally provided by physicians are provided by other licensed health professionals as instances of demedicalization, but rather as "deprofessionalization." It could be argued, however, that the transfer of services to nonphysicians requires a redefinition of the condition being treated as "nonmedical."

18. The number and circumstances of lay-assisted home births are difficult to study, and trends are not clear. Because lay midwives may be prosecuted in some states, they may not be identified on birth certificates, and estimates of the number of births they attend may be unreliable (Clayton 1991). One estimate is that at most 1 percent of births are attended by lay midwives (Butter and Kay 1988).

References

Abramovitz, M. 1988. *Regulating the Lives of Women: Social Welfare Policy from Colonial Times to the Present.* Boston: South End Press.

Adams, P. F., and Marano, M. A. 1995. Current estimates from the National Health Interview Survey, 1994. *Vital and Health Statistics,* series 10, no. 193.

Adamson, P. 1996. A failure of imagination. *The Progress of Nations.* New York: UNICEF.

Aday, L. A. 1993a. Indicators and predictors of health services utilization. In S. J. Williams and P. R. Torrens, eds., *Introduction to Health Services.* Albany: Delmar.

————. 1993b. *At Risk in America: The Health and Health Care Needs of Vulnerable Populations in the United States.* San Francisco: Jossey-Bass.

Aday, L. A., and Andersen, R. M. 1974. A framework for the study of access to medical care. *Health Services Research* 9:208–220.

Aday, L. A., Andersen, R., and Fleming, G. V. 1980. *Health Care in the U.S.: Equitable for Whom?* Beverly Hills: Sage.

Alan Guttmacher Institute. 1994. *Uneven and Unequal: Insurance Coverage and Reproductive Health Services.* New York: Alan Guttmacher Institute.

Alpha Center. 1995. The Medicaid expansions for pregnant women and children. Washington, D.C.: Alpha Center.

Altman, R. 1996. *Waking Up, Fighting Back: The Politics of Breast Cancer.* Boston: Little, Brown.

American Association of Health Plans (AAHP). 1996. *1995 AAHP HMO PPO Trends Report.* Washington, D.C.: AAHP.

American Cancer Society. 1993. *Guidelines for the Cancer-Related Checkup: An Update.* Atlanta: American Cancer Society.

American Civil Liberties Union (ACLU). 1995. Hospital mergers: The threat to reproductive health services. *Reproductive Rights Update.* Washington, D.C.: American Civil Liberties Union.

American College of Nurse-Midwives. 1995. *Nurse Midwifery Today: A Handbook of State Legislation*. Washington, D.C.: American College of Nurse-Midwives.

American College of Obstetricians and Gynecologists (ACOG). 1993. *The obstetrician-gynecologist and primary-preventive health care*. Washington, D.C.: ACOG.

———. 1995. *Statement on decreasing length of hospital stay following delivery*. Washington, D.C.: ACOG.

American Hospital Association (AHA). 1990. *Why Women's Health*. Chicago: American Hospital Association, Section for Maternal and Child Health.

———. 1993. *American Hospital Association Hospital Statistics: 1993–94 Edition*. Chicago: American Hospital Association.

American Medical Association (AMA). 1991. *Women in Medicine in America: In the Mainstream*. Chicago: American Medical Association.

———. 1993. *Physician Characteristics and Distribution in the U.S., 1993 Edition*. Chicago: American Medical Association.

———. 1994a. *Public Opinion on Health Care Issues*. Chicago: American Medical Association.

———. 1994b. *Physician Characteristics and Distribution in the U.S., 1994 Edition*. Chicago: American Medical Association.

———. 1997. *Physician Characteristics and Distribution in the U.S., 1996–1997 Edition*. Chicago: American Medical Association.

American Psychiatric Association. 1987. *Quick Reference to the Diagnostic Criteria from DSM-III-R*. Washington, D.C.: American Psychiatric Association.

Andersen, M. L. 1993. *Thinking about Women: Sociological Perspectives on Sex and Gender*. 3d ed. New York: Macmillan.

Andersen, R. M. 1995. Revisiting the behavioral model and access to medical care: Does it matter? *Journal of Health and Social Behavior* 36:1–10.

Annas, G. J. 1994. Women, health care, and the law: Birth, death, and in between. In E. Friedman, ed., *An Unfinished Revolution: Women and Health Care in America*, chap. 3. New York: United Hospital Fund of New York.

Apple, R. D., ed. 1990. *Women, Health, and Medicine in America: A Historical Handbook*. New Brunswick, N.J.: Rutgers University Press.

Asbell, B. 1995. *The Pill: A Biography of the Drug that Changed the World*. New York: Random House.

Auerbach, J. D., and Figert, A. E. 1995. Women's health research: Public policy and sociology. *Journal of Health and Social Behavior* Extra issue, 115–131.

Ayanian, J. Z., and Epstein, A. M. 1991. Differences in the use of procedures between women and men hospitalized for coronary heart disease. *New England Journal of Medicine* 325:221–225.

Baker, P. 1990. The domestication of politics: Women and American political society, 1780–1920. In L. Gordon, ed., *Women, the State, and Welfare*, chap. 3. Madison: University of Wisconsin Press.

Bartman, B. A., Moy, E., and Clancy, C. 1994. Characteristics of women's usual source of care: How do internists compare with other primary care physicians? *Journal of General Internal Medicine* 9:47.

Bartman, B. A., and Weiss, K. B. 1993. Women's primary care in the United States: A study of practice variation among physician specialties. *Journal of Women's Health* 2:261–268.

Bashur, R. L., Homan, R. K., and Smith, D. G. 1994. Beyond the uninsured: Problems in access to care. *Medical Care* 32:409–419.

Bayne-Smith, M. 1996. Health and women of color: A contextual overview. In *Race, Gender, and Health*, chap. 1. Thousand Oaks, Calif.: Sage.

Beauchamp, T. L., and Childress, J. F. 1994. *Principles of Biomedical Ethics*. 4th ed. New York: Oxford University Press.

Bell, S. E. 1987. Changing ideas: The medicalization of menopause. *Social Science and Medicine* 24:535–542.

Bem, S. L. 1993. *The Lenses of Gender: Transforming the Debate on Sexual Inequality*. New Haven: Yale University Press.

Benson, V., and Marano, M. A. 1994. Current estimates from the National Health Interview Survey, 1992. *Vital and Health Statistics*, series 10, no. 189. Hyattsville, Md.: Public Health Service.

Berg, C. J., Atrash, H. K., Koonin, L. M., and Tucker, M. 1996. Pregnancy-related mortality in the United States, 1987–1990. *Obstetrics and Gynecology* 88:161–167.

Bergthold, L. A. 1995. Medical necessity: Do we need it? *Health Affairs* 14:180–190.

Bernstein, A. B. 1996. Women's health in HMOs: What do we know and what do we need to find out? *Women's Health Issues* 6:51–59.

Bernstein, A. B., Dial, T. H., and Smith, M. D. 1995. Women's reproductive health services in health maintenance organizations. *Western Journal of Medicine* 163(suppl.):15–18.

Bertakis, K. D., Helms, L. J., Callahan, E. J., Azari, R., and Robbins, J. A. 1995. The influence of gender on physician practice style. *Medical Care* 33:407–416.

Bickell, N. A., Earp, J. A., Garrett, J. M., and Evans, A. T. 1994. Gynecologists' sex, clinical beliefs, and hysterectomy rates. *American Journal of Public Health* 84:1649–1652.

Bickell, N. A., Pieper, K. S., Lee, K. L., et al. 1992. Referral patterns for coronary artery disease treatment: Gender bias or good clinical judgment? *Annals of Internal Medicine* 116:791–797.

Blendon, R. J., Brodie, M., and Benson, J. 1995. What happened to America's support for the Clinton health plan? *Health Affairs* 14:7–23.

Blumer, H. 1971. Social problems as collective behavior. *Social Problems* 18:298–306.

Blustein, J. 1995. Medicare coverage, supplemental insurance, and the use of mammography by older women. *New England Journal of Medicine* 332:1138–1143.

Bogdan, J. C. 1990. Childbirth in America, 1650 to 1990. In R. D. Apple, ed.,

Women, Health, and Medicine in America: A Historical Handbook, chap. 4. New Brunswick, N.J.: Rutgers University Press.

Bolt, C. 1993. *The Women's Movements in the United States and Britain from the 1790s to the 1920s.* Amherst: University of Massachusetts Press.

Borst, C. G. 1995. *Catching Babies: The Professionalization of Childbirth, 1870–1920.* Cambridge: Harvard University Press.

Borum, M. L. 1996. Patient and physician gender may influence colorectal cancer screening by resident physicians. *Journal of Women's Health* 5:363–368.

Boston Women's Health Book Collective. 1984. *The New Our Bodies, Ourselves: A Book by and for Women.* New York: Simon and Schuster.

———. 1992. *The New Our Bodies, Ourselves: A Book by and for Women.* Updated and Expanded for the 1990s. New York: Touchstone.

Bowman, K. H. 1996. Attitudes toward abortion. In M. D. Smith, D. J. Besharov, K. Gardiner, and T. Hoff, eds., *What's Happening to Abortion Rates?,* pp. 47–60. Menlo Park, Calif.: Henry J. Kaiser Family Foundation.

Brandt, A. M. 1987. *No Magic Bullet: A Social History of Venereal Disease in the United States Since 1880.* Expanded ed. New York: Oxford University Press.

Braus, P. 1997. *Marketing Health Care to Women: Meeting New Demands for Products and Services.* Ithaca, N.Y.: American Demographics Books.

Brindis, C. 1994. Integrating reproductive health services within primary care: Policy options and opportunities. Women's Health and Primary Care: A Workshop to Build a Research and Policy Agenda. Conference proceedings. Washington, D.C.: George Washington University Center for Health Policy Research.

Brock, D. W. 1989. Justice, health care, and the elderly. *Philosophy and Public Affairs* 18:297–312.

Brodie, J. F. 1994. *Contraception and Abortion in 19th-Century America.* Ithaca: Cornell University Press.

Brodie, M. 1996. Americans' political participation in the 1993-94 national health care reform debate. *Journal of Health Politics, Policy and Law* 21:99–128.

Brody, E. M. 1994. Women as unpaid caregivers: The price they pay. In E. Friedman, ed., *An Unfinished Revolution: Women and Health Care in America,* chap. 5. New York: United Hospital Fund of New York.

Brown, E. R., Wyn, R., Cumberland, W. G., et al. 1995. Women's health-related behaviors and use of clinical preventive services: A report to the Commonwealth Fund. Los Angeles: UCLA Center for Health Policy Research.

Brown, P. 1995. Naming and framing: The social construction of diagnosis and illness. *Journal of Health and Social Behavior* Extra issue, 34–52.

Brown, S. A., and Grimes, D. E. 1993. *Nurse Practitioners and Certified Nurse-Midwives: A Meta-Analysis of Studies on Nurses in Primary Care Roles.* Washington, D.C.: American Nurses Association.

Brown, S. S., ed. 1988. *Prenatal Care: Reaching Mothers, Reaching Infants.* Washington, D.C.: National Academy Press.

————. 1994. Health care reform. *Women's Health Issues* 4:127–129.

Brown, S. S., and Eisenberg, L., eds. 1995. *The Best Intentions: Unintended Pregnancy and the Well-Being of Children and Families.* Washington, D.C.: National Academy Press.

Brumberg, J. J. 1989. *Fasting Girls: The History of Anorexia Nervosa.* New York: Penguin.

Buchmueller, T. C. 1996. Marital status, spousal coverage, and the gender gap in employer-sponsored health insurance. *Inquiry* 33:308–316.

Buechler, S. M. 1990. *Women's Movements in the United States: Woman Suffrage, Equal Rights, and Beyond.* New Brunswick, N.J.: Rutgers University Press.

Burt, M. A. 1993. *Publicly Supported Family Planning in the United States: Legislative and Policy History, Implications for the 1990s.* Washington, D.C.: The Urban Institute.

Butter, I. H., Carpenter, E.S., Kay, B. J., and Simmons, R. S. 1987. Gender hierarchies in the health labor force. *International Journal of Health Services* 17:133–149.

Butter, I. H., and Kay, B. J. 1988. State laws and the practice of lay midwifery. *American Journal of Public Health* 9:1161–1169.

Bynum, W. F. 1994. *Science and the Practice of Medicine in the Nineteenth Century.* Cambridge: Cambridge University Press.

Cafferata, G. L., and Meyers, S. M. 1990. Pathways to psychotropic drugs: Understanding the basis of gender differences. *Medical Care* 28:285–300.

Calhoun, C. 1995. "New social movements" of the early nineteenth century. In M. Traugott, ed., *Repertoires and Cycles of Collective Action,* pp. 173–215. Durham, N.C.: Duke University Press.

Callahan, D. 1988. *Setting Limits: Medical Goals in an Aging Society.* New York: Simon and Schuster.

Campaign for Women's Health. 1992. Health care reform: A critical issue. Washington, D.C.: Older Women's League.

————. 1993. A model benefits package for women in health care reform. Washington, D.C.: Older Women's League.

Campbell, J. C., and Landenburger, K. 1995. Violence against women. In C. I. Fogel and N. F. Woods, eds., *Women's Health Care: A Comprehensive Handbook,* chap. 18. Thousand Oaks, Calif.: Sage.

Carlson, K. J., and Eisenstat, S. A., eds. 1995. *Primary Care of Women.* St. Louis: Mosby.

Cassard, S. D., Weisman, C. S., Plichta, S. B., and Johnson, T. L. 1997. Physician gender and women's preventive services. *Journal of Women's Health* 6:199–207.

Cassedy, J. H. 1991. *Medicine in America: A Short History.* Baltimore: Johns Hopkins University Press.

Cathell, D. W. 1916. *The Physician Himself and Things That Concern His Reputation and Success.* Philadelphia: F. A. Davis.

Cayleff, S. E. 1987. *Wash and Be Healed: The Water-Cure Movement and Women's Health.* Philadelphia: Temple University Press.

Center for Public Integrity. 1994. *Well-Healed: Inside Lobbying for Health Care Reform.* Washington, D.C.: Center for Public Integrity.

Centers for Disease Control and Prevention (CDC). 1995a. Update: Acquired immunodeficiency syndrome—United States, 1994. *Morbidity and Mortality Weekly Report* 44:65–67.

————. 1995b. Trends in length of stay for hospital deliveries—United States, 1970–1992. *Morbidity and Mortality Weekly Report* 44:335–337.

Chafetz, J. S. 1991. The gender division of labor and the reproduction of female disadvantage: Toward an integrated theory. In R. L. Blumberg, ed., *Gender, Family, and Economy: The Triple Overlap*, chap. 3. Newbury Park, Calif.: Sage.

Chafetz, J. S., Dworkin, A. G., and Swanson, S. 1990. Social change and social activism: First-wave women's movements around the world. In G. West and R. L. Blumberg, eds., *Women and Social Protest*, chap. 16. New York: Oxford University Press.

Chandra, A. 1995. Health aspects of pregnancy and childbirth: United States, 1982–88. *Vital and Health Statistics*, series 23, no. 18. Hyattsville, Md.: National Center for Health Statistics.

Chavkin, W. 1996. Topics of our times: Public health on the line—abortion and beyond. *American Journal of Public Health* 86:1204–1206.

Chesler, E. 1992. *Woman of Valor: Margaret Sanger and the Birth Control Movement in America.* New York: Simon and Schuster.

Chez, R. A. 1993. Women's health care centers: Barriers or opportunities? *Women's Health Issues* 3:110–114.

Clancy, C. M., and Massion, C. T. 1992. American women's health care: A patchwork quilt with gaps. *Journal of the American Medical Association* 268:1918–1920.

Clarke, E. H. 1873. *Sex in Education: A Fair Chance for the Girls.* Boston: James R. Osgood.

Clayton, E. W. 1991. Women and advances in medical technologies: The legal issues. In J. Rodin and A. Collins, eds., *Women and New Reproductive Technologies: Medical, Psychosocial, Legal, and Ethical Dilemmas*, chap. 7. Hillsdale, N.J.: Lawrence Erlbaum Associates.

Cleary, P. D., Mechanic, D., and Greenley, J. R. 1982. Sex differences in medical care utilization: An empirical investigation. *Journal of Health and Social Behavior* 23:106–119.

Collins, K. S., and Simon, L. J. 1996. Women's health and managed care: Promises and challenges. *Women's Health Issues* 6:39–44.

Collins, K. S., Rowland, D., Salganicoff, A., and Chait, E. 1994. Assessing and improving women's health. In C. Costello and A. J. Stone, eds., *The American Woman 1994–95: Where We Stand—Women and Health*, chap. 1. New York: W. W. Norton.

Commonwealth Fund Commission on Women's Health. 1994. *Health Care Reform: What is at Stake for Women?* New York: Commonwealth Fund.

———. 1996a. Violence against women in the United States: A comprehensive background paper. New York: Commonwealth Fund.

———. 1996b. *Prevention and Women's Health: A Shared Responsibility.* New York: Commonwealth Fund.

Coney, S. 1994. *The Menopause Industry: How the Medical Establishment Exploits Women.* Alameda, Calif.: Hunter House.

Connell, R. W. 1987. *Gender and Power: Society, the Person, and Sexual Politics.* Stanford: Stanford University Press.

———. 1995. *Masculinities.* Berkeley: University of California Press.

Conrad, P. 1992. Medicalization and social control. *Annual Review of Sociology* 18:209–232.

Corey, C. R., and Freeman, H. E. 1990. Use of telephone interviewing in health care research. *Health Services Research* 25:129–144.

Cornelius, L., Beauregard, K. and Cohen, J. 1991. Usual sources of medical care and their characteristics. *National Medical Expenditure Survey Research Findings 11.* Rockville, Md.: Agency for Health Care Policy and Research.

Costello, C., and B. K. Krimgold, eds., 1996. *The American Woman 1996–97: Women and Work.* New York: W. W. Norton.

Costello, C., and Stone, A. J., eds., 1994. *The American Woman 1994–95: Where We Stand—Women and Health.* New York: W. W. Norton.

Cott, N.F. 1977. *The Bonds of Womanhood: "Women's Sphere" in New England, 1780–1835.* New Haven: Yale University Press.

———. 1984. Passionless: An interpretation of Victorian sexual ideology, 1790–1850. In J. W. Leavitt, ed., *Women and Health in America: Historical Readings,* chap. 4. Madison: University of Wisconsin Press.

———. 1986. *Root of Bitterness: Documents of the Social History of American Women.* Boston: Northeastern University Press.

———. 1987. *The Grounding of Modern Feminism.* New Haven: Yale University Press.

Coughlin, T. A., Ku, L., and Holahan, J. 1994. *Medicaid Since 1980: Costs, Coverage, and the Shifting Alliance Between the Federal Government and the States.* Washington, D.C.: Urban Institute Press.

Council on Ethical and Judicial Affairs of the American Medical Association. 1991. Gender disparities in clinical decision making. *Journal of the American Medical Association* 266:559–562.

Council on Graduate Medical Education. 1995. *Fifth Report: Women and Medicine.* Rockville, Md.: U.S. Department of Health and Human Services.

Culliton, B. J. 1991. NIH push for women's health. *Nature* 353:383.

Cypress, B. K. 1980. Characteristics of visits to female and male physicians. *Vital and Health Statistics,* series 13, no. 49. Hyattsville, Md.: U.S. Department of Health and Human Services.

————. 1984. Patterns of ambulatory care in obstetrics and gynecology. *Vital and Health Statistics,* series 13, no. 76. Hyattsville, Md.: U.S. Department of Health and Human Services.

Dally, A. G. 1991. *Women under the Knife: A History of Surgery.* London: Hutchinson Radius.

Dan, A. J., ed. 1994. *Reframing Women's Health: Multidisciplinary Research and Practice.* Thousand Oaks, Calif.: Sage.

Daniels, C. R. 1993. *At Women's Expense: State Power and the Politics of Fetal Rights.* Cambridge: Harvard University Press.

Daniels, N. 1985. *Just Health Care.* New York: Cambridge University Press.

Daniels, N., Light, D. W., and Caplan, R. L. 1996. *Benchmarks of Fairness for Health Care Reform.* New York: Oxford University Press.

Davis, K. 1995. Editorial: The federal budget and women's health. *American Journal of Public Health* 85:1051–1053.

Davis, K., Collins, K. S., and Morris, C. 1994. Managed care: Promise and concerns. *Health Affairs* 13:178–185.

Dearing, R. H., Gordon, H. A., Sohner, D. M., and Weidel, L. C. 1987. *Marketing Women's Health Care.* Rockville, Md.: Aspen.

DeBruin, D. A. 1994. Justice and the inclusion of women in clinical studies: A conceptual framework. In A. C. Mastroianni, R. Faden, and D. Federman, eds., *Women and Health Research: Ethical and Legal Issues of Including Women in Clinical Studies,* vol. 2., pp. 127–150. Washington, D.C.: National Academy Press.

Delbanco, S., and Smith, M. D. 1995. Reproductive health and managed care: An overview. *Western Journal of Medicine* 163(suppl.):1–6.

Dey, A. N. 1996. Characteristics of elderly home health care users: Data from the 1993 National Home and Hospice Care Survey. *Advance Data from Vital and Health Statistics,* no. 272. Hyattsville, Md.: National Center for Health Statistics.

Dial, T. H., Palsbo, S. E., Bergsten, C., Gabel, J. R., and Weiner, J. 1995. Clinical staffing in staff- and group-model HMOs. *Health Affairs* 14:168–180.

Dickersin, K., and Schnaper, L. 1996. Reinventing medical research. In K. L. Moss, ed., *Man-Made Medicine: Women's Health, Public Policy, and Reform,* chap. 3. Durham, N.C.: Duke University Press.

Donaldson, M. S., Yordy, K. D., Lohr, K. N., and Vanselow, N. A., eds. 1996. *Primary Care: America's Health in a New Era.* Washington, D.C.: National Academy Press.

Donegan, J. B. 1984. "Safe delivered," but by whom? Midwives and men-midwives in early America. In J. W. Leavitt, ed., *Women and Health in America: Historical Readings,* chap. 21. Madison: University of Wisconsin Press.

Donovan, P. 1993. Testing positive: Sexually transmitted disease and the public health response. New York: Alan Guttmacher Institute.

Doress-Worters, P. B., and Siegal, D. L. 1994. *The New Ourselves, Growing Older: Women Aging with Knowledge and Power.* New York: Simon and Schuster.

Doyal, L. 1983. Women, health, and the sexual division of labor: A case study of the women's health movement in Britain. *International Journal of Health Services* 13:373–387.

———. 1995. *What Makes Women Sick: Gender and the Political Economy of Health*. New Brunswick, N.J.: Rutgers University Press.

Drachman, V. G. 1976. *Women Doctors and the Women's Medical Movement: Feminism and Medicine 1850–1895*. Ph.D. diss., State University of New York at Buffalo.

———. 1984. *Hospital with a Heart: Women Doctors and the Paradox of Separatism at the New England Hospital 1862–1969*. Ithaca: Cornell University Press.

Drew, E. 1994. *On the Edge: The Clinton Presidency*. New York: Touchstone.

Duffy, J. 1993. *From Humors to Medical Science: A History of American Medicine*. 2d ed. Urbana: University of Illinois Press.

Dunn, D., Almquist, E. M., and Chafetz, J. S. 1993. Macrostructural perspectives on gender inequality. In P. England, ed., *Theory on Gender/Feminism on Theory*, chap. 4. New York: Aldine De Gruyter.

Eagan, A. B. 1994. The women's health movement and its lasting impact. In E. Friedman, ed., *An Unfinished Revolution: Women and Health Care in America*, chap. 2. New York: United Hospital Fund.

Edmunds, M. 1995. Policy research: Balancing rigor with relevance. *Women's Health: Research on Gender, Behavior, and Policy* 1:97–119.

Ehrenreich, B., and English, D. 1973a. *Complaints and Disorders: The Sexual Politics of Sickness*. New York: Feminist Press.

———. 1973b. *Witches, Midwives, and Nurses: A History of Women Healers*. New York: Feminist Press.

———. 1978. *For Her Own Good: 150 Years of the Experts' Advice to Women*. New York: Doubleday.

Eisenberg, D. M., Kessler, R. C., Foster, C., Norlock, F. E., Calkins, D. R., and Delbanco, T. 1993. Unconventional medicine in the United States: Prevalence, costs, and patterns of use. *New England Journal of Medicine* 328:246–252.

Eisenstein, Z. R. 1988. *The Female Body and the Law*. Berkeley: University of California Press.

Ellerbrock, T. V., Buch, T. J., Chamberland, M. E., and Oxtoby, M. J. 1991. Epidemiology of women with AIDS in the United States, 1981 through 1990. *Journal of the American Medical Association* 265:2971–2975.

Erickson, J. 1995. Breast cancer activists seek voice in research decisions. *Science* 269:1508–1509.

Eyler, A. E., Gorenflo, D. W., and Musser, K. 1996. Physician gender and productivity in a managed care setting. *Journal of Women's Health* 5:221–224.

Eysmann, S. B., and Douglas, P. S. 1992. Reperfusion and revascularization strategies for coronary artery disease in women. *Journal of the American Medical Association* 268:1903–1907.

Faden, R., Kass, N., and McGraw, D. 1996. Women as vessels and vectors: Lessons from the HIV epidemic. In S. M. Wolf, ed., *Feminism and Bioethics: Beyond Reproduction*, chap. 9. New York: Oxford University Press.

Falik, M. M., and Collins, K. S., eds. 1996. *Women's Health: The Commonwealth Fund Survey.* Baltimore: Johns Hopkins University Press.

Family Planning Advocates of New York State. 1996. *Merger Watch: Hospital Mergers: The Hidden Crisis for Family Planning, an Activist's Guide.* Albany: Family Planning Advocates.

Fee, E. 1975. Women and health care: A comparison of theories. *International Journal of Health Services* 5:397–415.

————. 1978. Science and the "woman question" 1860–1920: A study of English scientific periodicals. Ph.D. diss., Princeton University.

Feinberg, M. 1996. The Boston Women's Health Book Collective celebrates its 25th anniversary. *Network News* 21:1,4.

Feinstein, J. S. 1993. The relationship between socioeconomic status and health: A review of the literature. *Milbank Quarterly* 71:279–322.

Ferraro, S. 1993. You can't look away anymore: The anguished politics of breast cancer. *New York Times Magazine*, 15 August.

Fiebach, N. H., Viscoli, C. M., and Horwitz, R. I. 1990. Differences between women and men in survival after myocardial infarction: Biology or methodology? *Journal of the American Medical Association* 263:1092–1096.

Figert, A. E. 1996. *Women and the Ownership of PMS: The Structuring of a Psychiatric Disorder.* New York: Aldine DeGruyter.

Fish, V. K. 1990. The struggle over women's education in the nineteenth century: A social movement and countermovement. In G. West and R. L. Blumberg, eds., *Women and Social Protest*, chap. 14. New York: Oxford University Press.

Fisher, L. D., Kennedy, W., Davis, K. B., et al. 1982. Association of sex, physical size, and operative mortality after coronary artery bypass in the Coronary Artery Surgery Study (CASS). *Journal of Thoracic Cardiovascular Surgery* 84:334–341.

Fogel, C. I., and Woods, N. F., eds. 1995. *Women's Health Care: A Comprehensive Handbook.* Thousand Oaks, Calif.: Sage.

Forrest, J. D. 1993. Timing of reproductive life stages. *Obstetrics and Gynecology* 82:105–111.

Forrest, J. D. 1994. Epidemiology of unintended pregnancy and contraceptive use. *American Journal of Obstetrics and Gynecology* 170:1485–1488.

Forrest, J. D., and Henshaw S. K. 1993. Providing controversial health care: Abortion services since 1973. *Women's Health Issues* 3:152–157.

Franks, P., and Clancy, C. M. 1993. Physician gender bias in clinical decision-making: Screening for cancer in primary care. *Medical Care* 31:213–218.

Freeman, J. 1990. From protection to equal opportunity: The revolution in women's legal status. In L. A. Tilly and P. Gurin, eds., *Women, Politics, and Change*, chap. 19. New York: Russell Sage Foundation.

Freidson, E. 1973. *Profession of Medicine: A Study of the Sociology of Applied Knowledge*. New York: Dodd, Mead.

Freiman, M. P., and Marder, W. D. 1984. Changes in the hours worked by physicians, 1970–80. *American Journal of Public Health* 74:1348–1352.

Fugh-Berman, A. 1996. *Alternative Medicine: What Works*. Tucson: Odonian Press.

Gabay, M., and Wolfe, S. M. 1995. *Encouraging the Use of Nurse-Midwives: A Report for Policymakers*. Washington, D.C.: Public Citizen.

Gabel, J. R., Dial, T. H., Hobart, J., et al. 1994. *HMO Industry Profile: 1994 Edition*. Washington, D.C.: Group Health Association of America.

Gallup Organization. 1993. A Gallup study of women's attitudes toward the use of OB/GYN for primary care. Princeton: Gallup Organization.

Gamble, V. N., and Blustein, B. E. 1994. Racial differences in medical care: Implications for research on women. In A. C. Mastroianni, R. Faden, and D. Federman, eds., *Women and Health Research: Ethical and Legal Issues of Including Women in Clinical Studies*, vol. 2, pp. 174–191. Washington, D.C.: National Academy Press.

Garrow, D. J. 1994. *Liberty and Sexuality: The Right to Privacy and the Making of Roe v. Wade*. New York: MacMillan.

Gelb, J., and Palley, M. L. 1996. *Women and Public Policies: Reassessing Gender Politics*. Charlottesville: University Press of Virginia.

Geller, S. E., Burns, L. R., and Brailer, D. J. 1996. The impact of nonclinical factors on practice variations: The case of hysterectomies. *Health Services Research* 30:729–750.

German, P. S., Burton, L. C., Shapiro, S., et al. 1995. Extended coverage of preventive services for the elderly: Response and results in a demonstration population. *American Journal of Public Health* 85:379–386.

Giddens, A. 1979. *Central Problems in Social Theory: Action, Structure and Contradiction in Social Analysis*. Berkeley: University of California Press.

———. 1986. *The Constitution of Society: Outline of the Theory of Structuration*. Berkeley: University of California Press.

Gilman, C. P. 1994. *The Yellow Wallpaper*. Washington, D.C.: Orchises.

Ginzberg, L. D. 1990. *Women and the Work of Benevolence: Morality, Politics, and Class in the Nineteenth-Century United States*. New Haven: Yale University Press.

Glied, S., and Kofman, S. 1995. Women and mental health: Issues for health reform. Background paper for the Commonwealth Fund Commission on Women's Health. New York: Commonwealth Fund.

Goldin, C. 1990. *Understanding the Gender Gap: An Economic History of American Women*. New York: Oxford University Press.

Gonen, J. S. 1993. Women's rights vs. 'fetal rights': Politics, law and reproductive hazards in the workplace. In J. C. Merrick and R. H. Blank, eds., *The Politics of Pregnancy: Policy Dilemmas in the Maternal-Fetal Relationship*, pp. 175–190. Binghamton, N.Y.: Haworth.

Gordon, L. 1990a. *Woman's Body, Woman's Right: Birth Control in America.* New York: Penguin.

———. 1990b. The new feminist scholarship on the welfare state. In *Women, the State, and Welfare,* chap. 1. Madison: University of Wisconsin Press.

———. 1994. *Pitied but Not Entitled: Single Mothers and the History of Welfare, 1890–1935.* New York: Free Press.

Grason, H., and Guyer, B. 1995. Rethinking the organization of children's programs: Lessons from the elderly. *Milbank Quarterly* 73:565–597.

Graves, E. J. 1995. 1993 summary: National Hospital Discharge Survey. *Advance Data from Vital and Health Statistics,* no. 264. Hyattsville, Md.: National Center for Health Statistics.

Greenland, P., Reicher-Reiss, H., Goldbourt, U., and Behar, S. 1991. In-hospital and 1-year mortality in 1,524 women after myocardial infarction: Comparison with 4,315 men. *Circulation* 83:484–491.

Grimes, D. A. 1993. Editorial: Over-the counter oral contraceptives—an immodest proposal? *American Journal of Public Health* 83:1092–1094.

Group Health Association of America (GHAA). 1995. *National Directory of HMOs.* Washington, D.C.: GHAA.

Gusfield, J. R. 1981. *The Culture of Public Problems: Drinking-Driving and the Symbolic Order.* Chicago: University of Chicago Press.

Hall, E. 1991. Gender, work control and stress: A theoretical discussion and an empirical test. In J. V. Johnson and G. Johansson, eds., *The Psychosocial Work Environment: Work Organization, Democratization and Health,* pp. 89–108. Amityville, N.Y.: Baywood.

Hall, J. A., Palmer, H., Orav, E. J., et al. 1990. Performance quality, gender, and professional role: A study of physicians and nonphysicians in 16 ambulatory care practices. *Medical Care* 28:489–501.

Hall, J. A., Irish, J. T., Roter, D. L., Ehrlich, C. M., and Miller, L. H. 1994. Satisfaction, gender, and communication in medical visits. *Medical Care* 32:1216–1231.

Haller, J. S., Jr., and Haller, R. M. 1974. *The Physician and Sexuality in Victorian America.* Urbana: University of Illinois Press.

Hannan, E. L., Arani, D. T., Johnson, L. W., et al. 1992a. Percutaneous transluminal coronary angioplasty in New York State: Risk factors and outcomes. *Journal of the American Medical Association* 268:3092–3097.

Hannan, E. L., Bernard, H. R., Kilburn, H. C., and O'Donnell, J. F. 1992b. Gender differences in mortality rates for coronary artery bypass surgery. *American Heart Journal* 123:866–872.

Hannan, M. T., and Freeman, J. 1989. *Organizational Ecology.* Cambridge: Harvard University Press.

Harrison, M. 1992. Women's health as a specialty: A deceptive solution. *Journal of Women's Health* 1:101–106.

Hartmann, H. I., Kuriansky, J. A., and Owens, C. L. 1996. Employment and women's health. In M. M. Falik and K. S. Collins, eds., *Women's Health: The Commonwealth Fund Survey,* chap. 11. Baltimore: Johns Hopkins University Press.

Health Insurance Association of America (HIAA). 1996. *Source Book of Health Insurance.* Washington, D.C.: HIAA.

Hellinger, F. J. 1993. The use of health services by women with HIV infection. *Health Services Research* 28:543–561.

Henshaw, S. K. 1995. Factors hindering access to abortion services. *Family Planning Perspectives* 27:54–59.

Henshaw, S. K., and Torres, A. 1994. Family planning agencies: Services, policies and funding. *Family Planning Perspectives* 26:52–59, 82.

Henshaw, S. K., and Van Vort, J. 1994. Abortion services in the United States, 1991 and 1992. *Family Planning Perspectives* 26:100–106.

Herz, D. E., and Wootton, B. H. 1996. Women in the workforce: An overview. In C. Costello and B. Kivimae, eds., *The American Woman 1996–97: Women and Work,* chap. 1. New York: W. W. Norton.

Hess, B. B., and Ferree, M. M., eds. 1987. *Analyzing Gender: A Handbook of Social Science Research.* Newbury Park, Calif.: Sage.

Hibbard, J. H., and Pope, C. R. 1986. Another look at sex differences in the use of medical care: Illness orientation and the types of morbidities for which services are used. *Women and Health* 11:21–36.

Hilgartner, S., and Bosk, C. L. 1988. The rise and fall of social problems: A public arenas model. *American Journal of Sociology* 94:53–78.

Hing, E., Kovar, M. G., and Rice, D. P. 1983. Sex differences in health and use of medical care: United States, 1979. *Vital and Health Statistics,* series 3, no. 24. Washington, D.C.: U.S. Government Printing Office.

Hoffman, E., and Johnson, D. 1995. Women's health and managed care: Implications for the training of primary care physicians. *Journal of the American Medical Women's Association* 50:17–19.

Holahan, J., Winterbottom, C., and Rajan, S. 1995. A shifting picture of health insurance coverage. *Health Affairs* 14:253–264.

Holmes, M. M., Resnick, H. S., Kilpatrick, D. G., and Best, C. L. 1996. Rape-related pregnancy: Estimates and descriptive characteristics from a national sample of women. *American Journal of Obstetrics and Gynecology* 175:320–325.

Horton, J. A., ed. 1995. *The Women's Health Data Book: A Profile of Women's Health in the United States.* 2d ed. Washington, D.C.: Jacobs Institute of Women's Health.

Horton, J. A., Cruess, D. F., and Pearse, W. H. 1993. Primary and preventive care services provided by obstetrician-gynecologists. *Obstetrics and Gynecology* 82:723–726.

Horton, J. A., Murphy, P., and Hale, R. W. 1994. Obstetrician-gynecologists as primary care providers: A national survey of women. *Primary Care Update ObGyns* 1:212–215.

Howes, J., and Allina, A. 1994. Women's health movements. *Social Policy,* summer:6–14.

Hubbard, R. 1990. *The Politics of Women's Biology.* New Brunswick, N.J.: Rutgers University Press.

Hughes, D., and Simpson, L. 1995. The role of social change in preventing low birth weight. *The Future of Children* 5:87–102.

Jacobi, M. P. 1925. Modern female invalidism. In Women's Medical Association of New York City, *Mary Putnam Jacobi, M.D.: A Pathfinder in Medicine.* New York: G. P. Putnam's Sons.

Jacobson, J. L. 1993. Women's health: The price of poverty. In M. Koblinsky, J. Timyan, and J. Gay, eds., *The Health of Women: A Global Perspective,* chap. 1. Boulder: Westview Press.

Jecker, N. S. 1994. Can an employer-based health insurance system be just? In J. A. Morone and G. S. Belkin, eds., *The Politics of Health Care Reform: Lessons from the Past, Prospects for the Future,* pp. 259–275. Durham, N.C.: Duke University Press.

Joffe, C. 1995. *Doctors of Conscience: The Struggle to Provide Abortion before and after Roe v. Wade.* Boston: Beacon Press.

Johns, L. 1994. Obstetrics-gynecology as primary care: A market dilemma. *Health Affairs* 13:194–200.

Johnson, H., and Broder, D. S. 1996. *The System: The American Way of Politics at the Breaking Point.* Boston: Little, Brown.

Johnson, K. 1992. Women's health: Developing a new interdisciplinary specialty. *Journal of Women's Health* 1:95–99.

Johnson, T. L., and Fee, E. 1994. Women's participation in clinical research: From protectionism to access. In A. C. Mastroianni, R. Faden, and D. Federman, eds., *Women and Health Research: Ethical and Legal Issues of Including Women in Clinical Studies,* vol. 2, pp, 1–10. Washington, D.C.: National Academy Press.

Johnston, H., Laraña, E., and Gusfield, J. R. 1994. Identities, grievances, and new social movements. In *New Social Movements: From Ideology to Identity,* chap. 1. Philadelphia: Temple University Press.

Kadar, A. G. 1994. The sex-bias myth in medicine. *Atlantic Monthly* 274:66–70.

Kaiser Commission on the Future of Medicaid. 1995. The Medicaid program at a glance. Washington, D.C.: Henry J. Kaiser Family Foundation.

Kaiser Family Foundation. 1995a. Abortion delivery in the United States: New survey raises questions about what current trends and non-surgical alternatives may mean for the future. News Release. Washington, D.C.: Henry J. Kaiser Family Foundation.

———. 1995b. The Medicare program. Washington, D.C.: Henry J. Kaiser Family Foundation.

Kanter, R. M. 1977. *Men and Women of the Corporation.* New York: Basic Books.

Kaplan, L. 1995. *The Story of Jane: The Legendary Underground Feminist Abortion Service.* New York: Pantheon Books.

Kelsey, S. F., James, M., Holubkov, A. L., et al. 1993. Results of percutaneous transluminal coronary angioplasty in women: 1985–1986 National Heart, Lung, and Blood Institute's Coronary Angioplasty Registry. *Circulation* 87:720-727.

Kerber, L. K. 1986. *Women of the Republic: Intellect and Ideology in Revolutionary America.* New York: W. W. Norton.

———. 1995. A constitutional right to be treated like American ladies: Women and the obligations of citizenship. In L. K. Kerber, A. Kessler-Harris, and K. K. Sklar, eds., *U.S. History as Women's History: New Feminist Essays*, chap. 1. Chapel Hill: University of North Carolina Press.

Kessler, R. C., McGonagle, K. A., Zhao, S., et al. 1994. Lifetime and 12-month prevalence of DSM-III-R psychiatric disorders in the U.S. *Archives of General Psychiatry* 51:8–19.

Kessler-Harris, A. 1995. The paradox of motherhood: Night work restrictions in the United States. In U. Wikander, A. Kessler-Harris, and J. Lewis, eds., *Protecting Women: Labor Legislation in Europe, the United States, and Australia, 1880–1920*, chap. 12. Urbana: University of Illinois Press.

Kett, J. F. 1968. *The Formation of the American Medical Profession: The Role of Institutions, 1780–1860.* New Haven: Yale University Press.

Khan, S. S., Nessim, S., Gray, R., et al. 1990. Increased mortality of women in coronary artery bypass surgery: Evidence of referral bias. *Annals of Internal Medicine* 112:561–567.

Khoury, A. J., Summers, L., and Weisman, C. S. Forthcoming. Characteristics of current hospital-sponsored and non-hospital birth centers. *Maternal and Child Health Journal.*

King, C. R. 1992. Abortion in nineteenth-century America: A conflict between women and their physicians. *Women's Health Issues* 2:32–39.

———. 1993. *Children's Health in America.* New York: Twayne.

Kingdon, J. W. 1995. *Agendas, Alternatives, and Public Policies.* 2nd ed. New York: HarperCollins.

Kirp, D. L., Yudof, M. G., and Franks, M. S. 1986. *Gender Justice.* Chicago: University of Chicago Press.

Kirschstein, R. L. 1991. Research on women's health. *American Journal of Public Health* 81:291–293.

Klandermans, B. 1992. The social construction of protest and multiorganizational fields. In A. D. Morris and C. M. Mueller, eds., *Frontiers in Social Movement Theory*, chap. 4. New Haven: Yale University Press.

Koblinsky, M., Timyan, J., and Gay, J., eds. 1993. *The Health of Women: A Global Perspective.* Boulder: Westview Press.

KPMG Peat Marwick LLP. 1995. *Health Benefits in 1995.* San Francisco: KPMG.

Kronenberg, F., Mallory, B., and Downey, J. A. 1994. Rehabilitation medicine and alternative therapies: New words, old practices. *Archives of Physical Medicine and Rehabilitation* 75:928–929.

Kreuter, M. W., Strecher, V. J., Harris, R., Kobrin, S. C., and Skinner, C. S. 1995. Are patients of women physicians screened more aggressively? A prospective study of physician gender and screening. *Journal of General Internal Medicine* 10:119–125.

Krumholz, H. M., Douglas, P. S., Lauer, M. S., and Pasternak, R. C. 1992. Selection of patients for coronary angiography and coronary revascularization early after myocardial infarction: Is there evidence for a gender bias? *Journal of Internal Medicine* 116:785–790.

Ku, L. 1993. *Publicly Supported Family Planning in the United States: Financing of Family Planning Services.* Washington, D.C.: The Urban Institute and Child Trends.

Ladd-Taylor, M. 1990. Women's health and public policy. In R. D. Apple, ed., *Women, Health and Medicine in America*, chap. 15. New Brunswick, N.J.: Rutgers University Press.

Lader, L. 1995. *A Private Matter: RU 486 and the Abortion Crisis.* New York: Prometheus Books.

Laurence, L., and Weinhouse, B. 1994. *Outrageous Practices: The Alarming Truth About How Medicine Mistreats Women.* New York: Fawcett Columbine.

Leader, S., and Perales, P. J. 1995. Provision of primary-preventive health care services by obstetrician-gynecologists. *Obstetrics and Gynecology* 85:391–395.

Leavitt, J. W., ed. 1984. *Women and Health in America: Historical Readings.* Madison: University of Wisconsin Press.

———. 1986. *Brought to Bed: Childbearing in America, 1750 to 1950.* New York: Oxford University Press.

Leigh, W. A. 1995. Women and the 1993–1994 health reform debate: Issues and questions. *Women's Health: Research on Gender, Behavior, and Policy* 1:177–196.

Lemcke, D. P., Pattison, J., Marshall, L. A., and Cowley, D. S. 1995. *Primary Care of Women.* Norwalk, Conn.: Appleton and Lange.

Lemp, G. F., Hirozawa, A. M., Cohen, J. B., et al. 1992. Survival for women and men with AIDS. *Journal of Infectious Diseases* 166:74–79.

Leppa, C. J. 1995. Women as health care providers. In C. I. Fogel and N. F. Woods, eds., *Women's Health Care: A Comprehensive Handbook*, chap. 2. Thousand Oaks, Calif.: Sage.

Lesser, A. J. 1985. The origin and development of maternal and child health programs in the United States. *American Journal of Public Health* 75:590–598.

Link, B. G, and Phelan, J. 1995. Social conditions as fundamental causes of disease. *Journal of Health and Social Behavior* Extra issue, 80–94.

Lipkind, K. L. 1996. National Hospital Ambulatory Medical Care Survey: 1993 Outpatient Department Summary. *Advance Data from Vital and Health Statistics*, no. 276. Hyattsville, Md.: National Center for Health Statistics.

Lipson, D. J., and Naierman, N. 1996. Effects of health system changes on safety-net providers. *Health Affairs* 15:33–48.

Lock, M. 1993. *Encounters with Aging: Mythologies of Menopause in Japan and North America.* Berkeley: University of California Press.

Looker, P. 1993. Women's health centers: History and evolution. *Women's Health Issues* 3:95–100.

Loop, F. D., Golding, L. R., MacMillan, J. P., et al. 1983. Coronary artery surgery in women compared with men: Analyses of risks and long-term results. *Journal of the American College of Cardiology* 1:383–390.

Loudon, I. 1992. *Death in Childbirth: An International Study of Maternal Care and Maternal Mortality 1800–1950.* Oxford: Clarendon Press.

Louis Harris and Associates. 1993. *The Health of American Women.* New York: Louis Harris and Associates, Inc.

Love, S. M. 1995. *Dr. Susan Love's Breast Book.* 2d ed. Reading, Mass.: Addison-Wesley.

Luker, K. 1984. *Abortion and the Politics of Motherhood.* Berkeley: University of California Press.

Lupton, D. 1994. *Medicine as Culture: Illness, Disease and the Body in Western Societies.* Thousand Oaks, Calif.: Sage.

Lurie, N., Slater, J., McGovern, P., et al. 1993. Preventive care for women: Does the sex of the physician matter? *New England Journal of Medicine* 329:478–482.

Lynaugh, J. E. 1990. Institutionalizing women's health care in nineteenth- and twentieth-century America. In R. D. Apple, ed., *Women, Health, and Medicine in America: A Historical Handbook,* chap. 10. New Brunswick, N.J.: Rutgers University Press.

———. 1994. Women and nursing: A historical perspective. In E. Friedman, ed., *An Unfinished Revolution: Women and Health Care in America,* chap. 10. New York: United Hospital Fund of New York.

MacKay, H. T., and MacKay, A. P. 1995. Abortion training in obstetrics and gynecology residency programs in the United States, 1991–1992. *Family Planning Perspectives* 27:112–115.

MacKinnon, C. A. 1989. *Toward a Feminist Theory of the State.* Cambridge: Harvard University Press.

Mahowald, M. B. 1993. *Women and Children in Health Care: An Unequal Majority.* New York: Oxford University Press.

———. 1996. On treatment of myopia: Feminist standpoint theory and bioethics. In S. M. Wolfe, ed., *Feminism and Bioethics: Beyond Reproduction,* chap. 3. New York: Oxford University Press.

Makuc, D. M., Freid, V. M., and Parsons, P. E. 1994. Health insurance and cancer screening among women. *Advance Data from Vital and Health Statistics,* no. 254. Hyattsville, Md.: National Center for Health Statistics.

Mandel, R. B., and Dodson, D. L. 1992. Do women officeholders make a difference? In P. Ries and A. J. Stone, eds., *The American Woman 1992–93: A Status Report—Women and Politics,* chap. 3. New York: W. W. Norton.

Mann, C. 1995. Women's health research blossoms. *Science* 269:766–770.

Marieskind, H. I. 1975. The women's health movement. *International Journal of Health Services* 5:217–223.

———. 1980. *Women in the Health System: Patients, Providers, and Programs.* St. Louis: C. V. Mosby.

Marmot, M. G., Bobak, M., and Smith, G. D. 1995. Explanations for social inequalities in health. In B. C. Amick, S. Levine, A. R. Tarlov, and D. C. Walsh, eds., *Society and Health*, chap. 6. New York: Oxford University Press.

Marsh, M., and Ronner, W. 1996. *The Empty Cradle: Infertility in America from Colonial Times to the Present.* Baltimore: Johns Hopkins University Press.

Mastroianni, A. C., Faden, R., and Federman, D., eds. 1994. *Women and Health Research: Ethical and Legal Issues of Including Women in Clinical Studies,* vol 1. Washington, D.C.: National Academy Press.

Mayer, J. P. 1988. *Alexis de Tocqueville: Democracy in America.* New York: Harper-Perennial.

Maynard, C., Litwin, P. E., Martin, J. S., and Weaver, D. 1992. Gender differences in the treatment and outcome of acute myocardial infarction: Results from the Myocardial Infarction Triage and Intervention Registry. *Archives of Internal Medicine* 152:972–976.

McAdam, D. 1994. Culture and social movements. In E. Laraña, H. Johnston, and J. R. Gusfield, eds., *New Social Movements: From Ideology to Identity,* chap. 2. Philadelphia: Temple University Press.

———. 1995. "Initiator" and "spin-off" movements: Diffusion processes in protest cycles. In M. Traugott, ed., *Repertoires and Cycles of Collective Action,* pp. 217–239. Durham, N.C.: Duke University Press.

McCann, C. R. 1994. *Birth Control Politics in the United States, 1916–1945.* Ithaca: Cornell University Press.

McCarthy, J. D. 1994. Activists, authorities, and media framing of drunk driving. In E. Laraña, H. Johnston, and J. R. Gusfield, eds., *New Social Movements: From Ideology to Identity.* Philadelphia: Temple University Press.

McCarthy, J. D., and Zald, M. N. 1977. Resource mobilization and social movements: A partial theory. *American Journal of Sociology* 82:1212–41.

McCoy, H. V., Trapido, E. J., McCoy, C. B., Strickman-Stein, N., Engle, S., and Brown, I. 1992. Community activism relating to a cluster of breast cancer. *Journal of Community Health* 17:27–36.

Mechanic, D. 1978. Sex, illness, illness behavior, and the use of health services. *Social Science and Medicine* 12B:207–214.

Meckel, R. 1990. *Save the Babies: American Public Health Reform and the Prevention of Infant Mortality, 1850–1920.* Baltimore: Johns Hopkins University Press.

Meinert, C. L. 1995. The inclusion of women in clinical trials. *Science* 269:795–796.

Meyer, D. S., and Staggenborg, S. 1996. Movements, countermovements, and the structure of political opportunity. *American Journal of Sociology* 101:1628–1660.

Miller, C. A. 1988. Prenatal care outreach: An international perspective. In S. S. Brown, ed., *Prenatal Care: Reaching Mothers, Reaching Infants*, appendix B. Washington, D.C.: National Academy Press.

Miller, L. G. 1979. Pain, parturition, and the profession: Twilight sleep in America. In S. Reverby and D. Rosner, eds., *Health Care in America: Essays in Social History*, chap. 2. Philadelphia: Temple University Press.

Miller, R. H., and Luft, H. S. 1994. Managed care plan performance since 1980: A literature analysis. *Journal of the American Medical Association* 271:1512–1519.

Millman, M., ed. 1993. *Access to Health Care in America*. Washington, D.C.: National Academy Press.

Minow, M. 1990. *Making All the Difference: Inclusion, Exclusion, and American Law*. Ithaca: Cornell University Press.

Mohr, J. C. 1978. *Abortion in America: The Origins and Evolution of National Policy, 1800–1900*. Oxford: Oxford University Press.

———. 1984. Patterns of abortion and the response of American physicians, 1790–1930. In J. W. Leavitt, ed., *Women and Health in America: Historical Readings*, chap. 8. Madison: University of Wisconsin Press.

Moon, M. 1994. Women and long-term care. In C. Costello and A. J. Stone, eds., *The American Woman 1994–95: Where We Stand—Women and Health*, chap. 4. New York: W. W. Norton.

Morantz, R. M. 1977. Nineteenth century health reform and women: A program of self-help. In G. B. Risse, R. L. Numbers, and J. W. Leavitt, eds., *Medicine without Doctors: Home Health Care in American History*, pp. 73–93. New York: Science History Publications.

———. 1984. Making women modern: Middle-class women and health reform in 19th-century America. In J. W. Leavitt, ed., *Women and Health in America: Historical Readings*, chap. 24. Madison: University of Wisconsin Press.

———. 1985. The "connecting link": The case for the woman doctor in 19th-century America. In J. W. Leavitt and R. L. Numbers, eds., *Sickness and Health in America: Readings in the History of Medicine and Public Health*, chap. 11. Madison: University of Wisconsin Press.

Morantz-Sanchez, R. M. 1985. *Sympathy and Science: Women Physicians in American Medicine*. New York: Oxford University Press.

———. 1990. Physicians. In R. D. Apple, ed., *Women, Health, and Medicine in America: A Historical Handbook*, chap. 19. New Brunswick, N.J.: Rutgers University Press.

Morgen, S., and Julier, A. 1991. Women's health movement organizations: Two decades of struggle and change. Eugene: University of Oregon Center for the Study of Women in Society.

Moscucci, O. 1990. *The Science of Woman: Gynaecology and Gender in England, 1800–1929*. Cambridge: Cambridge University Press.

Moses, E. B. 1994. *The Registered Nurse Population: Findings from the National*

Sample Survey of Registered Nurses, March 1992. Rockville, Md.: U.S. Department of Health and Human Services.

Mosher, W. D., and Pratt, W. F. 1990. Use of contraception and family planning services in the United States, 1988. *American Journal of Public Health* 80:1132–1133.

Muller, C. F. 1990. *Health Care and Gender.* New York: Russell Sage.

———. 1994. Women in allied health professions. In E. Friedman, ed., *An Unfinished Revolution: Women and Health Care in America,* chap. 12. New York: United Hospital Fund of New York.

Multiple Risk Factor Intervention Trial Group. 1977. Statistical design considerations in the NHLI Multiple Risk Factor Intervention Trial (MRFIT). *Journal of Chronic Diseases* 30:261–275.

Muncy, R. 1991. *Creating a Female Dominion in American Reform 1890–1935.* New York: Oxford.

Mundinger, M. O. 1994. Advanced-practice nursing: Good medicine for physicians? *New England Journal of Medicine* 330:211–214.

Murtaugh, C., Kemper, P., and Spillman, B. 1990. The risk of nursing home use in later life. *Medical Care* 28:952–961.

Nadel, M. V. 1990. National Institutes of Health: Problems in implementing policy on women in study populations. Statement before the Subcommittee on Health and Environment, Committee on Energy and Commerce, U.S. House of Representatives, 18 June.

Nathanson, C. A. 1975. Illness and the feminine role: A theoretical review. *Social Science and Medicine* 9:57–62.

———. 1991. *Dangerous Passage: The Social Control of Sexuality in Women's Adolescence.* Philadelphia: Temple University Press.

National Abortion and Reproductive Rights Action League (NARAL). 1996. *Who Decides? A State-by-State Review of Abortion and Reproductive Rights.* 1996 Supplement. Washington, D.C.: NARAL.

National Alliance of Breast Cancer Organizations (NABCO). 1994. Mission statement. New York: NABCO.

National Center for Health Statistics (NCHS). 1995. *Health United States, 1994.* Hyattsville, Md.: Public Health Service.

———. 1996a. *Health United States, 1995.* Hyattsville, Md.: Public Health Service.

———. 1996b. *Healthy People 2000 Review, 1995–1996.* Hyattsville, Md.: Public Health Service.

National Committee for Quality Assurance. 1995. *Report Card Pilot Project.* Washington, D.C.: NCQA.

National Governors' Association. 1995. State Medicaid Coverage of Pregnant Women and Children: Summary 1995. Washington, D.C.: National Governors' Association.

National Institutes of Health (NIH). 1992. *Report of the National Institutes of*

Health: Opportunities for Research on Women's Health. Washington, D.C.: U.S. Department of Health and Human Services.

————. 1994. *Proceedings: Secretary's Conference to Establish a National Action Plan on Breast Cancer.* Bethesda, Md.: National Institutes of Health.

National Women's Law Center. 1994. How Women Fare under Clinton Health Care Reform. Washington, D.C.: National Women's Law Center.

Nelson, H. L, and Nelson, J. L. 1996. Justice in the allocation of health care resources: A feminist account. In S. M. Wolf, ed., *Feminism and Bioethics: Beyond Reproduction,* chap. 12. New York: Oxford University Press.

Norsigian, J. 1993. Women and national health care reform: A progressive feminist agenda. *Journal of Women's Health* 2:91–94.

Numbers, R. L. 1977. Do-it-yourself the sectarian way. In G. B. Risse, R. L. Numbers, and J. W. Leavitt, eds., *Medicine without Doctors: Home Health Care in American History,* pp. 49–72. New York: Science History Publications.

Palmer, R. L., and Greenberg, S. K. 1936. *Facts and Frauds in Woman's Hygiene: A Medical Guide against Misleading Claims and Dangerous Products.* New York: Vanguard Press.

Parsons, P. E. 1994. Health reform update. *Network News* 19:2.

Petchesky, R. P. 1990. *Abortion and Woman's Place: The State, Sexuality, and Reproductive Freedom.* Boston: Northeastern University Press.

Pew Health Professions Commission. 1995. *Critical Challenges: Revitalizing the Health Professions for the Twenty-First Century.* San Francisco: University of California at San Francisco Center for the Health Professions.

Pew Research Center for the People and the Press. 1994. *The Public, Their Doctors, and Health Care Reform: Part II. Gloomy Doctors and "Scared Public" Spurn Clinton Plan but Favor Reform Principles.* Washington, D.C.: Pew Research Center for the People and the Press.

Plichta, S. B. 1996. Violence and abuse: Implications for women's health. In M. M. Falik and K. S. Collins, eds., *Women's Health: The Commonwealth Fund Survey,* chap. 9. Baltimore: Johns Hopkins University Press.

Purdy, L. M. 1996. A feminist view of health. In S. M. Wolfe, ed., *Feminism and Bioethics: Beyond Reproduction,* chap. 6. New York: Oxford.

Rabinowitz, B. 1994. Comprehensive breast centers: Engendering physician involvement. *Journal of Oncology Management.* 3:52–55.

Radford, B., and Shaw, G. 1993. Antiabortion violence: Causes and effects. *Women's Health Issues* 3:144–151.

Raymond, J. G. 1993. *Women as Wombs: Reproductive Technologies and the Battle over Women's Freedom.* New York: HarperCollins.

Reagan, L. J. 1995. Linking midwives and abortion in the Progressive Era. *Bulletin of the History of Medicine.* 69:569–598.

Reed, J. 1978. *From Private Vice to Public Virtue: The Birth Control Movement and American Society Since 1830.* New York: Basic Books.

————. 1984. Doctors, birth control, and social values, 1830–1970. In J. W. Leavitt, ed., *Women and Health in America: Historical Readings*, chap. 9. Madison: University of Wisconsin Press.

Reisinger, A. L. 1995. Health insurance and access to care: Issues for women. Background paper prepared for the Commonwealth Fund Commission on Women's Health. New York: Commonwealth Fund.

————. 1996. Health insurance and women's access to health care. In M. M. Falik and K. S. Collins, eds., *Women's Health: The Commonwealth Fund Survey*, chap. 12. Baltimore: Johns Hopkins University Press.

Rhode, D. L. 1989. *Justice and Gender: Sex Discrimination and the Law*. Cambridge: Harvard University Press.

Riessman, C. K. 1983. Women and medicalization: A new perspective. *Social Policy* 14:3–18.

Robinson, J. C., Gardner, L. B., and Luft, H. S. 1993. Health plan switching in anticipation of increased medical care utilization. *Medical Care* 31:43–51.

Rodin, J., and Collins, A. 1991. The new reproductive technologies: Overview of the challenges and issues. In *Women and New Reproductive Technologies: Medical, Psychosocial, Legal, and Ethical Dilemmas*, chap. 1. Hillsdale, N.J.: Lawrence Erlbaum Associates.

Rodin, J., and Ickovics, J. R. 1990. Women's health: Review and research agenda as we approach the 21st century. *American Psychologist* 45:1018–1034.

Rodriguez-Trias, H. 1992. Women's health, women's lives, women's rights. *American Journal of Public Health* 82:663–664.

Rodwin, M. A. 1994. Patient accountability and quality of care: Lessons from medical consumerism and the patients' rights, women's health and disability rights movements. *American Journal of Law and Medicine* 20:147–167.

Rooks, J. P., Weatherby, N. L., Ernst, E. K. M., et al. 1989. Outcomes of care in birth centers: The National Birth Center Study. *New England Journal of Medicine* 321:1804–1811.

Rosen, G. 1993. *A History of Public Health*. Baltimore: Johns Hopkins University Press.

Rosenbaum, S., and Darnell, J. 1997. An Analysis of the Medicaid and health-related provisions of the Personal Responsibility and Work Opportunity Reconciliation Act of 1996 (P.L. 104–193). Washington, D.C.: Kaiser Commission on the Future of Medicaid.

Rosenbaum, S., Shin, P., Mauskopf, A., Fund, K., Stern, G., and Zuvekas, A. 1995. Beyond the freedom to choose: Medicaid, managed care, and family planning. *Western Journal of Medicine* 163[suppl.]:33–38.

Rosenberg, C. E. 1987. *The Care of Strangers: The Rise of America's Hospital System*. New York: Basic Books.

Rosenblatt, R. A., Hart, G., Gamliel, S., et al. 1995. Identifying primary care disciplines by analyzing the diagnostic content of ambulatory care. *Journal of the American Board of Family Practice* 8:34–45.

Ross, C. E., and Bird, C. E. 1994. Sex stratification and health lifestyle: Consequences for men's and women's perceived health. *Journal of Health and Social Behavior* 25:161–178.

Ross, C. E., and Mirowsky, J. 1995. Does employment affect health? *Journal of Health and Social Behavior* 36:230–243.

Rosser, S. V. 1994. *Women's Health—Missing from U.S. Medicine*. Bloomington: Indiana University Press.

Rossouw, J. E., Finnegan, L. P., Harlan, W. R., Pinn, V. W., Clifford, C., and McGowan, J. A. 1995. The evolution of the Women's Health Initiative: Perspectives from the NIH. *Journal of the American Medical Women's Association* 50:50–55.

Roter, D. L., and Hall, J. A. 1994. Examining gender-specific issues in patient-physician communications. Women's Health and Primary Care: A Workshop to Build a Research and Policy Agenda. Conference proceedings. Washington, D.C.: George Washington University Center for Health Policy Research.

Rothenberg, K. H. 1996. Feminism, law, and bioethics. *Kennedy Institute of Ethics Journal* 6:69–84.

Rothman, B. K. 1986. *The Tentative Pregnancy: Prenatal Diagnosis and the Future of Motherhood*. New York: Penguin.

———. 1991. *In Labor: Women and Power in the Birthplace*. New York: W. W. Norton.

Rothman, S. M. 1978. *Woman's Proper Place: A History of Changing Ideals and Practices, 1870 to the Present*. New York: Basic Books.

———. 1994. *Living in the Shadow of Death: Tuberculosis and the Social Experience of Illness in American History*. New York: Basic Books.

Rothstein, W. G. 1992. *American Physicians in the Nineteenth Century: From Sects to Science*. Baltimore: Johns Hopkins University Press.

Rovner, J. 1996. The safety net: What's happening to health care of last resort? *Advances* Special supplement.

Rowland, D., and Davis, K. 1994. Caring for women in older age. In E. Friedman, ed., *An Unfinished Revolution: Women and Health Care in America*, chap. 6. New York: United Hospital Fund of New York.

Rowland, D., and Hanson, K. 1996. Medicaid: Moving to managed care. *Health Affairs* 15:150–152.

Rowland, D., Rosenbaum, S., Simon, L., and Chait, E. 1995. *Medicaid and Managed Care: Lessons from the Literature*. Washington, D.C.: Kaiser Commission on the Future of Medicaid.

Rowland, R. 1992. *Living Laboratories: Women and Reproductive Technologies*. Bloomington: Indiana University Press.

Roy, J. M. 1990. Surgical gynecology. In R. D. Apple, ed., *Women, Health, and Medicine in America: A Historical Handbook*, chap. 7. New Brunswick, N.J.: Rutgers University Press.

Rupp, L. J., and Taylor, V. 1987. *Survival in the Doldrums: The American Women's Rights Movement, 1945 to the 1960s*. New York: Oxford University Press.

Russell, L. 1994. *Educated Guesses: Making Policy about Medical Screening Tests.* Berkeley: University of California Press.

Ruzek, S. B. 1978. *The Women's Health Movement: Feminist Alternatives to Medical Control.* New York: Praeger.

———. 1993. Towards a more inclusive model of women's health. *American Journal of Public Health* 83:6–7.

———. 1995a. Technology and perceptions of risk: Clinical, scientific, and consumer perspectives. *Executive Briefing.* Health Technology Assessment Information Service. Plymouth Meeting, Pa.: ECRI-WHO Collaborating Center for Technology Transfer.

———. 1995b. Caring, curing, and concern: Key concepts for an integrated model of women's health. Paper presented at the Society of Behavioral Medicine, annual scientific meeting, San Diego.

Ruzek, S. B., Clarke, A. E., and Olesen, V. L. 1997. What are the dynamics of differences? In S. B. Ruzek, V. L. Olesen, and A. E. Clarke, eds., *Women's Health: Complexities and Differences,* chap. 3. Columbus: Ohio State University Press.

Ruzek, S. B., Olesen, V. L., and Clarke, A. E., eds. 1997. *Women's Health: Complexities and Differences.* Columbus: Ohio State University Press.

Sabo, D., and Gordon, D. F., eds., 1995. *Men's Health and Illness: Gender, Power, and the Body.* Thousand Oaks, Calif.: Sage.

Samuels, S. E., and Smith, M. D., eds. 1994. *The Pill: From Prescription to Over the Counter.* Menlo Park, Calif.: Henry J. Kaiser Family Foundation.

Samuels, S. U. 1995. *Fetal Rights, Women's Rights: Gender Equality in the Workplace.* Madison: University of Wisconsin Press.

Sapiro, V. 1990. The gender basis of American social policy. In L. Gordon, ed., *Women, the State, and Welfare,* chap. 2. Madison: University of Wisconsin Press.

Schappert, S. M. 1993a. Office visits to psychiatrists: United States, 1989–90. *Advance Data from Vital and Health Statistics,* no. 237. Hyattsville, Md.: National Center for Health Statistics.

———. 1993b. Office visits to obstetricians and gynecologists: United States, 1989–90. *Advance Data from Vital and Health Statistics,* no. 223. Hyattsville, Md.: National Center for Health Statistics.

———. 1996. National Ambulatory Medical Care Survey: 1994 Summary. *Advance Data from Vital and Health Statistics,* no. 273. Hyattsville, Md.: National Center for Health Statistics.

Schaps, M. J., Linn, E. S., Wilbanks, G. D., and Wilbanks, E. R. 1993. Women-centered care: Implementing a philosophy. *Women's Health Issues* 3:52–54.

Schlesinger, M., and Lee, T. 1994. Is health care different? Popular support of federal health and social policies. In J. A. Morone and G. S. Belkin, eds., *The Politics of Health Care Reform: Lessons from the Past, Prospects for the Future.* Durham, N.C.: Duke University Press.

Scholten, C. M. 1984. "On the importance of the obstetrick art": Changing customs of childbirth in America, 1760–1825. In J. W. Leavitt, ed., *Women and Health in America: Historical Readings*, chap. 10. Madison: University of Wisconsin Press.

Schondelmeyer, S. W., and Johnson, J. A. 1994. Economic implications of switching from prescription status. In S. E. Samuels and M. D. Smith, eds., *The Pill: From Prescription to Over the Counter*, pp. 189–235. Menlo Park, Calif.: Henry J. Kaiser Family Foundation.

Schroeder, P., and Snowe, O. 1994. The politics of women's health. In C. Costello and A. J. Stone, eds., *The American Woman 1994–95: Where We Stand—Women and Health*, pp. 91–108. New York: W. W. Norton.

Scott, W. R. 1995. *Institutions and Organizations*. Thousand Oaks, Calif.: Sage.

Seaman, B. 1995. *The Doctors' Case against the Pill*. 25th anniversary ed. Alameda, Calif.: Hunter House.

Seltzer, V. L., and Pearse, W. H. 1995. *Women's Primary Health Care: Office Practice and Procedures*. New York: McGraw-Hill.

Shapiro, R. Y., Jacobs, L. R., and Harvey, L. K. 1995. Toward a dynamic and pluralistic understanding of individual motivation: The case of health care reform. Paper presented at the Annual Meeting of the Midwest Political Science Association, Chicago, April 6–8.

Sharpe, V. A., and Faden, A. I. 1996. Appropriateness in patient care: A new conceptual framework. *Milbank Quarterly* 74:115–138.

Sherman, L. A., Temple, R., and Merkatz, R. B. 1995. Women in clinical trials: An FDA perspective. *Science* 269:793–795.

Sherwin, S. 1992. *No Longer Patient: Feminist Ethics and Health Care*. Philadelphia: Temple University Press.

———. 1996. Feminism and bioethics. In S. M. Wolf, ed., *Feminism and Bioethics: Beyond Reproduction*, chap. 1. New York: Oxford University Press.

Shock, N. W., Greulich, R. C., Andres, R., Arenberg, D., Costa, P. T., Lakatta, E. G., and Tobin, J. D. 1984. *Normal Human Aging: The Baltimore Longitudinal Study of Aging*. Washington, D.C.: U.S. Government Printing Office.

Short, P. F. 1996. Medicaid's role in insuring low-income women. New York: Commonwealth Fund.

Shortell, S. M., Gillies, R. R., Anderson, D. A., et al. 1996. *Remaking Health Care in America: Building Organized Delivery Systems*. San Francisco: Jossey-Bass.

Shorter, E. 1991. *Women's Bodies: A Social History of Women's Encounter with Health, Ill-Health, and Medicine*. New Brunswick, N.J.: Transaction.

Showalter, E. 1985. *The Female Malady: Women, Madness, and English Culture, 1830–1980*. New York: Penguin.

Shryock, R. H. 1966. *Medicine in America: Historical Essays*. Baltimore: Johns Hopkins Press.

Singh, S., Benson, R. B., and Frost, J. J. 1994. Impact of the Medicaid eligibility expansions on the coverage of deliveries. *Family Planning Perspectives* 26: 31–33.

Singh, S., Forrest, J. D., and Torres, A. 1989. *Prenatal Care in the United States: A State and County Inventory,* vol. I. New York: Alan Guttmacher Institute.

Sklar, K. K. 1995. *Florence Kelley and the Nation's Work: The Rise of Women's Political Culture, 1830–1900.* New Haven: Yale University Press.

Skocpol, T. 1992. *Protecting Soldiers and Mothers: The Political Origins of Social Policy in the United States.* Cambridge: Harvard University Press.

―――. 1995. *Social Policy in the United States: Future Possibilities in Historical Perspective.* Princeton: Princeton University Press.

―――. 1996. *Boomerang: Clinton's Health Security Effort and the Turn against Government in U.S. Politics.* New York: W. W. Norton.

Skocpol, T., and Ritter, G. 1995. Gender and the origins of modern social policies in Britain and the United States. In T. Skocpol, *Social Policy in the United States: Future Possibilities in Historical Perspective,* chap. 3. Princeton: Princeton University Press.

Smelser, N. 1962. *Theory of Collective Behavior.* New York: Free Press.

Smith-Rosenberg, C. 1985. *Disorderly Conduct: Visions of Gender in Victorian America.* New York: Oxford University Press.

Smith-Rosenberg, C., and Rosenberg, C. 1984. The female animal: Medical and biological views of woman and her role in nineteenth-century America. In J. W. Leavitt, ed., *Women and Health in America: Historical Readings,* chap. 1. Madison: University of Wisconsin Press.

Smyke, P. 1991. *Women and Health.* London: Zed Books.

Snow, D. A., and Benford, R. D. 1992. Master frames and cycles of protest. In A. D. Morris and C. M. Mueller, eds., *Frontiers in Social Movement Theory.* Chap. 6. New Haven: Yale University Press.

Sofaer, S., and Abel, E. 1990. Older women's health and financial vulnerability: Implications of the Medicare benefit structure. *Women and Health* 16:47–67.

Soffa, V. M. 1994. *The Journey beyond Breast Cancer: From the Personal to the Political.* Rochester, Vt.: Healing Art Press.

Spector, M., and Kitsuse, J. I. 1987. *Constructing Social Problems.* New York: Aldine DeGruyter.

Speert, H. 1980. *Obstetrics and Gynecology in America: A History.* Chicago: American College of Obstetricians and Gynecologists.

Stage, S. 1979. *Female Complaints: Lydia Pinkham and the Business of Women's Medicine.* New York: W. W. Norton.

Staggenborg, S. 1991. *The Pro-Choice Movement: Organization and Activism in the Abortion Conflict.* New York: Oxford University Press.

Starfield, B. 1992. *Primary Care: Concept, Evaluation, and Policy.* New York: Oxford University Press.

Starr, P. 1982. *The Social Transformation of American Medicine.* New York: Basic Books.

————. 1994. *The Logic of Health Care Reform: Why and How the President's Plan Will Work*. Rev. and expanded ed. New York: Penguin.

Steering Committee of the Physicians' Health Study Research Group. 1989. Final report on the aspirin component of the ongoing physicians' health study. *New England Journal of Medicine* 321:129–135.

Steingart, R. M., Packer, M., Hamm, P., et al. 1991. Sex differences in the management of coronary artery disease. *New England Journal of Medicine* 325: 226–230.

Stevens, R. 1971. *American Medicine and the Public Interest*. New Haven: Yale University Press.

Stone, R., Cafferata, G. L., and Sangl, J. 1987. Caregivers of the frail elderly: A national profile. *Gerontologist* 27:616–626.

Stussman, B. J. 1996. National Hospital Ambulatory Medical Care Survey: 1993 emergency department summary. *Advance Data from Vital and Health Statistics*, No. 271. Hyattsville, Md.: National Center for Health Statistics.

Sulmasy, D. P., Haller, K., Weisman, C., et al. 1996. End-of-life decisions in AIDS differ by exposure category. *Journal of General Internal Medicine* 11:118.

Tarrow, S. 1993. Cycles of collective action: Between moments of madness and the repertoire of contention. *Social Science History* 17:281–307.

————. 1994. *Power in Movement: Social Movements, Collective Action and Politics*. Cambridge: Cambridge University Press.

Taylor, V. 1989. Social movement continuity: The women's movement in abeyance. *American Sociological Review* 54:761–775.

Thomas, S. 1994. *How Women Legislate*. New York: Oxford University Press.

Thompson, J. E., Walsh, L. V., and Merkatz, I. R. 1990. The history of prenatal care: Cultural, social and medical contexts. In I. R. Merkatz and J. E. Thompson, eds., *New Perspectives on Prenatal Care*, chap. 2. New York: Elsevier.

Tilly, C. 1995. Contentious repertoires in Great Britain, 1758–1834. In M. Traugott, ed., *Repertoires and Cycles of Collective Action*, pp. 15–42. Durham, N.C.: Duke University Press.

Tobin, J. N., Wassertheil-Smoller, S., Wexler, J. P., Steingart, R. M., Budner, N., Lense, L., and Washspress, J. 1987. Sex bias in considering coronary bypass surgery. *Annals of Internal Medicine* 107:19–25.

Tong, R. 1996. Feminist bioethics: Toward developing a "feminist" answer to the surrogate motherhood question. *Kennedy Institute of Ethics Journal* 6:37–52.

Traugott, M. 1995. Barricades as repertoire: Continuities and discontinuities in the history of French contention. In *Repertoires and Cycles of Collective Action*, pp. 43–56. Durham, N.C.: Duke University Press.

Trussell, J., Steward, F., Potts, M., et al. 1993. Should oral contraceptives be available without prescription? *American Journal of Public Health* 83:1094–1099.

Turner, B. J., Amsel, Z., Lustbader, E., et al. 1992. Breast cancer screening: Effect of physician specialty, practice setting, year of medical school graduation, and sex. *American Journal of Preventive Medicine* 8:78–85.

Turner, B. J., Markson, L. E., McKee, L. J., et al. 1994. Health care delivery, zidovudine use, and survival of women and men with AIDS. *Journal of Acquired Immune Deficiency Syndromes* 7:1250–1262.

Turner, R. H., and Killian, L. M. 1987. *Collective Behavior.* 3d ed. Englewood Cliffs, N.J.: Prentice-Hall.

Ulrich, L. T. 1990. *A Midwife's Tale: The Life of Martha Ballard, Based on Her Diary, 1785–1812.* New York: Vintage Books.

United Nations. 1995. *The World's Women 1995: Trends and Statistics.* New York: United Nations.

———. 1996. *The United Nations and the Advancement of Women, 1945–1996.* New York: United Nations.

U.S. Bureau of the Census. 1995. *Statistical Abstract of the United States: 1995.* Washington, D.C.: U.S. Government Printing Office.

U.S. Congress Office of Technology Assessment. 1986. *Nurse Practitioners, Physician Assistants, and Certified Nurse-Midwives: A Policy Analysis.* Washington, D.C.: U.S. Government Printing Office.

U.S. General Accounting Office (GAO). 1992. *Women's Health: FDA Needs to Ensure More Study of Gender Differences in Prescription Drug Testing.* Washington, D.C.: Government Printing Office.

———. 1995. *Mammography Services: Initial Impact of New Federal Law Has Been Positive.* Washington, D.C.: U.S. General Accounting Office.

U.S. Preventive Services Task Force. 1989. *Guide to Clinical Preventive Services: An Assessment of the Effectiveness of 169 Interventions.* Baltimore: Williams and Wilkins.

———. 1996. *Guide to Clinical Preventive Services.* 2d ed. Baltimore: Williams and Wilkins.

U.S. Public Health Service (USPHS). 1985. Women's health: Report of the Public Health Service task force on women's health issues, vol. I. *Public Health Reports* 100:1–106.

Verbrugge, L. M. 1985. Gender and health: An update on hypotheses and evidence. *Journal of Health and Social Behavior* 26:156–182.

———. 1989. The twain meet: Empirical explanation of sex differences in health and mortality. *Journal of Health and Social Behavior* 30:282–304.

———. 1990. Pathways of health and death. In R. D. Apple, ed., *Women, Health, and Medicine in America: A Historical Handbook,* chap. 2. New Brunswick, N.J.: Rutgers University Press.

Verbrugge, M. H. 1979. The social meaning of personal health: The Ladies' Physiological Institute of Boston and Vicinity in the 1850s. In S. Reverby and D. Rosner, eds., *Health Care in America: Essays in Social History,* chap. 3. Philadelphia: Temple University Press.

Vertinsky, P. A. 1994. *The Eternally Wounded Woman: Women, Doctors, and Exercise in the Late Nineteenth Century.* Urbana: University of Illinois Press.

Waldron, I. 1995. Contributions of changing gender differences in behavior and social roles to changing gender differences in mortality. In D. Sabo and D. F. Gordon, eds., *Men's Health and Illness: Gender, Power, and the Body,* chap. 2. Thousand Oaks, Calif.: Sage.

Wallis, L. A. 1993. Why a curriculum on women's health? *Journal of Women's Health* 2:55–60.

Walsh, D. C., Sorensen, G., and Leonard, L. 1995. Gender, health, and cigarette smoking. In B.C. Amick, S. Levine, A.R. Tarlov, and D.C. Walsh, eds., *Society and Health,* chap. 5. New York: Oxford University Press.

Walsh, L. V., and Boggess, J. H. 1996. Findings of the American College of Nurse-Midwives Annual Membership Surveys, 1993 and 1994. *Journal of Nurse-Midwifery* 41:230–235.

Walsh, M. R. 1977. *Doctors Wanted: No Women Need Apply.* New Haven: Yale University Press.

Walters, R. G. 1997. *American Reformers, 1815–1860.* New York: Hill and Wang.

Wardwell, W. I. 1994. Alternative medicine in the United States. *Social Science and Medicine* 38:1061–1068.

Weaver, W. D., White, H. D., Wilcox, R. G., et al. 1996. Comparisons of characteristics and outcomes among women and men with acute myocardial infarction treated with thrombolytic therapy. *Journal of the American Medical Association* 275:777–782.

Weiner, J. P. 1994. Forecasting the effects of health reform on U.S. physician workforce requirement: Evidence from HMO staffing patterns. *Journal of the American Medical Association* 272:222–230.

Weiner, J. P., and de Lissovoy, G. 1993. Razing a Tower of Babel: A taxonomy for managed care and health insurance plans. *Journal of Health Politics, Policy and Law* 18:75–103.

Weinick, R. M., and Beauregard, K. M. 1997. Women's use of preventive screening services: A comparison of HMO versus fee-for-service enrollees. *Medical Care Research and Review* 54:176–199.

Weisman, C. S. 1996. Women's use of health care. In M. M. Falik and K. S. Collins, eds., *Women's Health: The Commonwealth Fund Survey,* chap. 1. Baltimore: Johns Hopkins University Press.

Weisman, C. S., Cassard, S. D., and Plichta, S. B. 1995. Types of physicians used by women for regular health care: Implications for services received. *Journal of Women's Health* 4:407–416.

Weisman, C. S., Celentano, D. D., Teitelbaum, M. A., and Klassen, A. C. 1989. Cancer screening services for the elderly. *Public Health Reports* 104:209–214.

Weisman, C. S., Curbow, B., and Khoury, A. J. 1995. The National Survey of

Women's Health Centers: Current models of women-centered care. *Women's Health Issues* 5:103–117.

———. 1996. Women's health centers and managed care. *Women's Health Issues* 6:255–263.

———. 1997. Case Studies of Women's Health Centers: Innovations and Issues in Women-Centered Care. New York: Commonwealth Fund.

Weisman, C. S., Levine, D. M., Steinwachs, D. M., and Chase, G. A. 1980. Male and female physician career patterns: Specialty choices and graduate training. *Journal of Medical Education.* 55:813–825.

Weisman, C. S., Nathanson, C. A., Teitelbaum, M. A., Chase, G. A., and King, T. M. 1986a. Abortion attitudes and performance among male and female obstetrician-gynecologists. *Family Planning Perspectives* 18:67–73.

Weisman, C. S., and Teitelbaum, M. A. 1985. Physician gender and the physician-patient relationship: Recent evidence and relevant questions. *Social Science and Medicine* 20:1119–1127.

Weisman, C. S., and Teitelbaum, M. A. 1989. Women and health care communication. *Patient Education and Counseling.* 13:183–199.

Weisman, C. S., Teitelbaum, M. A., Nathanson, C. A., et al. 1986b. Sex differences in the practice patterns of recently trained obstetrician-gynecologists. *Obstetrics and Gynecology* 67:776–781.

Weiss, K. B., and Solloway, M. 1994. *Women's Health and Primary Care: A Workshop to Build a Research and Policy Agenda. Conference Proceedings.* Washington, D.C.: George Washington University.

Weissman, J. S., and Epstein, A. M. 1994. *Falling through the Safety Net: Insurance Status and Access to Health Care.* Baltimore: Johns Hopkins University Press.

Weissman, M. M., and Olfson, M. 1995. Depression in women: Implications for health care research. *Science* 269:799–801.

Welter, B. 1983. The cult of true womanhood: 1820–1860. In M. Gordon, ed., *The American Family in Social-Historical Perspective.* 3d ed., chap. 19. New York: St. Martin's Press.

Wertz, R. W., and Wertz, D. C. 1989. *Lying-In: A History of Childbirth in America.* New Haven: Yale University Press.

West, G., and Blumberg, R. L. 1990. Reconstructing social protest from a feminist perspective. In *Women and Social Protest,* chap. 1. New York: Oxford University Press.

Wikler, D., and Wikler, N. J. 1991. Turkey-baster babies: The demedicalization of artificial insemination. *Milbank Quarterly* 69:5–40.

Wilensky, G. R., and Cafferata, G. L. 1983. Women and the use of health services. *American Economic Review* 73:128–133.

Wilson, R. A. 1966. *Feminine Forever.* New York: M. Evans and Company.

Wingard, D. L. 1984. The sex differential in morbidity, mortality, and lifestyle. *Annual Review of Public Health* 5:433–458.

Wise, P. H. 1995. Infant mortality: Confronting disciplinary fragmentation in research and policy. In B. P. Sachs, R. Beard, E. Papiernik, and C. Russell, eds., *Reproductive Health Care for Women and Babies,* chap. 22. New York: Oxford University Press.

Witt, L., Paget, K. M., and Matthews, G. 1994. *Running As a Woman: Gender and Power in American Politics.* New York: Free Press.

Women's Legal Defense Fund. 1996. What the new health insurance reform law means for women and their families. Washington, D.C.: Women's Legal Defense Fund.

Women's Policy, Inc. 1996a. Special report: First session of the 104th Congress. Washington, D.C.: Women's Policy, Inc.

————. 1996b. The Women's Health Equity Act of 1996: Legislative summary and overview. Washington, D.C.: Women's Policy, Inc.

Women's Research and Education Institute. 1994a. *Women's Health Care Costs and Experiences.* Washington, D.C.: Women's Research and Education Institute.

————. 1994b. *Coverage for Reproductive and Preventive Services in the Major Health Reform Proposals and Medicaid.* Washington, D.C.: Women's Research and Education Institute.

Wood, A. D. 1984. "The fashionable diseases": Women's complaints and their treatment in nineteenth-century America. In J. W. Leavitt, *Women and Health in America: Historical Readings,* chap. 16. Madison: University of Wisconsin Press.

Woodwell, D. A. 1995. Characteristics of prepaid plan visits to office-based physicians: United States, 1991. *Advance Data from Vital and Health Statistics,* no. 269. Hyattsville, Md.: National Center for Health Statistics.

Woodwell, D. A., and Schappert, S. M. 1995. National Ambulatory Medical Care Survey: 1993 summary. *Advance Data from Vital and Health Statistics,* no. 270. Hyattsville, Md.: National Center for Health Statistics.

Worcester, N., and Whatley, M. H. 1988. The response of the health care system to the Women's Health Movement: The selling of women's health centers. In S. V. Rosser, ed., *Feminism within the Science and Health Care Professions: Overcoming Resistance,* chap. 7. Oxford: Pergamon Press.

————. 1992. The selling of HRT: Playing on the feat factor. *Feminist Review* 41:1–26.

Wyn, R., and Brown, E. R. 1996. Women's health: Key issues in access to insurance coverage and to services among non-elderly women. In R. M. Andersen, T. H. Rice, and G. F. Kominski, eds., *Changing the U.S. Health Care System: Key Issues in Health Services, Policy, and Management,* chap. 11. San Francisco: Jossey-Bass.

Wyn, R., Brown, E. R., and Yu, H. 1996. Women's use of preventive health services. In M. M. Falik and K. S. Collins, eds., *Women's Health: The Commonwealth Fund Survey,* chap. 2. Baltimore: Johns Hopkins University Press.

Yin, R. K. 1994. *Case Study Research: Design and Methods.* 2d edition. Thousand Oaks, Calif.: Sage.

Young, I. M. 1990. *Justice and the Politics of Difference.* Princeton: Princeton University Press.

Zimmerman, M. K. 1987. The women's health movement: A critique of medical enterprise and the position of women. In B. B. Hess and M. M. Ferree, eds., *Analyzing Gender: A Handbook of Social Science Research,* chap. 16. Newbury Park, Calif.: Sage.

Zola, I. K. 1972. Medicine as an institution of social control. *Sociological Review* 20:487–504.

Index

Carol S. Weisman is Professor of Health Management and Policy in the School of Public Health at The University of Michigan. She received her B.A. from Wellesley College and her Ph.D. in Social Relations from the Johns Hopkins University. She was a member of the faculty of the Johns Hopkins University for twenty-two years, and from 1988 to 1997 was Professor of Health Policy and Management in the Johns Hopkins School of Hygiene and Public Health. A Robert Wood Johnson Foundation Investigator Award in Health Policy Research supported the project culminating in this book.

As sociologist and health services researcher, Dr. Weisman has a longstanding interest in the organization and quality of health services for women and in women as health care providers. She is the author of over sixty articles in professional journals and several book chapters. In addition to her research and teaching, she has worked with a number of organizations on women's health issues, including Planned Parenthood of Maryland and the Jacobs Institute of Women's Health, in Washington, D.C. She is associate editor of *Women's Health Issues*, the official journal of the Jacobs Institute.

Library of Congress Cataloging-in-Publication Data

Weisman, Carol Sachs.
    Women's health care : activist traditions and institutional change / Carol S. Weisman.
        p.   cm.
    Includes bibliographical references and index.
    ISBN 0-8018-5825-9 (alk. paper). — ISBN 0-8018-5826-7 (pbk. : alk. paper)
    1. Women's health services — Political aspects — United States.   2. Women — Health and
hygiene — United States.   3. Health care reform — United States.   I. Title.
RA564.85.W435   1998   97-34492
362.1'98'0973 — DC21   CIP